T4-AJQ-880

Primary Care Orthopaedics

Primary Care Orthopaedics

VICTORIA R. MASEAR, M.D.
Associate Professor
Director, Division of Orthopaedic Surgery
Department of Surgery
University of Alabama at Birmingham
Birmingham, Alabama

ILLUSTRATED BY:
W. Owen Bradley, III

DEPT Family Health Center Residency Program
ST. CLARE'S HOSPITAL
600 McCLELLAN STREET
SCHENECTADY. N.Y. 12304

W.B. SAUNDERS COMPANY
A Division of Harcourt Brace & Company
PHILADELPHIA   LONDON   TORONTO
MONTREAL   SYDNEY   TOKYO

W.B. SAUNDERS COMPANY
A Division of Harcourt Brace & Company

The Curtis Center
Independence Square West
Philadelphia, Pennsylvania 19106

Library of Congress Cataloging-in-Publication Data

Primary care orthopaedics / [edited by] Victoria R. Masear.
      p.   cm.
   ISBN 0–7216–5436–3
   1. Orthopedics.   2. Primary care (Medicine)   I. Masear, Victoria
R.
   [DNLM: 1. Orthopedics.   WE 168 P952 1996]
   RD732.P75   1996
   617.3—dc20
   DNLM/DLC   95-24470

PRIMARY CARE ORTHOPAEDICS   ISBN 0–7216–5436–3

Copyright © 1996 by W.B. Saunders Company.

All rights reserved. No part of this publication may be reproduced or transmitted in any form or by any means, electronic or mechanical, including photocopy, recording, or any information storage and retrieval system, without permission in writing from the publisher.

Printed in the United States of America.

Last digit is the print number: 9   8   7   6   5   4   3   2   1

Dedication

To my father for teaching me honesty and hard work and to my husband for his undying support.

Contributors

Jorge E. Alonso, M.D.
Assistant Professor of Surgery,
Division of Orthopaedic Surgery, and
  Assistant Professor of Biomedical Engineering,
University of Alabama at Birmingham,
Birmingham, Alabama
Chapter 4: Pelvic and Acetabulum Fractures
Chapter 8: Tibial Shaft Fractures
Chapter 9: Ankle Fractures

Ekkehard Bonatz, M.D.
Assistant Professor,
Division of Orthopaedic Surgery,
Department of Surgery,
University of Alabama at Birmingham,
Birmingham, Alabama
Chapter 15: Bone and Soft Tissue Injuries of
  the Hand
Chapter 20: Vascular Injuries
Chapter 22: Overuse Syndromes of the Hand
  and Wrist
Chapter 23: Bite Injuries and Infections in the
  Hand and Foot

John Coen, M.D.
Major, Staff Surgeon,
United States Air Force Medical Corps,
William Beaumont Army Medical Center,
El Paso, Texas
Chapter 26: Developmental Conditions in
  Children
Chapter 26: Developmental Conditions in Adults

Michael J. Conklin, M.D.
Assistant Professor,
Section of Pediatric Orthopaedic
  Surgery,
Division of Orthopaedic Surgery,
Department of Surgery,
University of Alabama at Birmingham,
Birmingham, Alabama
Chapter 1: Orthopaedic Evaluation
Chapter 6: Femoral Shaft Fractures in
  Children
Chapter 27: Congenital Deformities

Daniel DiChristina, M.D.
Assistant Professor,
Department of Orthopedic Surgery,
State University of New York Health
  Science
Section of Sports Medicine,
  Center at Syracuse,
Syracuse, New York
Chapter 9: Ankle Sprains

Kimberly Morris Fagan, M.D.
Baptist Health System,
Clinical Assistant Professor,
Department of Medicine,
University of Alabama at Birmingham,
Birmingham, Alabama
Chapter 7: Knee Injuries in Sports

William P. Garth, Jr., M.D.
Associate Professor,
Division of Orthopaedic Surgery,
Department of Surgery, and Director, Section of
  Sports Medicine,
School of Medicine,
University of Alabama at Birmingham,
Birmingham, Alabama
Chapter 7: Knee Injuries in Sports
Chapter 9: Ankle Sprains
Chapter 22: Overuse Syndromes of the Upper
      and Lower Extremities

Cyrus Ghavam, M.D.
Fellow, Spine Surgery,
Charlotte Spine Center,
Charlotte, North Carolina
Chapter 3: Injuries to the Spinal Column

John Greco, M.D.
Resident, Division of Orthopaedic Surgery,
Department of Surgery,
University of Alabama at Birmingham,
Birmingham, Alabama
Chapter 2: Orthopaedic Emergencies and
      Infections

Kenneth A. Jaffe, M.D.
Assistant Professor of Surgery,
Division of Orthopaedic Surgery,
Department of Surgery,
University of Alabama at Birmingham,
Birmingham, Alabama
Chapter 2: Orthopaedic Emergencies and
      Infections
Chapter 5: Hip Fractures and Dislocations
Chapter 25: Tumors of the Musculoskeletal
      System

Glenn Jonas, M.D.
Hand Fellow, Division of Orthopaedic Surgery,
Department of Surgery,
University of Alabama at Birmingham,
Birmingham, Alabama
Chapter 14: Fractures and Ligament Injuries of
      the Wrist

John T. Killian, M.D.
Associate Professor and Director, Section of
  Pediatric Orthopaedic Surgery,
Division of Orthopaedic Surgery,
Department of Surgery,
University of Alabama at Birmingham,
Birmingham, Alabama
Chapter 5: Hip Fractures and Dislocations
Chapter 7: Fractures About the Pediatric Knee
Chapter 26: Developmental Conditions in
      Children

John S. Kirkpatrick, M.D.
Assistant Professor,
Division of Orthopaedic Surgery,
Department of Surgery,
University of Alabama at Birmingham,
Birmingham, Alabama
Chapter 3: Injuries to the Spinal Column
Chapter 17: Spinal Cord Injuries

Donald H. Lee, M.D.
Assistant Professor and Director, Section of
  Hand Surgery,
Division of Orthopaedic Surgery,
Department of Surgery,
University of Alabama at Birmingham,
Birmingham, Alabama
Chapter 11: Fractures and Dislocations of the
      Shoulder
Chapter 12: Injuries to the Humerus and
      Elbow
Chapter 13: Fractures of the Forearm
Chapter 21: Injuries to Muscles and Tendons

Victoria R. Masear, M.D.
Associate Professor and Director, Division of
  Orthopaedic Surgery,
Department of Surgery,
University of Alabama at Birmingham,
Birmingham, Alabama
Chapter 10: Fractures and Dislocations of the
      Foot
Chapter 14: Fractures and Ligament Injuries of
      the Wrist
Chapter 24: Chronic Pain Syndromes
Chapter 29: Casting and Splinting Techniques

Richard D. Meyer, M.D.
Associate Professor,
Division of Orthopaedic Surgery,
Department of Surgery,
Orthopaedic and Hand Surgery,
University of Alabama at Birmingham,
Birmingham, Alabama
Chapter 16: Injuries to the Peripheral Nerves
Chapter 18: Injuries to the Brachial Plexus
Chapter 19: Nerve Entrapment

Scott Morris, M.D.
Resident, Division of Orthopaedic Surgery,
Department of Surgery,
University of Alabama at Birmingham,
Birmingham, Alabama
Chapter 5: Hip Fractures and Dislocations

Jean E. Oakes, M.D.
Orthopaedic and Hand Surgeon,
Baptist Montclair Hospital,
Birmingham, Alabama
Chapter 21: Injuries to Muscles and
              Tendons

P. Lauren Savage, Jr.
Resident, Division of Orthopaedic Surgery,
Department of Surgery,
University of Alabama at Birmingham,
Birmingham, Alabama
Chapter 29: Casting and Splinting Techniques

Stuart Stephenson, M.D.
Assistant Professor,
Division of Orthopaedic Surgery,
Department of Surgery,
University of Alabama at Birmingham,
Birmingham, Alabama
Chapter 6: Femoral Shaft Fractures in Adults

Chapter 7: Fractures About the Adult Knee
Chapter 28: Arthritis and Degenerative
              Conditions

J. R. Tamarapalli, M. D.
Research Scientist,
Division of Orthopaedic Surgery,
Department of Surgery,
University of Alabama at Birmingham,
Birmingham, Alabama
Chapter 19: Nerve Entrapment

Jeff Wade, M.D.
Resident,
Division of Orthopaedic Surgery,
Department of Surgery,
University of Alabama at Birmingham,
Birmingham, Alabama
Chapter 2: Orthopaedic Emergencies and
              Infections

Preface

In this age of managed care, primary care practitioners are asked to treat a large variety of orthopaedic conditions. The goal of this textbook is to familiarize medical students and primary care practitioners with the most common orthopaedic conditions and injuries. This textbook outlines those conditions and includes their history, diagnosis, and treatment. An in-depth description of the treatment is given for those conditions that can be treated nonoperatively. Suggestions are also given as to which conditions should be referred for subspecialty care and/or surgery.

The text is most useful for primary care physicians encountering common orthopaedic problems. It is also a valuable aid for pediatricians, family practitioners, emergency room physicians, internists treating musculoskeletal conditions, and medical students and residents. The text emphasizes those conditions that are most common in an orthopaedic practice. Congenital, developmental, and traumatic conditions and tumors of the musculoskeletal system are included. Of paramount importance is an understanding of musculoskeletal anatomy. It is highly recommended that the reader refer to an anatomy textbook for each anatomical region. The musculoskeletal physical examination is covered in detail in Chapter 1. Chapter 2 includes a review of the most common orthopaedic emergencies and their care and treatment. The bulk of the text is devoted to individual anatomical regions and the conditions that affect these regions. The final chapter deals with splinting and casting techniques. The text does not give a detailed description of surgical techniques except those that can be performed in an emergency room setting. For those conditions requiring surgery in the operative room, referral to a subspecialist is recommended.

The most useful education that I received in my medical training was a good knowledge of anatomy, as taught by James J. Hill, Jr., M.D. I soon came to realize that the treatment of musculoskeletal conditions and injuries must be accompanied by a working knowledge of anatomy. This text teaches some basic anatomy to broaden the scope of treatment for musculoskeletal conditions and injuries.

VICTORIA R. MASEAR, M.D.

Contents

C H A P T E R 1

Orthopaedic Evaluation
1
Michael J. Conklin

C H A P T E R 2

Orthopaedic Emergencies and Infections
35
Kenneth Jaffe
John Greco
Jeff Wade

C H A P T E R 3

Injuries to the Spinal Column
50
John S. Kirkpatrick
Cyrus Ghavam

C H A P T E R 4

Pelvic and Acetabulum Fractures
63
Jorge E. Alonso

C H A P T E R 5

Hip Fractures and Dislocations
72
Kenneth Jaffe
John T. Killian
Scott Morris

C H A P T E R 6

Fractures of the Femur
81

Part I: Femoral Shaft Fractures in Adults
81
Stuart Stephenson

Part II: Femoral Shaft Fractures in Children
83
Michael J. Conklin

C H A P T E R 7

Fractures and Ligamentous Injuries of the Knee
88

Part I: Knee Injuries in Sports
88
William P. Garth, Jr.
Kimberly Morris Fagan

Part II: Fractures About the Pediatric Knee
101
John Killian

Part III: Fractures About the Adult Knee
106
Stuart Stephenson

CHAPTER 8
Tibial Shaft Fractures
110
Jorge E. Alonso

CHAPTER 9
Fractures and Ligamentous Injuries of the Ankle
117

Part I: Ankle Sprains
117
Daniel DiChristina
William P. Garth, Jr.

Part II: Ankle Fractures
122
Jorge E. Alonso

CHAPTER 10
Fractures and Dislocations of the Foot
128
Victoria R. Masear

CHAPTER 11
Fractures and Dislocations of the Shoulder
142
Donald H. Lee

CHAPTER 12
Injuries to the Humerus and Elbow
156
Donald H. Lee

CHAPTER 13
Fractures of the Forearm
165
Donald H. Lee

CHAPTER 14
Fractures and Ligament Injuries of the Wrist
169
Glenn Jonas
Victoria R. Masear

CHAPTER 15
Bone and Soft Tissue Injuries of the Hand
185
Ekkehard Bonatz

CHAPTER 16
Injuries to the Peripheral Nerves
199
Richard D. Meyer

CHAPTER 17
Spinal Cord Injuries
206
John S. Kirkpatrick

CHAPTER 18
Injuries to the Brachial Plexus
208
Richard D. Meyer

CHAPTER 19
Nerve Entrapment
212
J. R. Tamarapalli
Richard D. Meyer

C H A P T E R 20

Vascular Injuries
221
Ekkehard Bonatz

C H A P T E R 21

Injuries to Muscles
and Tendons
227
Jean E. Oakes
Donald H. Lee

C H A P T E R 22

Overuse Syndromes
236

Part I: Overuse Syndromes
of the Upper and
Lower Extremities
236
William P. Garth, Jr.

Part II: Overuse Syndromes
of the Hand and Wrist
246
Ekkehard Bonatz

C H A P T E R 23

Bite Injuries and
Infections in the Hand
and Foot
250
Ekkehard Bonatz

C H A P T E R 24

Chronic Pain Syndromes
258
Victoria R. Masear

C H A P T E R 25

Tumors of the
Musculoskeletal System
263
Kenneth Jaffe

C H A P T E R 26

Developmental
Conditions
289

Part I: Developmental
Conditions in Children
289
John T. Killian
John Coen

Part II: Developmental
Conditions in Adults
299
John Coen

C H A P T E R 27

Congenital Deformities
304
Michael Conklin

C H A P T E R 28

Arthritis and
Degenerative Conditions
329
Stuart Stephenson

C H A P T E R 29

Casting and
Splinting Techniques
337
P. Lauren Savage, Jr.
Victoria R. Masear

Index
347

CHAPTER 1

Orthopaedic Evaluation

Michael Conklin

A thorough history and a physical examination are an indispensable part of the evaluation of musculoskeletal disorders. A detailed history and physical examination will guide the physician in the judicious use of radiographs and laboratory tests.

Before embarking on a discussion of the musculoskeletal physical examination, a review of some commonly used anatomic terms is in order.

Abduction Moving a body part away from the midline.
Adduction Moving a body part toward the midline.
Coronal The coronal plane is also known as the frontal plane and can be used to describe the plane that is visualized when viewing the trunk or extremity from an anteroposterior or posteroanterior projection.
Lateral That aspect of a body part that is away from the midline.
Medial That aspect of a body part that is toward the midline.
Prone The prone position, when referring to the body as a whole, is the face-down position. "Prone" or "pronation" can also be used to refer to the hand and forearm. This is the palm-down position.
Radial Often used to describe the lateral aspect of the hand or forearm with the hand in the anatomic position. The radial side of

the hand or forearm can also be thought of as the thumb side.
Sagittal The plane that is visualized when viewing the trunk or extremities from the side.
Supine The supine position, when referring to the body as a whole, is the face-up position. When referring to the hands and forearm, it is the palms-up position.
Transverse The plane that would be visualized if one could take an axial cross-section through the trunk or extremities. A good example of a transverse cut is the axial images of the trunk visualized on CAT scan.
Ulnar The ulnar side of the hand or forearm is the small finger side.
Valgus An angular deformity in which the apex of the deformity points toward the midline. "Knock-knees" are an example of valgus lower extremities.
Varus An angular deformity in which the apex of the deformity points away from the midline. "Bowlegs" are an example of varus lower extremities.

HISTORY

The orthopaedic history follows the format of any other medical work-up. This includes the chief complaint, history of present illness, past medical history, past surgical history, medicines, allergies, family history, social and industrial history, review of systems, and, in pediatric cases, birth and developmental history.

Chief Complaint

The chief complaint is that symptom or symptoms that have brought the patient to seek medical attention.

History of Present Illness

The history of present illness is an in-depth exploration of the symptoms described in the chief complaint. Common orthopaedic symptoms include the following:

Pain

The following characteristics of pain should be explored:

Location. The patient should describe *precisely* the location of pain. It may be helpful to encourage the patient to "point with one finger" to the area most painful.

Radiation. Is the pain localized or does it radiate? Do certain activities or positions cause radiation? Be sure to determine exactly how far the pain radiates (e.g., does low back pain radiate only to thigh level or does it radiate all the way to the foot?).

Quality. Is the pain sharp, dull, stabbing, aching?

Timing. When did the pain first begin and what was the patient doing at the time? Is the pain constant or intermittent? Is there daily variation in the pain? Does the pain awaken the patient?

Severity. Some patients are stoic whereas others tend to exaggerate their symptoms; therefore, it is inadequate simply to ask a patient, "How severe is the pain?" The physician should specifically ask, "Does the pain interfere with your daily activities?" "Does the pain interfere with your work?" "Is the pain severe enough to require medication, and if so, have you taken acetaminophen (Tylenol), aspirin, anti-inflammatories, or narcotics for the pain?"

Aggravation / Relief. What activities worsen the pain? Do walking, sitting, or specific positions exacerbate the pain? What gives relief? Do lying, sitting down, leaning forward, or other specific positions alleviate the pain? Do specific medications or treatments such as heat or splinting seem to relieve the pain?

Previous Treatment. Has any previous treatment been rendered and what effect has it had on the pain? This could include anything from activity restrictions to splinting, bracing, casting, medication, or surgery.

Course. Is the pain worsening or improving with time?

Trauma

Patients will frequently present with a history of trauma, major or minor. Obviously, those patients presenting with acute major trauma will undergo initial evaluation according to the format of the primary and secondary survey described in Chapter 2. Patients presenting with minor trauma or remote major trauma with persistent complaints related to this should be evaluated in the following fashion:

Mechanism. A specific mechanism of injury should be sought. This encompasses a specific description of a motor vehicle accident, including the position of the patient in the vehicle (e.g., front seat, rear seat, driver), whether or not the patient was restrained, the speed of the vehicle, and the orientation of the impact in relationship to the patient. For other mechanisms such as a fall, it is important to know not only the height of the fall but the way in which the patient landed and how the upper extremities were positioned in an attempt to break the fall. In the case of gunshot wounds, the history is frequently difficult to obtain due to the patient's unwillingness to disclose information but still should be carefully sought. The caliber of the weapon, the number of shots fired, and the position of the patient relative to the assault are important.

Timing. The exact time of the injury should be noted.

Symptoms. Symptoms related to the injury, such as pain, swelling, deformity, numbness, or weakness, should be noted.

Deformity

Deformity is a frequent complaint and can be either congenital or acquired.

Timing. When was the deformity first noted, and has it worsened or improved over time?

Disability. What effect does the deformity have on daily activities?

Inheritance. Do similar deformities run in the family?

Mass

Location. Where is the mass? Are there any other masses?

Onset. When was the mass first noted? Was it associated with any systemic symptoms, illnesses, or injury?

Size. What has been the progression of the mass over time? Has it gotten larger or smaller?

Associated Symptoms. Is the mass associated with pain, numbness, or paralysis?

Paralysis

Both motor paralysis and numbness are frequent orthopaedic complaints.

Location. The specific location of numbness or the muscle group or groups involved in paralysis should be sought.

Timing. The timing of the onset, as well as whether it was insidious or sudden, should be sought. Have the symptoms worsened or improved with time?

Severity. How much does the numbness or weakness interfere with activities?

Bowel and Bladder. Is there a change in bowel or bladder habits? The physician should specifically seek a history of urgency, hesitancy, stress incontinence, or frequent urinary tract infections. In regard to bowel control, both loss of control and constipation can be symptoms associated with a neurologic deficit.

Gait Disturbance

Both gait abnormality and a delay in ambulation are frequent presenting complaints in the pediatric population. Frequently they are neuromuscular in origin. In the adult population, gait disturbance may be secondary to neuromuscular, degenerative, or post-traumatic causes. Inquire about the quality of the gait abnormality, the timing of onset, and the course. Note the use of ambulatory aids such as walkers, crutches, canes, or bracing.

Past Medical History

This review should include past medical history; past surgical history; medications; drug or other allergies; and habits: alcohol, tobacco, drugs, and exercise.

Family History

The physician should inquire whether relatives have suffered from a similar orthopaedic or musculoskeletal complaint. A family history is particularly germane in regard to congenital deformities and syndromes.

Social History

The social history may have a major impact in regard to the presenting complaints as well as treatment decisions. It includes a work history, an economic history, and other social factors. In the pediatric population, the social situation is frequently intimately related to the presenting problem (e.g., abuse cases) and frequently will influence treatment decisions. A school history is also important in this population.

Birth History

In the pediatric population, both a prenatal and perinatal history are indispensable. The birth history should include timing of gestation, birth weight, mode of delivery (i.e., vaginal or cesarean section), presentation (i.e., breech or vertex), and APGAR scores. Perinatal medical problems also should be explored. Prenatal care and history of maternal drug use are important.

Developmental History

This is particularly important in evaluating pediatric neuromuscular disorders. Rolling over, development of head control, crawling, sitting independently, pulling to stand, and ambulation are important motor milestones. Intellectual milestones include but are not limited to language development.

At the conclusion of the orthopaedic history, the physician should have a rough differential in mind. This will guide the physician to detail the physical examination along specific lines.

PHYSICAL EXAMINATION

The musculoskeletal examination will be discussed in general terms. More specific details may be found in chapters relating to individual anatomic areas. The orthopaedic physical examination can be divided into the following subcategories.

Inspection

Note the appearance of the extremity in regard to color, swelling, or deformity. The deformity may be angular or rotational or involve a length or size discrepancy.

Palpation

This requires a knowledge of normal bone, muscle, and tendon anatomy. Abnormalities may be noted in regard to swelling, masses, joint effusion, tenderness, or bone crepitance.

Range of Motion Examination

Both active and passive range of motion (ROM) maneuvers should be conducted. In checking passive ROM, the examiner moves the joint. Active ROM is the arc of motion that can be achieved by the patient using his or her own muscle power. Decreased passive ROM indicates muscle or joint contracture, tendon tightness, or an intrinsic joint abnormality. Decreased active ROM in the face of normal passive ROM indicates that the joint is normal but that an abnormality exists in the muscle, tendon, or nerves, or in patient cooperation.

Neurologic Examination

This involves motor, sensory, and reflex examinations, including, where indicated, testing for pathologic and primitive reflexes. Likewise, special tests such as Romberg's test for ataxia and position and vibratory sense testing (posterior column disease or peripheral neuropathies) may be called for.

Motor strength is graded zero through five. A grade of five indicates normal muscle strength and a complete ROM against gravity with full resistance added by the examiner. A grade of four indicates complete ROM

against gravity and that some, although not full, resistance can be overcome by the muscle. A grade of three indicates that the muscle will move the joint through a complete ROM against gravity but that no resistance can be tolerated. A grade of two indicates a complete ROM only when gravity is eliminated as a factor. A grade of one indicates that a muscle contraction is palpable, but no range of joint motion is seen. A grade of zero indicates no evidence of muscle contractility.

Sensation is evaluated for both dermatomal distribution (Fig. 1–1) and peripheral nerve function.

Vascular Examination

Palpation of peripheral pulses, observation of capillary refill, and observation of color are accomplished.

Posture

On first encountering the patient, the general appearance is observed, with particular attention to posture. The patient is asked to stand. Observe the ease with which the patient moves from a sitting to a standing position. Difficulties in movement are noted. The standing posture of the spine is observed in both the coronal (anterior/posterior) and sagittal (lateral) planes. In the sagittal plane, there should be a gentle cervical lordosis, thoracic kyphosis, and lumbar lordosis (Fig. 1–2). In the coronal plane, the spinous processes should fall in a straight line.

Lower extremity position is evaluated. In the coronal plane, the physician should look for varus or valgus alignment (Fig. 1–3). Normal knee alignment is 5° to 7° of valgus. In the sagittal plane, balance should be observed. The hips and knees should be fully extended, and the foot should be at a right angle to the leg. If this is so, an imaginary plumb line dropped from the spinous process of C7 should fall through the center of the pelvis and through the hip joints, the knee, and the ankle.

Gait

The patient is asked to walk and is observed from the side, front, and back. A thorough discussion of the gait examination is beyond

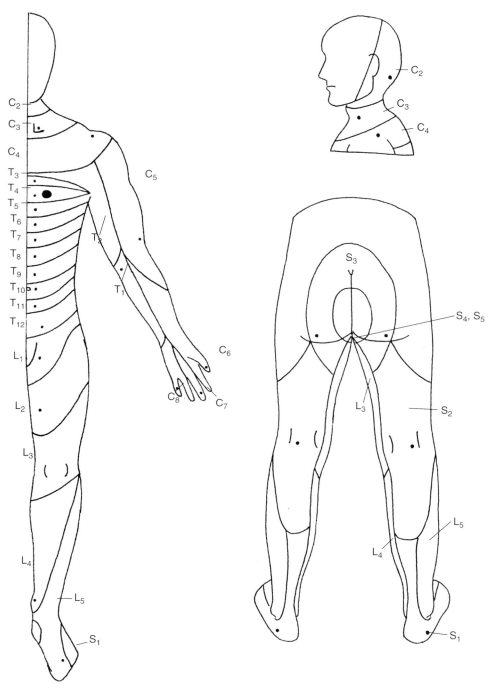

Figure 1–1. Dermatomal distribution.

the scope of this book, and the reader is encouraged to consult the reference material; however, a few key points will be mentioned. Gait is broken down into a swing phase and a stance phase, with 60 percent of the gait being spent in stance phase (Fig. 1–4). When a patient shortens the stance phase on one extremity secondary to pain, this is called an "antalgic" gait. Think of it in terms of how a patient would walk if he or she had a thumb-tack in the foot. Patients with a neuromuscu-lar abnormality commonly walk with the foot

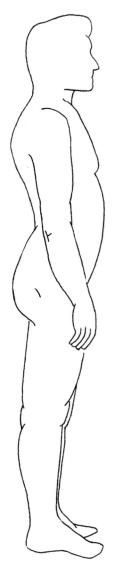

Figure 1–2. Spinal posture showing normal cervical lordosis, thoracic kyphosis and lumbar lordosis.

are an important part of the neurologic examination.

A patient who uses any ambulatory aids such as a walker or cane should be observed with and without the aids, if possible. Likewise, a patient using lower extremity braces should be observed with and without the braces when possible.

This is a convenient time to perform a Gower's test in the patient with neuromuscular disease. Ask the patient to sit on the floor and then to arise from this seated position. If the patient uses the hands to "crawl" up the legs, this is a positive Gower's test and indicates proximal muscle (hip extensor and quadriceps) weakness.

Other aspects of the examination conducted with the patient standing, such as the scoliosis examination, are done at the conclusion of the gait examination but are discussed in their respective sections.

The patient is next asked to assume a seated position on the examination table. I cannot stress enough the importance of observing a patient in regard to ease of movement from one position to another. Many subtle clues can be gleaned from observing the patient when he or she is least aware of observation. This can be very important in the uncooperative child or in an adult for whom there are questions of disability or malingering.

THE CERVICAL SPINE

Inspection

The cervical spine should be inspected for alignment in the sagittal and coronal planes. Normally a gentle cervical lordosis is observed. The cervical spine should be straight in the coronal plane, and the midline of the occiput should be centered over the vertebra prominens (C7 or T1). In observing the patient from the front, there should be no head tilt or chin rotation such as one might see in torticollis (Chapter 27).

The level of the shoulders is observed. Shoulder asymmetry may indicate Sprengel's deformity (Chapter 27) or scoliosis (Chapter 26).

Palpation

The bone elements are palpated in the midline posteriorly for alignment and tender-

plantar-flexed (in equinus) (Fig. 1–5). Patients with degenerative or painful conditions of the hip will walk with a Trendelenburg lurch (Fig. 1–6). This is manifested as a trunk shift over the stance phase limb when the patient is viewed from the front or the back.

The gait examination should always be conducted with the patient barefoot, as the foot frequently assumes a different position when weight-bearing. The patient is asked to walk on the toes and to walk on the heels. These gross tests for calf muscle strength and anterior tibial muscle strength, respectively,

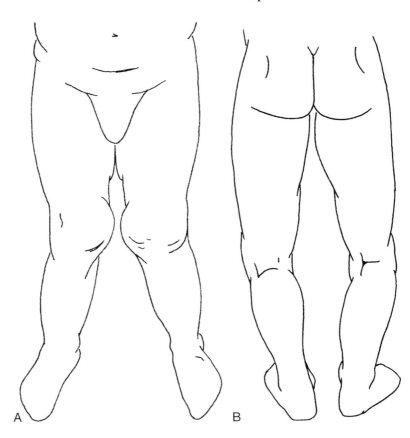

Figure 1–3. *A,* Genu valgus: apex of deformity points toward the midline. *B,* Genu varus: apex of angle is away from the midline.   A   B

ness. In cases of trauma, the cervical collar can be gently opened, the head carefully stabilized, and palpation carried out. The sternocleidomastoid muscles are palpated for spasm or fibrosis (Fig. 1–7).

Range of Motion

The range of motion in regard to flexion/ extension, lateral bend, and rotation is carried out. The normal flexion/extension arc is 80° to 90° (Fig. 1–8). The lateral bend is 60° to 70° total arc (Fig. 1–9), with normal rotation being 65° to 75° to each side (Fig. 1–10).

Neurologic Examination

A complete neurologic examination of the upper extremities is intimately related to the cervical spine examination. This involves careful testing of motor strength, sensation,

and reflexes, which will be discussed in detail in Chapter 3.

THORACOLUMBOSACRAL SPINE

Inspection

In ambulatory patients, examination of the spine is begun with the patient in the standing position, with feet together and arms hanging freely at the sides. The spine is observed from the side for sagittal plane deformity. Any accentuation (Fig. 1–11) of the normal thoracic kyphosis or lumbar lordosis is noted. The spine is observed from the back for coronal plane deformity (scoliosis) (Fig. 1–12). An imaginary plumb line dropped from the vertebra prominens should pass through the midsacral line or gluteal cleft. The level of the shoulders and scapulae is observed for symmetry, and the pelvis is inspected for obliquity. Obliquity of the pel-

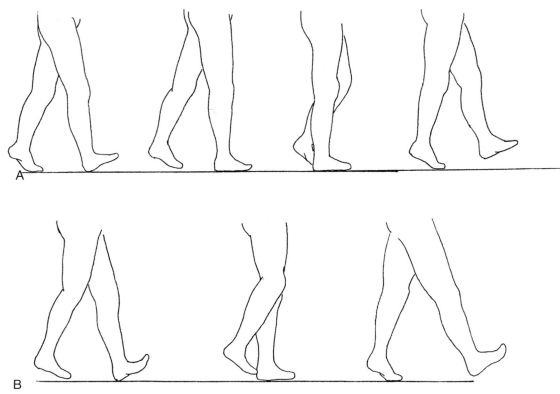

Figure 1-4. Normal gait. *A,* Stance phase, right foot (60 percent of gait cycle). *B,* Swing phase, right foot (40 percent of gait cycle).

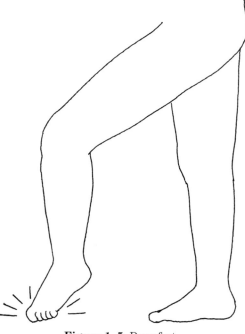

Figure 1-5. Drop foot.

vis may be secondary to leg length discrepancy, and blocks are placed beneath the foot on the short side until the pelvis is level (the spine examination is thus carried out both with and without a level pelvis).

The spinous processes are inspected and should fall in a straight line. The ribs and scapulae are inspected for rotation. They are usually more prominent on the convex side of a scoliosis. The distance from the side of the trunk to the arms is inspected for symmetry. The patient is asked to bend forward with the arms hanging freely as if to touch the toes. The examiner should sight up the spine from a posterior position, looking for malrotation of the ribs, scapulae, or lumbar paraspinal musculature (Fig. 1-13). When viewed from the side with the patient bent over, the spine should show a long, gentle kyphosis, and the lumbar lordosis should flatten out. A sharp angular kyphosis should be noted, as well as a failure of the normal lumbar lordosis to flatten with forward bending.

The skin is inspected for cutaneous stigmata such as café-au-lait spots, hairy patches, and skin dimpling.

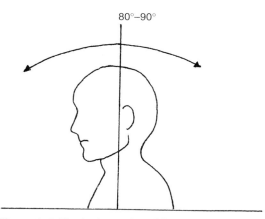

Figure 1–8. Flexion/extension of the cervical spine, normally 80 to 90 degrees total arc.

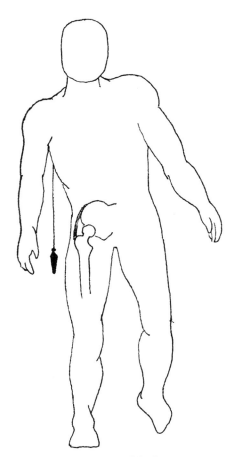

Figure 1–6. Trendelenburg gait.

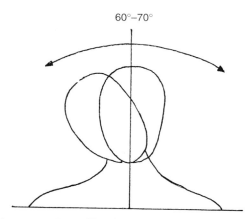

Figure 1–9. Lateral bend of the cervical spine, normally 60 to 70 degrees total arc.

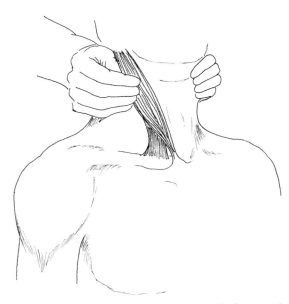

Figure 1–7. Palpation of the sternocleidomastoid muscle.

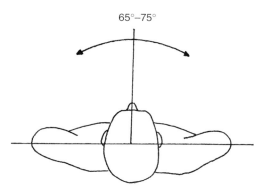

Figure 1–10. Rotation of the cervical plane, normally 65 to 75 degrees to either side.

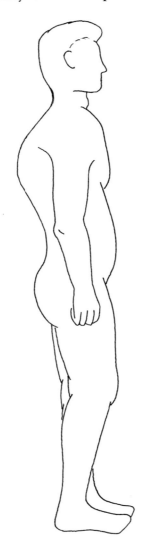

Figure 1–11. Increased thoracic kyphosis.

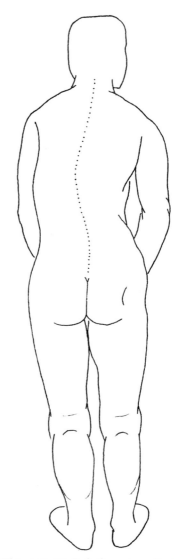

Figure 1–12. Left thoracic scoliosis.

Palpation

The spinous processes are palpated in the midline to evaluate alignment as well as to check for tenderness. In cases of trauma, the patient will be lying in a supine position. The examiner should be able to palpate the bone anatomy carefully with minimal movement of the patient, or the patient may be "log rolled" onto the side.

The back musculature is palpated with attention to tenderness, masses, or increased tone. The paraspinal musculature in the low back may be firm or hard in cases of muscular spasm. Trapezius and rhomboid muscle spasm or tenderness is seen in fibromyalgia.

Range of Motion

The range of motion is evaluated in regard to forward flexion, extension, lateral bend, and rotation. Flexion can be quantified in two ways. One is by measuring the distance from C7 to the sacrum, with the patient both standing and in forward bend (Fig. 1–14). This distance will increase with the patient in forward bend. Spinal flexion can also be quantified by the level to which the fingertips will reach (e.g., fingertips to midleg, fingertips to toes). The pelvis is stabilized by the examiner, the patient is asked to extend (bend backward), and the degrees of extension are recorded. Again with the pelvis sta-

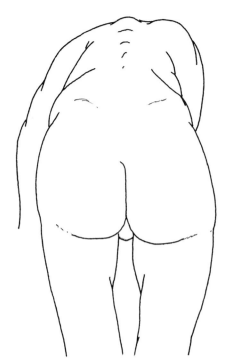

Figure 1–13. Prominence of ribs and scapula secondary to right thoracic scoliosis.

bilized, the patient is asked to bend first to the right and then to the left, and the range of motion is recorded. Lastly, with the pelvis stabilized, the patient is asked to rotate first to the right and then to the left (Fig. 1–15). The degrees of rotation of the shoulders relative to the pelvis are recorded. Any pain response elicited during the range of motion examination is noted.

Neurologic Examination

A complete neurologic examination of the trunk and lower extremities, including motor, sensory, and reflex examinations, is conducted as described later in this chapter. All muscle groups to the lower extremities are graded from zero to five; this includes hip flexors, extensors, adductors and abductors, knee flexors and extensors, ankle and toe flexors and extensors, and foot eversion and inversion. Sensation to all dermatomes (see Fig. 1–1) is recorded. Knee and ankle jerk reflexes are evaluated, as well as the Babinski and clonus tests. After the age of 1 year, more than one to two beats of clonus is suspicious for an upper motor neuron lesion. Abdominal reflexes should be tested to all

four quadrants, as well as truncal sensation. Asymmetry of the abdominal reflex or truncal numbness may be the only manifestation of a thoracic syringomyelia or other cord lesion in the thoracic spine.

Conclude the neurologic examination with a rectal examination. Rectal tone, volitional squeeze, and perianal sensation are evaluated.

THE SHOULDER AND CLAVICULAR REGION

Inspection

While viewing the patient from the front, the contour of the clavicle is inspected. Normally the clavicle is shaped in a "lazy S," with the medial aspect of the clavicle convex anteriorly and the lateral aspect concave anteriorly. The clavicle is subcutaneous and is easily visualized. The sternoclavicular joint is inspected for swelling, deformity, and symmetry.

The contour of the shoulder is noted. There will be a relative loss of the ball of the shoulder in patients with deltoid atrophy. An anterior fullness will be noted in anterior dislocation. Inspecting from posteriorly, one should note the spine of the scapula running from medial to lateral and terminating in the acromion process. The supraspinatus and infraspinatus muscles lie above and below the spine, respectively. A relative emptiness of the supraspinatus or infraspinatus fossae may be seen in patients with atrophy secondary to peripheral nerve or brachial plexus injuries.

Palpation

Starting medially at the sternoclavicular joint, palpate for swelling, tenderness, instability, fullness, or relative absence of the medial edge of the clavicle. Palpate laterally along the clavicle, noting crepitance, tenderness, or swelling. Palpate the acromioclavicular joint for tenderness or swelling. The clavicle should lie in the same superior/inferior plane as the acromion, and any superior displacement of the clavicle should be noted. Specific examination of the glenohumeral joint is covered in detail in Chapter 11, but palpation of the humeral head should prove it to be in its normal location in the glenoid.

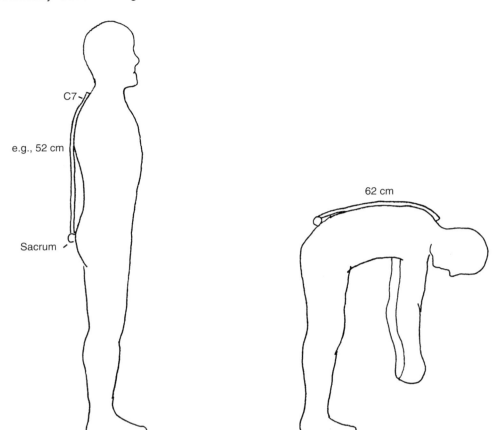

Figure 1–14. Quantification of spinal flexion.

Palpate the rotator cuff just distal to the anterior tip of the acromion. Palpate the deltoid muscle anteriorly and laterally. Palpate the supraspinatus and infraspinatus muscles posteriorly. Note any asymmetry.

Range of Motion

With the patient standing, the arm is brought straight anteriorly; the maximum position achieved is recorded as forward flexion (Fig. 1–16). Normally, flexion should be not less than 120°. With the patient's arm at the side, the extremity is then moved straight posteriorly to check extension. Normal extension is to 30° to 45°. The arm is brought straight lateral and superior, and this is recorded as abduction (Fig. 1–17). Abduction is effectively examined while the examiner stands behind the patient so that upward rotation of the scapula can be observed. Initial abduction is checked with the patient's shoulder in neutral rotation. After 120°, the arm must be

externally rotated to achieve further abduction. Normal abduction approaches 180°. Shoulder rotation is examined with the elbow flexed 90° at the patient's side (Fig. 1–18). The straight anterior position is neutral rotation. The forearm is then internally and externally

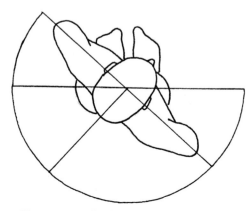

Figure 1–15. Evaluation of spinal rotation.

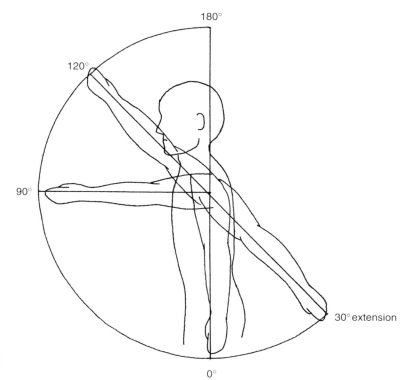

Figure 1–16. Shoulder flexion and extension, normally 180 and 30 degrees, respectively.

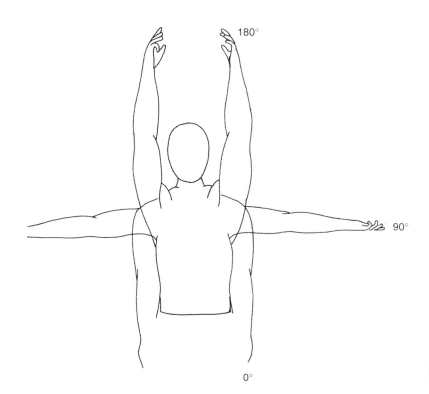

Figure 1–17. Shoulder abduction, normally 180 degrees.

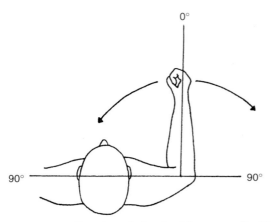

Figure 1–18. Rotation of the shoulder, normally 55 degrees internally and 45 degrees externally.

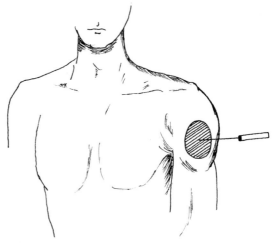

Figure 1–20. Sensory distribution of axillary nerve (C5).

rotated from the neutral position. Normal internal rotation is 55°; external rotation is 45°.

Special Tests

The impingement sign and impingement test are special evocative maneuvers used to evaluate subacromial impingement and rotator cuff pathology and will be described in detail in Chapters 21 and 22.

Neurologic Examination

With the patient's elbow at the side, flexed 90°, and the forearm pointing straight anteriorly, the examiner attempts alternately to resist internal and external rotation of the hand to evaluate strength of the internal and external rotators, respectively. Deltoid (C5) strength is evaluated by resisted abduction, rhomboid (C5) strength by the ability to retract the scapula, and the strength of the serratus anterior (C5, 6, 7) by having the patient push against a wall and evaluating for winging of the scapula (Fig. 1–19).

The sensory distribution of the axillary nerve is over the lateral aspect of the deltoid (Fig. 1–20). Axillary neuropraxia may be seen after anterior shoulder dislocation.

The remainder of the neurologic examination is covered in depth in Chapter 17.

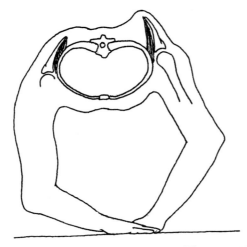

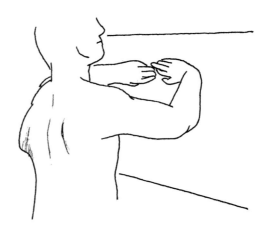

Figure 1–19. Winging of left scapula.

ARM, ELBOW, AND FOREARM

Inspection

The patient is observed from an anterior position with the extremity hanging freely at the side. The angle that the upper arm makes with the forearm is spoken of as the carrying angle. Normally this is 5° to 15° of valgus. An increased valgus carrying angle can be seen after lateral condyle fractures of the elbow (Fig. 1–21). A decreased carrying angle or cubitus varus is a common sequela of supracondylar humerus fractures in children (Fig. 1–22). The extremity is observed from the side for flexion or extension contractures of the elbow.

Inspect the contour of the biceps muscle anteriorly and of the triceps muscle posteriorly. In the forearm, inspect the flexor and extensor muscle masses volarly and dorsally, respectively.

Palpation

The humerus is enclosed in muscle for most of its length until it becomes subcutaneous

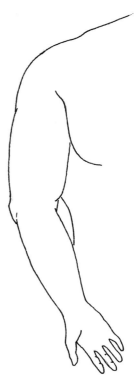

Figure 1–22. Cubitus varus.

at the medial and lateral epicondyles. Nevertheless, it can be palpated with deep pressure for crepitance or pain. The medial epicondyle is palpable on the medial side of the distal aspect of the humerus. The ulnar nerve runs in the ulnar groove just posterior to the medial epicondyle.

The lateral epicondyle is palpable subcutaneously on the lateral aspect of the distal humerus. Palpation may disclose tenderness after lateral condyle fracture or in cases of "tennis elbow."

The olecranon is palpable as the bone point of the elbow and is the most proximal aspect of the ulna. On flexion, the medial epicondyle, lateral epicondyle, and olecranon form an equilateral triangle posteriorly. In posterior elbow dislocation, the apex of the triangle, the olecranon, is displaced posteriorly in relationship to the other two points. In supracondylar fracture of the humerus, the relationship of the triangle is preserved and all three points are displaced posteriorly in relationship to the proximal fragment of the humerus.

Palpating distally from the lateral epicondyle, the examiner's finger will fall into a subtle depression that is the radiocapitellar

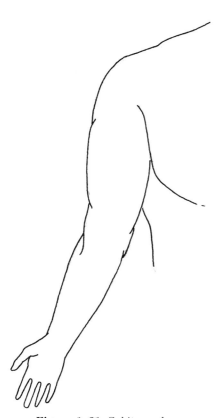

Figure 1–21. Cubitus valgus.

joint. The radial head is just distal to this and is more easily identified by feeling for rotation when the forearm is pronated and supinated. Just posterior to the radial head, between it and the olecranon, is a relative soft spot or depression. This is the best place to palpate the elbow joint for hemarthrosis or effusion, which will feel like a fullness or fluctuance.

Range of Motion

As the elbow is a hinge joint, only flexion and extension are allowed. Extension of the elbow to a straight arm position is spoken of as 0°. Normal extension is to 0°, with mild hyperextension being common in women or patients with hyperlaxity. Normal flexion is 150° (Fig. 1–23). With the patient's elbow at the side and flexed 90°, the hand is placed straight ahead with the palm facing the trunk and the thumb pointing up. This is the neutral position. The hand is then turned palm down and palm up to check pronation and supination, respectively. Alternatively, a straight object such as a dowel or pencil can be placed in the closed fist and used as a caliper with which to check pronation and supination (Fig. 1–24). Normal pronation and supination are approximately 80° each.

Neurologic Examination

Motor Testing

Elbow flexion (biceps, brachialis—musculocutaneous nerve—C5,6). The patient actively flexes the elbow while the examiner resists.

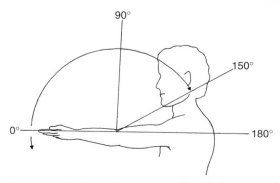

Figure 1–23. Elbow flexion, normally 150 degrees and extension of zero degrees.

Elbow extension (triceps—radial nerve—C7). The patient actively extends the elbow while the examiner resists.

Wrist extension (extensor carpi radialis longus, extensor carpi radialis brevis, extensor carpi ulnaris—radial nerve—C6,7). Stabilize the patient's distal forearm in one hand, then ask the patient to extend the wrist actively against resistance from the examiner's other hand.

Wrist flexion (flexor carpi radialis—median nerve—C7; flexor carpi ulnaris—ulnar nerve—C8). With the forearm supinated, stabilize the distal forearm in one hand and ask the patient to flex the wrist fully while resistance is applied.

Finger extension (extensor digitorum communis, extensor indicis, extensor digiti minimi—radial nerve—C7). The patient is asked to extend the fingers actively while the examiner attempts to push them into flexion.

Finger flexion (flexor digitorum superficialis—median nerve—C8; flexor digitorum profundus—ulnar nerve and anterior interosseous branch of median nerve—C8). While stabilizing the metacarpophalangeal joint and proximal interphalangeal joint in extension, ask the patient to flex the distal interphalangeal joint. This tests the flexor digitorum profundus tendon. Now stabilize the other fingers in extension and ask the patient to flex the remaining finger. This tests the flexor digitorum superficialis tendon to that finger.

Sensory Examination

Sensation to the posterior arm and posterior forearm is supplied by branches of the radial nerve. Sensation to the medial arm is supplied by the medial brachial cutaneous nerve. The volar-medial forearm is supplied by the medial antebrachial cutaneous nerve while the volar-lateral forearm is supplied by the lateral antebrachial cutaneous nerve (terminal branch of the musculocutaneous nerve). Note the dermatomal distribution to the upper extremity (see Fig. 1–1).

Reflexes

Biceps reflex (musculocutaneous nerve—C5). The elbow should be flexed with the patient's hand supported and the arm relaxed. The examiner grasps the patient's elbow, placing a thumb over the biceps tendon. The thumb is then struck briskly with a reflex hammer.

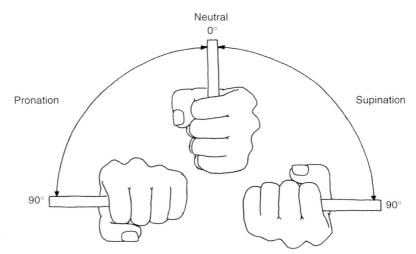

Figure 1–24. Forearm pronation and supination, normally 80
degrees each.

The biceps should contract, causing elbow
flexion.
  Brachioradialis reflex (radial nerve—C6).
The patient flexes the elbow and rests the
forearm on the thigh. The musculotendinous
junction of the brachioradialis on the radial
aspect of the forearm is then struck with a
reflex hammer. This may elicit wrist extension, radial deviation, or elbow flexion.
  Triceps reflex (radial nerve—C7). The
examiner should support the patient's arm,
with the forearm hanging in a flexed position,
and briskly strike the triceps tendon just
superior to the olecranon. Elbow extension
will be seen.

WRIST AND HAND

Inspection

Evaluate the alignment of the hand on the
distal forearm in the coronal plane. It should
be centered on the forearm, with the longitudinal axis of the third metacarpal aligned
with the radius and ulna. Likewise, from a
lateral view the hand should be well centered
on the distal forearm, and the wrist should
be slightly extended in the resting position.
Normally, the hand has a gentle transverse
arch concave volarly. Note the "attitude" of
the hand (Fig. 1–25). In the resting position,
the fingers and thumb are gently flexed, with
the amount of flexion increasing as one
moves from index to little finger. Evaluate
the thenar and hypothenar eminences and
compare them with the opposite hand for
symmetry.

  Inspect the nails and nail beds. The nail
beds are pink, with a small, pale, crescent-
shaped area at the nail base, the lunula. The
nail beds may be pale when a person is ane-
mic. Nails may be abnormally shaped, such
as spoon nails in fungal infection or clubbing
of the nails in chronic hypoxemic conditions.
Ecchymosis beneath the nail indicates a nail
bed laceration (see Chapter 15).

Palpation

Begin palpation at the radial styloid process
at the lateral aspect of the wrist. A depression just distal to the radial styloid process
is noted—the "anatomic snuff box." This
overlies the scaphoid bone. The wrist is composed of eight carpal bones arranged in two
rows: the proximal row from radial to ulnar
is composed of the scaphoid, lunate, triquetrum, and pisiform. The distal row is the trapezium, trapezoid, capitate, and hamate. The
bone prominence on the ulnar/volar aspect
of the wrist is the pisiform, a sesamoid bone
at the insertion of the flexor carpi ulnaris.
On the ulnar aspect of the wrist lies the ulnar
styloid. Just distal to the ulnar styloid lies
the triangular fibrocartilage and the ulnocar-
pal ligaments, which may be a source of soft
tissue injury.
  Move around to the dorsum of the wrist
along the ulnar side. Note that in the anatomic position the ulnar styloid lies slightly
posterior. Palpate around the prominence of
the distal ulna until the palpating finger
drops onto the distal radius, which has a relatively flat surface dorsally. Between the two

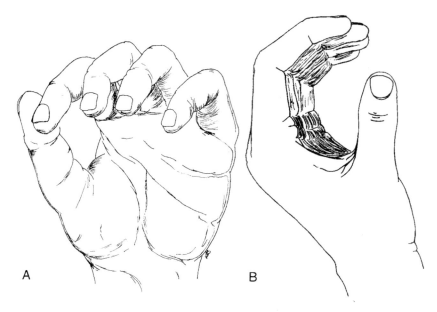

Figure 1–25. Front and side views of the "attitude" of the hand.

is the distal radioulnar joint. Palpate the joint for swelling or tenderness. The subtle prominence on the dorsal surface of the distal radius is Lister's tubercle. Ask the patient to extend the thumb and note the extensor pollicis longus tendon coursing around Lister's tubercle. Just ulnar to Lister's tubercle palpate distally on the radius until the examining finger falls into a depression, which is the radiocarpal joint. Volarly flex the wrist to expose the lunate to palpation. Just distal to the lunate the capitate is palpable. Soft tissue palpation should proceed along the extensor tendons. From radial to ulnar, these are the abductor pollicis longus, extensor pollicis brevis, extensor carpi radialis longus and brevis, extensor pollicis longus, extensor digitorum communis, extensor indicis, extensor digiti minimi, and extensor carpi ulnaris.

Note any localized swelling along the dorsum of the wrist. This is a common location for a ganglion cyst.

The flexor tendons can be palpated volarly. From ulnar to radial, they are the flexor carpi ulnaris, flexor digitorum profundus and superficialis, palmaris longus, and flexor carpi radialis. The flexor pollicis longus tendon lies deep and radial in the carpal tunnel. The median nerve lies just ulnar to the flexor carpi radialis tendon within the carpal tunnel. The ulnar nerve runs through Guyon's canal between the pisiform and the hamate. Gently tapping on the median or ulnar nerve

at the wrist may elicit pain or paresthesias along the nerve distribution, a positive Tinel's test.

Palpate metacarpals one through five. They are most accessible to palpation dorsally. Likewise, palpate the proximal, middle, and distal phalanges. Note that the thumb has only two phalanges, proximal and distal. Palpate the metacarpophalangeal (MCP), proximal interphalangeal (PIP), and distal interphalangeal (DIP) joints. Be precise about palpation and note whether tenderness is found volarly, dorsally, radially, or ulnarly. Note any increase in size of the joints, and determine by palpation whether it is bone or soft tissue in origin.

Range of Motion

To evaluate wrist flexion and extension, note the angle that the long axis of the forearm makes with the long axis of the hand on the lateral view (Fig. 1–26). Normal wrist extension is 70° and flexion 80°. Evaluate ulnar and radial deviation of the wrist by noting the angle the long axis of the hand makes with the forearm when viewing from anterior (coronal plane). Normal ulnar and radial deviation is 30° and 20°, respectively (Fig. 1–27).

Thumb range of motion is complex. Note that thumb flexion involves moving the

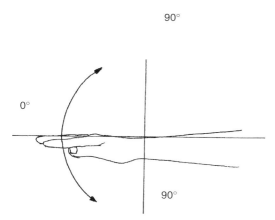

Figure 1–26. Wrist flexion (80 degrees) and extension (70 degrees).

thumb toward the base of the little finger MCP joint. This tests flexion of the thumb carpometacarpal joint (CMC), MCP joint, and IP joint (Fig. 1–28). Extension of the thumb occurs in the opposite direction, as in the "thumbs up" sign. Normal CMC extension and MCP extension are to neutral position, while the thumb interphalangeal joint hyperextends 20 degrees. Palmar abduction/adduction of the thumb (Fig. 1–29) is normally zero to 70°. Thumb opposition is a complex motion occurring primarily at the CMC joint. The patient should be able actively to oppose the thumb tip to the tips of all the fingers.

Normal finger MCP motion is from 30° hyperextension to 90° of flexion. Normal PIP motion is from neutral to 100° flexion, while DIP motion is from 10° of hyperextension to

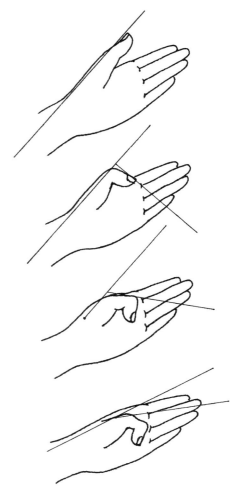

Figure 1–28. Thumb flexion. Interphalangeal joint, 20 degrees hyperextension to 80 degrees flexion. Metacarpophalangeal joint, 0 to 60 degrees flexion. Carpometacarpal joint, 0 to 40 degrees.

80° of flexion. Finger abduction is evaluated by asking the patient to spread the fingers. Note the angle that the index and the little digit make with the long axis of the third metacarpal. Normally this is approximately

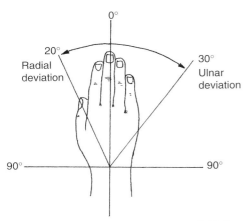

Figure 1–27. Radial deviation of wrist of 20 degrees and ulnar deviation of 30 degrees.

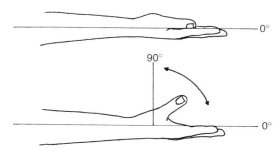

Figure 1–29. Palmar abduction/adduction of thumb.

20° each. To evaluate adduction, the patient is asked to cross the fingers.

Neurologic Examination

Motor Examination

Much of the motor examination of the hand has been described along with examination of the forearm. Many of the muscles originate there. Intrinsic muscles of the hand are supplied by the median and ulnar nerves; representative tests for median and ulnar intrinsics are described here.

The *abductor pollicis brevis muscle* (median nerve) is the most proximal muscle of the hypothenar eminence and overlies the thumb metacarpal. The patient is asked to abduct the thumb actively while the examiner palpates the abductor pollicis for contraction.

The *first dorsal interosseous muscle* (ulnar nerve) lies in the first web space just radial to the index metacarpal. The examiner should palpate the muscle while asking the patient to abduct the index finger actively against resistance.

The examiner should palpate the *abductor digiti minimi* (ulnar nerve) along the ulnar border of the small finger metacarpal and ask the patient to abduct the small finger actively.

Sensory Examination

Note the sensory distribution of the median, ulnar, and radial nerves to the hand (Fig. 1–30). Note the dermatomal distribution (Fig. 1–1).

The thumb and each of the fingers receive two digital nerves, one on the radial and one on the ulnar side. For this reason, when evaluating distal sensation it is important to perform the two-point discrimination test to both the radial and ulnar aspects of the fingertip. This is performed with either a caliper or paper clip. The patient is asked to shut his or her eyes. The examiner touches the patient with either one or two blunt points at a time. It is important not to apply deep pressure but rather to touch lightly. The patient is asked to state whether one or two points are being used. A patient should be able to tell two points when they are 5 mm or more apart.

THE HIP AND PELVIS

Inspection

The initial examination of the hip and pelvis begins with the examination of posture and gait. The pelvis is inspected for obliquity. When the examiner views from a posterior direction, the height of the iliac crests is noted. If they are not level, blocks are placed underneath the foot on the short side. The thickness of the blocks required to level the pelvis is recorded.

Inspect the skin for abrasions, ecchymosis, swelling, birthmarks, skin dimpling, or sinus tracts. In the infant, inspect the symmetry of the skin folds along the groin, thigh, and gluteal regions. Asymmetry may be seen in developmental dysplasia of the hip or longitudinal deficiencies of the lower extremity (Chapter 27). Inspect the buttocks and thigh musculature for symmetry.

With the patient lying supine, apparent and true leg lengths are measured. Apparent leg length is measured from the umbilicus to the tip of the medial malleolus. The true leg length is measured from the anterior/superior iliac spine to the tip of the medial malleolus.

Palpation

Palpation is conducted with the patient either standing or lying down. Beginning at the anterior superior iliac spines (ASIS), palpate superiorly and posteriorly along the iliac crest to the posterior superior iliac spines (PSIS). Between these two landmarks lies the iliac crest. This is a point of origin and insertion for a number of muscles, including the gluteus musculature and the internal and external oblique muscles of the abdomen. The ASIS is the point of origin for the sartorius muscle. Palpate anteriorly and inferiorly from the ASIS in line with the inguinal ligament until a bone prominence is reached just lateral to the midline in the groin. This is the pubic tubercle. Deep palpation in this area will disclose tenderness in pubic rami fractures. Palpate medially from the PSIS. The examining finger overlies the sacrum. The sacroiliac joints are not accessible to direct palpation. Tenderness to deep palpation or swelling in this area may be elicited in posterior pelvic ring injuries.

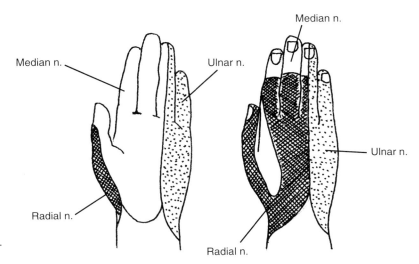

Figure 1–30. Sensory distribution of the hand.

Place the thumb on the PSIS. Spread the thumb and long finger widely with the long finger straight inferiorly. The bone prominence in the middle of the buttock at the approximate level of the gluteal fold is the ischial tuberosity.

With the long finger on the ischial tuberosity, rotate the hand so that the thumb points laterally and somewhat superiorly. It will lie over the bony prominence of the greater trochanter. This may be more easily appreciated by internally and externally rotating the thigh and noting the movement of the trochanter. Palpate the buttock musculature between the trochanter and iliac crest. The gluteus maximus (hip extensor) lies posteriorly, while the gluteus medius, gluteus minimus, and tensor fascia lata (hip abductors) lie laterally.

The structures of the femoral triangle are palpable just beneath the inguinal ligament. Find the pulse of the femoral artery and assess its strength. Though not palpable, the femoral nerve lies just lateral while the femoral vein lies just medial to the artery. Just medial to the femoral vein are the inguinal lymph nodes, which should be assessed for adenopathy.

Just medial to the structures of the femoral triangle lie the adductor muscles. Note the adductor longus tendon, the most obvious tendon in the groin. Palpate distally from here along the medial thigh to assess the adductor muscle group.

Anteriorly on the thigh palpate the quadriceps, or knee extensors. The rectus femoris is straight anterior and superficial, running from the anterior inferior iliac spine to the quadriceps tendon. The vastus medialis and vastus lateralis lie medial and lateral, respectively. The vastus intermedius is deep to the rectus femoris and is not accessible to direct palpation.

Palpate the hamstring musculature in the posterior thigh. The semitendinosus and semimembranosus muscles lie in the posteromedial thigh, while the biceps femoris muscle lies posterolaterally. Spasm, tenderness, or atrophy is noted.

Range of Motion

With the patient lying supine and the knee flexed, the hip is flexed to its maximum degree, with the opposite hip in full extension to prevent flexion of the pelvis. Normal hip flexion is 135°. The Thomas test for hip flexion contracture is carried out (Fig. 1–31). With the patient lying supine, place one hand beneath the lumbar spine. Both hips are then flexed until the lumbar lordosis is flattened. The hip being tested is gradually brought into extension. When the hip will no longer extend or when further extension of the hip causes a return of the lumbar lordosis, the angle that the thigh makes with the examining table is noted. This is the amount of hip flexion contracture.

Check hip abduction with the hip in both flexion and extension (Fig. 1–32). Normal abduction in extension is 45°.

With the hip in mild flexion and the knee in extension, the lower extremity is brought

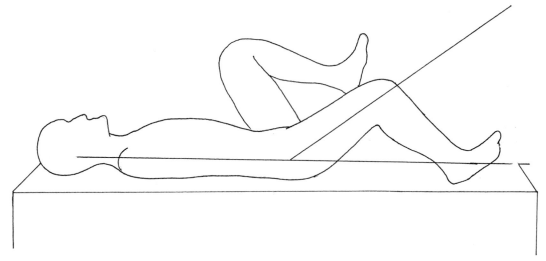

Figure 1–31. Thomas test for hip flexion contracture. The lumbar lordosis has been eliminated by flexion of the contralateral hip.

across the midline (legs crossed) to its maximum degree to check hip adduction. Normal adduction is 20° to 30°.

Internal and external rotation of the hip are tested in both flexion and extension (Fig. 1–33). Normal values are 45° of external and 35° of internal rotation.

Neurologic Examination

Motor Examination

The hip flexors, extensors, adductors, and abductors are tested and graded from zero to five.

Flexors (iliopsoas—L1, 2, 3). Sitting on the edge of the examining table with the knees flexed 90°, the patient is asked to flex the hip actively. The examiner should resist with downward pressure on the distal femur.

Adductors (obturator nerve—L2, 3, 4). With the patient lying on the side and the hip and knee fully extended, the examiner places one hand on the down extremity for stabilization: with the other hand on the up leg, the examiner attempts to abduct the thigh while the patient is asked to resist.

Abductors (superior gluteal nerve–L4, 5, S1). Lying on the side with the hip and knee fully extended, the patient is asked to abduct

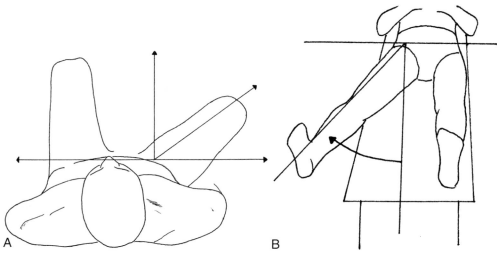

Figure 1–32. *A*, Testing of hip abduction with hip in flexion. *B*, Hip abduction tested with hip in extension.

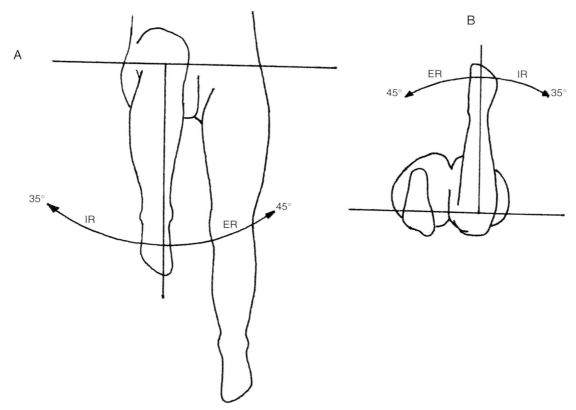

Figure 1–33. Evaluation of hip internal (IR) and external (ER) rotation with hip in flexion (A) and extension (B).

the hip while the examiner places downward pressure on the leg.

Hip extensors (inferior gluteal nerve—L5, S1, S2). Lying prone with the knees slightly bent, the patient is asked to extend the hip while the examiner applies downward pressure to the distal thigh.

If the patient cannot perform active range of motion against gravity, as just described, gravity is removed as a factor in this way: the hip abductors and adductors are tested with the patient supine; the hip flexors and extensors are tested with the patient lying on her or his side.

Sensory Examination

Sensation to the skin overlying the buttocks is supplied by the cluneal nerves (L1, 2, 3). Sensation to the lateral thigh is supplied by the lateral femoral cutaneous nerve. Sensation to the anterior thigh is supplied by the anterior femoral cutaneous nerve. The posterior aspect of the thigh is supplied by the posterior femoral cutaneous nerve.

In addition to peripheral nerve sensation, evaluate sensation in regard to dermatomal distribution (see Fig. 1–1).

Special Tests

Trendelenburg Test

This test evaluates the strength of the gluteus medius muscle. It may also be positive in patients with hip joint pathology. Stand behind the patient with the patient standing erect. Place one hand on the top of each iliac crest posteriorly. Ask the patient to lift the right foot. Normally, the right iliac crest should elevate with contraction of the left gluteus medius, shifting the center of gravity over the left lower extremity (Fig. 1–34). Failure to do so is significant for left gluteus medius weakness or left hip joint pathology. Repeat the test by asking the patient to lift the left foot with the right foot on the ground.

Ortolani and Barlow Maneuvers

These are discussed in Chapter 27.

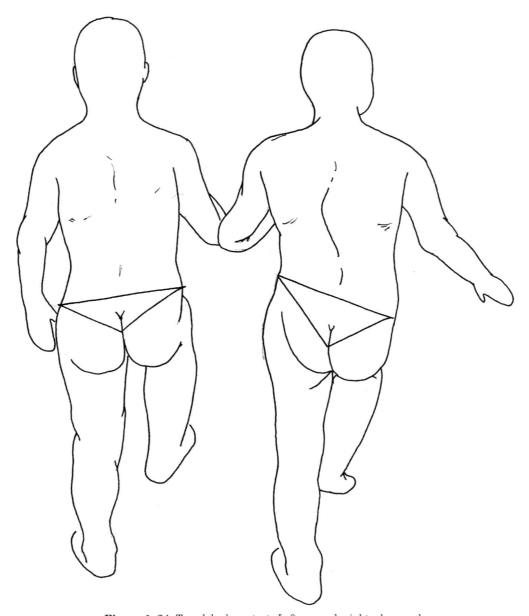

Figure 1–34. Trendelenburg test. *Left,* normal; *right,* abnormal.

Galeazzi Sign

This is discussed in Chapter 27.

KNEE AND LEG

Inspection

Examination of the knee and leg begins with the patient standing as part of the posture examination. While the examiner views from the anterior direction, the knee and lower extremity of the patient are evaluated for varus or valgus (see Fig. 1–3). The patient is viewed from the side for hyperextension or flexion of the knee.

Ask the patient to lie supine on the examining table. The knee should be in full extension. When viewed from above, varus and valgus deformity are noted. Varus deformity is quantified by measuring the distance between the knees with the medial malleoli together. Valgus deformity is quantified by measuring the distance between the medial malleoli with the knees together. Note the distal quadriceps musculature and quadriceps tendon as they converge to insert on the superior pole of the patella. Asymmetry indicates quadriceps atrophy. The patella should be readily visible except in the very obese patient. It should lie centrally in the patellofemoral groove. Note any asymmetry in height of the patella. Note localized swelling or masses about the knee.

Inspect the leg for deformity or asymmetry. Normally, the tibia is straight from the knee to the ankle in both the coronal and sagittal planes. Inspect the anterior, lateral, and posterior compartment musculature for asymmetry.

Palpation

Ask the patient to sit on the edge of the examining table with the knees flexed 90°. Palpate the patella. Palpate the quadriceps tendon and its insertion into the superior pole. Palpate the origin of the patellar tendon on the inferior pole of the patella, the patellar tendon proper, and its insertion into the tibial tubercle. Palpate the relative soft spot on either side of the patellar tendon just beneath the patella. This is the knee joint line. Palpate from anterior to posterior along the medial and lateral joint lines. Palpate the lateral collateral ligament from the lateral femoral condyle to the fibular head. Palpate the medial collateral ligament from the medial femoral condyle to the anteromedial aspect of the tibia.

Turn the patient prone to palpate the popliteal region. Note that the medial and lateral hamstring tendons and the medial and lateral head of the gastrocnemius form a diamond shape: the popliteal fossa. Localized swelling in the popliteal fossa may be due to a popliteal cyst or tumor. Assess the popliteal pulse in the middle of the popliteal fossa.

Palpate the tibia, which is subcutaneous along its entire medial border. Palpate the fibula, which is subcutaneous in its proximal aspect (fibular head) and its distal aspect (lateral malleolus). The shaft of the fibula lies deep to the peroneal musculature but can be assessed for tenderness with deep palpation. The common peroneal nerve can be palpated as it courses around the neck of the fibula by rolling it between the fingers. Just lateral to the anterior crest of the tibia, palpate the anterior compartment musculature (tibialis anterior, extensor hallucis longus, and extensor digitorum longus). Palpate the lateral compartment musculature (peroneus longus and brevis) just lateral and posterior to the anterior compartment overlying the shaft of the fibula. Palpate the calf musculature. The gastrocnemius is proximal and superficial. The soleus muscle lies deep to the gastrocnemius, and its muscle belly extends more distally. Palpate the Achilles tendon.

Range of Motion

Passive range of motion is examined with the patient lying supine. As the knee is a hinge joint, only flexion and extension are allowed. Normal knee flexion is to 130°, and normal extension is from 0 to 10° of hyperextension (Fig. 1–35). With the patient sitting on the side of the examining table and the knee flexed to 90°, ask him to extend the knee actively. Note any extensor lag (discrepancy between passive and active extension) that may indicate quadriceps weakness or disruption of the patellar tendon.

Neurologic Examination

Motor Testing

Knee extension (quadriceps—femoral nerve—L2, 3, 4). With the patient seated on the edge of the examining table and the knee flexed 90°, ask her to extend the knee actively while downward pressure is applied on the distal leg. Normally the patient should be able to extend the knee completely in spite of maximum pressure.

Knee flexion (hamstrings—sciatic nerve—L5, S1). While the patient is lying prone, have him flex the knee actively while pressure is applied to the distal leg in an attempt to resist flexion.

Ankle extension (dorsiflexion) (tibialis anterior—deep peroneal nerve—L4, 5). With the patient's knee bent over the side of the table, the examiner places a hand on the dorsum of the patient's foot. The patient is then asked to dorsiflex the foot actively while the examiner resists.

Great toe extension (extensor hallucis longus—deep peroneal nerve—L5). The patient is asked to extend the great toe actively while the examiner resists.

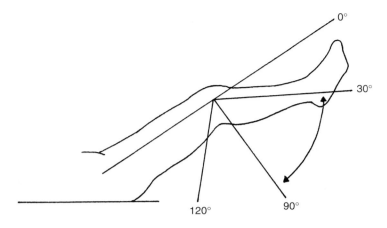

Figure 1–35. Knee flexion (130 degrees) and extension (zero degrees).

Lesser toe extension (extensor digitorum longus—deep peroneal nerve—L5). The patient is asked to actively extend her lesser toes while the examiner resists.

Ankle plantar flexion (gastrocnemius, soleus—tibial nerve—S1, 2). The examiner's hand is placed against the plantar surface of the foot. The patient is asked to plantar flex the foot actively while the examiner resists.

Great toe flexion (flexor hallucis longus—tibial nerve—L5). The patient is asked to flex the great toe actively while the examiner resists.

Lesser toe flexion (flexor digitorum longus—tibial nerve—L5). The patient is asked to plantar flex (curl) the toes actively while the examiner resists.

Foot inversion (tibialis posterior—tibial nerve—L5). The patient is asked to actively invert (supinate) the foot while the examiner resists with laterally directed pressure on the medial aspect of the foot.

Foot eversion (peroneus longus and brevis—superficial peroneal nerve—S1). The patient is asked to evert (pronate) the foot while the examiner applies medially directed pressure to the lateral aspect of the foot.

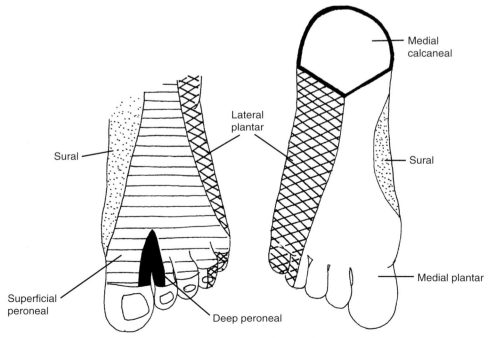

Figure 1–36. Sensory distribution of the foot.

Sensory Examination

For the sensory examination of the knee, leg, and foot, the reader is referred to the sensory dermatomes (see Fig. 1–1) and the peripheral nerve supply to the foot (Fig. 1–36).

Reflexes

Knee jerk (patellar tendon) reflex (L4). With the knee bent over the side of the table and the leg hanging free, the patellar tendon is struck briskly with a reflex hammer. Side to side asymmetry is noted as well as any asymmetry between the upper and lower extremity reflexes.

Special Testing

Knee Ligamentous Stability

These tests will be discussed in detail in Chapter 7.

McMurray's Test

Discussed in detail in Chapter 7.

FOOT AND ANKLE

Inspection

Examination of the foot begins with examination of the shoe. Note the wear pattern of the shoe. Increased wear of the medial aspect of the shoe or broken medial contours are seen in patients with flat feet. Increased lateral wear is seen in patients who walk on inverted or supinated feet. Patients who walk with a foot drop will scuff the toe portion of the shoe.

The patient is asked to remove the shoes, and the standing position of the foot is noted. When viewed from the side, the foot should be at a right angle to the leg. Plantar flexion of the foot with the heel lifted off the ground is called equinus (Fig. 1–37). Dorsiflexion of the foot with the forefoot lifted off the ground is calcaneus (Fig. 1–38). When viewed from the side, the foot should have a gentle medial longitudinal arch, with the entire lateral border resting on the floor. Flattening of the medial arch (pes planus) (Fig. 1–39) or exaggeration of the arch (pes cavus) (Fig. 1–40) should be noted.

View the foot from the back. The heel should have 5° of valgus. The position of the

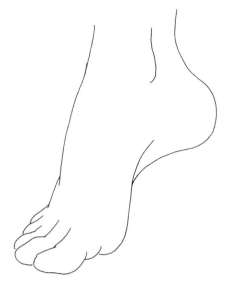

Figure 1–37. Equinus deformity.

forefoot is noted while viewing from the front. All five metatarsal heads should lie flat on the floor (Fig. 1–41A). The base of the first metatarsal is elevated in the arch, with only the head touching the floor. In contrast, the entire fifth metatarsal should lie on the floor. Turning in of the forefoot such that the medial rays are lifted is supination (Fig. 1–41B). Turning out of the forefoot with depression of the first metatarsal and, in more extreme cases, lifting of the lateral aspect of the forefoot is pronation (Fig.

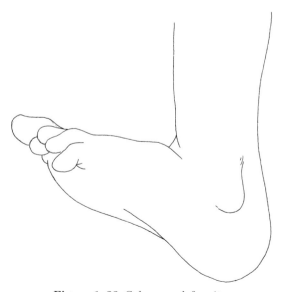

Figure 1–38. Calcaneus deformity.

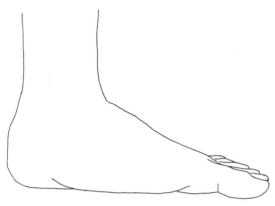

Figure 1–39. Pes planus (flat foot).

1–41*C*). Inspect the great and lesser toes for flexion or extension deformities. In the coronal plane, the toes should be straight. The great toe should lie in 10° of valgus in relationship to the first metatarsal.

The medial and lateral malleoli should be inspected for deformity.

Soft tissue inspection involves evaluation of color for pallor, rubor, or skin mottling. Calluses, corns, or ulcers are noted. Localized or generalized swelling is noted.

Palpation

Have the patient sit on the edge of the examining table with the leg hanging free. Palpate the tibia to its distal medial tip, the medial malleolus. Palpate the deltoid ligament, which fans out from the tip of the medial malleolus to the medial hindfoot. Palpate

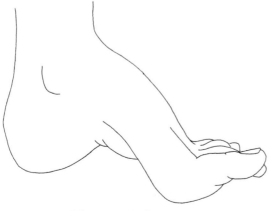

Figure 1–40. Pes cavus.

anteriorly and laterally on the medial malleolus to the ankle joint line, which is more easily identified by dorsiflexing and plantar flexing the foot. Palpate laterally along the ankle joint line, and anterior distal tibiofibular joint. Note tenderness or swelling. Note ankle effusion. Palpate the lateral malleolus. The anterior talofibular ligament runs from the anterior aspect of the lateral malleolus to the dorsolateral surface of the foot. Note any swelling or tenderness. Continue palpation along the lateral and posterior aspects of the lateral malleolus. Palpate the Achilles tendon and its insertion into the tuberosity of the calcaneus. Note tenderness or discontinuity.

Palpate the medial aspect of the foot. Note that the first bone prominence distal to the medial malleolus is the talar head. This is followed by the navicular, the medial cuneiform, and the base of the first metatarsal. Note excessive prominence of the talar head. The talar head is more prominent medially in pes planus. Palpate from medial to lateral on the dorsum of the medial cuneiform, middle cuneiform, lateral cuneiform, and cuboid bones. Palpate along the lateral aspect of the foot, from posterior to anterior, the calcaneus, cuboid, and the prominence of the base of the fifth metatarsal. Note swelling or tenderness. Deep palpation discloses a relative depression just distal to the anterior aspect of the lateral malleolus. This is the sinus tarsi between the calcaneus and the talus. It will feel relatively full in the club foot and will be deep or exaggerated in pes planus. Palpate dorsally along the shafts of the first through fifth metatarsals. Palpate the metatarsophalangeal (MTP) joints, the proximal, middle and distal phalanges, and the interphalangeal joints. Pay particular attention to the first MTP joint. Note any bone prominence along the medial aspect of the first metatarsal head and any valgus malalignment of the MTP joint.

Palpate the plantar surface of the foot from the anterior aspect of the tuberosity of the calcaneus, proceeding distally along the medial longitudinal arch. Note any tenderness. Palpate the plantar aspects of the metatarsal heads and note any tenderness.

Palpate the posterior tibial tendon as it courses around the medial malleolus to insert on the navicular. Just posterior to this lies the flexor digitorum longus tendon. The tibial nerve and posterior tibial artery lie posterior to these two tendons at the medial

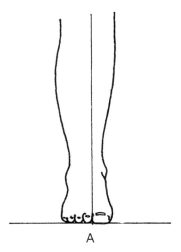

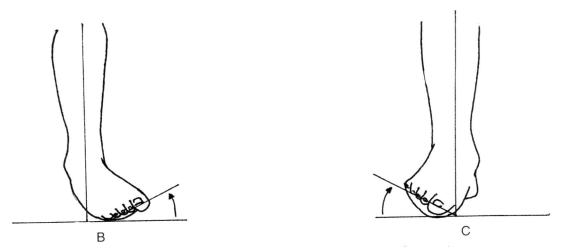

Figure 1–41. Forefoot alignment. *A*, Normal; *B*, supination; *C*, pronation.

malleolus. Just posterior to the neurovascular bundle lies the flexor hallucis longus tendon.

Palpate the tibialis anterior tendon coursing from just lateral to the crest of the tibia toward the base of the first metatarsal. Moving laterally, palpate the extensor hallucis longus tendon, the dorsalis pedis pulse, and the extensor digitorum longus tendons.

The peroneus longus and brevis tendons are accessible to palpation as they course around the lateral malleolus. Palpate the peroneus brevis to its insertion on the base of the fifth metatarsal.

Palpate the soft tissues between the metatarsal shafts for swelling or tenderness. Tenderness between the metatarsal heads (particularly the third and fourth) may indicate Morton's neuroma.

Range of Motion

Ankle extension (dorsiflexion) and plantar flexion are examined with the patient sitting on the edge of the examining table and the knee bent 90° (Fig. 1–42). Normal dorsiflexion is 20°, and plantar flexion is 50°.

Inversion and eversion are motions that occur primarily at the subtalar joint between the talus and calcaneus. Normal inversion and eversion are 5° in each direction. Grasp the distal tibia firmly and, with the other hand grasping the heel, attempt to invert and evert the foot.

The MTP joint is intimately involved in the toe-off phase of gait; therefore, first MTP pathology can lead to a functional deficit. Check the MTP joint for flexion and extension. Stabilize the distal aspect of the patient's first metatarsal and attempt first to push up or extend the great toe. Normal extension is to 70°. Attempt to flex the toe. Normal flexion is 45°.

Neurologic Examination

Motor Testing

Since the long flexors to the ankle and foot all originate in the leg, the motor examination has been described in the section on the knee and leg. Be aware, however, that the foot does have intrinsic muscles. These are difficult to test manually, but intrinsic muscle pathology, as seen in some neuromuscular disorders (Charcot-Marie-Tooth) or after foot compartment syndrome, may manifest as pes cavus or clawing (MP hyperextension and PIP/DIP flexion) of the toes.

Sensory Examination

The peripheral nerve sensory supply to the foot is as follows: the sural nerve supplies the dorsolateral aspect of the foot and ankle; the superficial peroneal nerve supplies the dorsum of the foot; the deep peroneal nerve supplies a small patch of skin on the dorsum of the foot at the base of the first web space; the saphenous nerve supplies the medial aspect of the foot; and the medial and lateral plantar nerve branches of the tibial nerve supply the medial and lateral aspects of the plantar surface of the foot, respectively (see Fig. 1–36).

The sensory examination of nerves to the foot and ankle also should proceed with the dermatomal distribution in mind (see Fig. 1–1).

Reflexes

Achilles Tendon Reflex. With the patient's leg dangling free, gently place the examining hand beneath the forefoot to dorsiflex the foot to a neutral position. Briskly tap the Achilles tendon with the reflex hammer. The ankle should plantar flex, with contraction of the gastrocsoleus.

Clonus Test. With the leg dangling freely and the knee bent 90°, the foot is quickly and forcibly dorsiflexed. The examiner should feel for a subtle and immediate "kick back" of the foot into plantar flexion, and count the number of beats. Any more than one to two beats of clonus is abnormal after the age of 1 year and may indicate an upper motor neuron lesion.

Babinski Reflex. A sharp object such as a key is run along the plantar surface of the foot, beginning at the calcaneus and proceeding distally along the lateral aspect. A positive

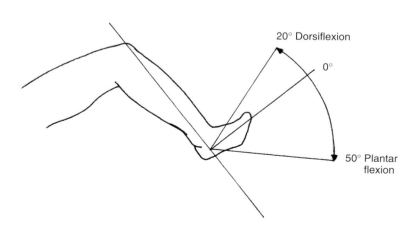

20° Dorsiflexion

0°

50° Plantar flexion

Figure 1–42. Ankle dorsiflexion (20 degrees) and plantar flexion (50 degrees).

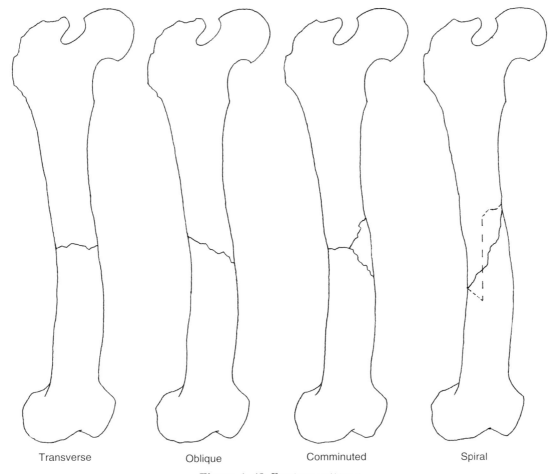

| Transverse | Oblique | Comminuted | Spiral |

Figure 1–43. Fracture patterns.

reaction is manifested as dorsiflexion of the great toe, with fanning of the lesser toes. After infancy, a positive Babinski is abnormal.

Special Tests

Thompson Test for Achilles Tendon Continuity

With the patient lying prone and the foot lying over the end of the examining table, the calf muscle is squeezed. The foot should plantar flex. Failure to do so may be secondary to discontinuity of the gastrocsoleus/Achilles tendon mechanism.

For specific testing of ankle stability, see Chapter 9.

Congenital deformities of the foot are discussed in detail in Chapter 27.

RADIOGRAPHIC EVALUATION

Although a detailed discussion of the radiographic evaluation of specific injuries is beyond the scope of this chapter and can be found in the appropriate chapters in this text, a few general comments are in order. The radiographic evaluation should be tailored to the specific findings on history and physical examination. If a specific area is suspected as being the site of pathology, it is imperative that x-ray views of that bone extend from the joint above to the joint below. This is particularly important in cases of trauma and tumor. It is likewise important that two perpendicular views, with the beam directed 90 degrees to each other, be obtained. An all too frequent example of cases when pathology can be missed by failure to do this involves the radiographic evaluation of the shoulder.

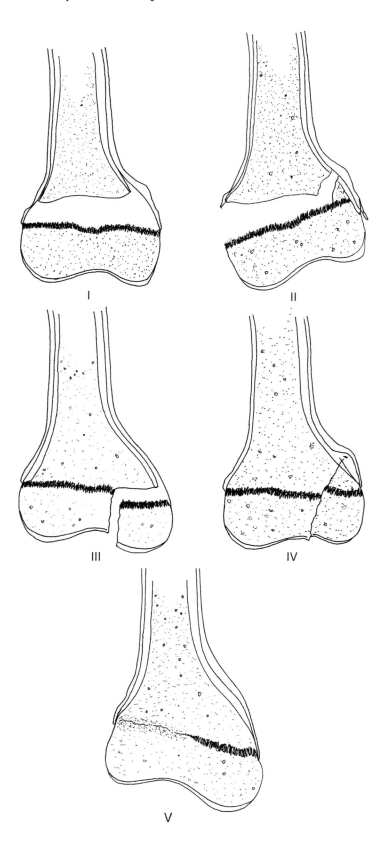

Figure 1–44. The Salter-Harris classification of growth plate (physeal) injuries. *Type I:* fracture line is through physis. *Type II:* fracture extends through physis and metaphysis. *Type III:* fracture extends through epiphysis (intra-articular and physis). *Type IV:* fracture extends through metaphyseal and epiphyseal regions (intra-articular). *Type V:* crush injury to physis.

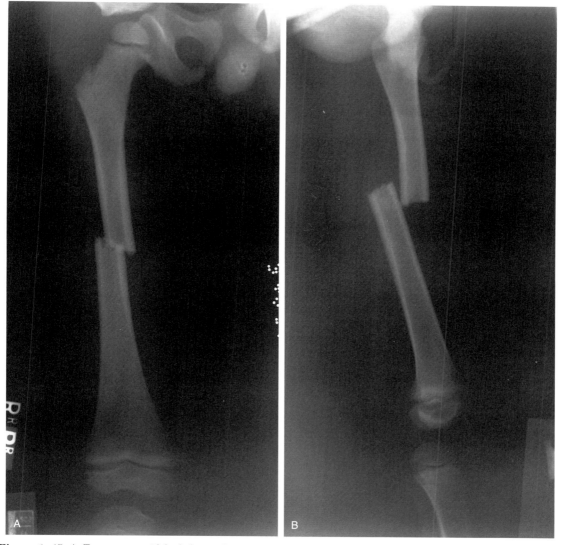

Figure 1–45. *A,* Transverse midshaft femur fracture in a 4-year-old child with 30 percent of lateral translation, 5 degrees of valgus, and 2 to 3 mm of shortening. *B,* One hundred percent posterior translation and twenty degrees of posterior angulation.

Oblique views are obtained as indicated to profile specific areas further. Common oblique views include the scaphoid view of the wrist, Judet views of the pelvis to evaluate acetabular fractures, mortise views of the ankle, and oblique views of the foot. Postreduction radiographs should always be obtained after the reduction of any fracture or dislocation. It is helpful to consult with the radiologist when deciding on special views or special studies. Special studies, including CT scan, magnetic resonance imaging, and bone scan, are discussed in this text when indicated.

CLASSIFICATION OF FRACTURES AND DISLOCATIONS

Fractures are first characterized by the bone involved (e.g., femur, ulna) and by that portion of the bone involved: epiphysis, metaphysis, or diaphysis. They are either intra-articular—that is, extending into the joint surface, or extra-articular—not involving the joint. Any intra-articular fracture must be critiqued for joint irregularity.

A fracture is classified as open or closed. In open fracture, a break in the skin communicates with the fracture site. This may range from a small, pin-point sized laceration to a massive soft tissue loss.

Various fracture patterns have been described for long bone fractures. These are transverse, oblique, spiral, and comminuted (Fig. 1–43). Greenstick and buckle fractures are incomplete fractures that occur in immature bones.

Fractures that involve the growth plate are common in children. These have been classified by Salter and Harris into five types, as depicted in Figure 1–44. A Salter-Harris I fracture courses transversely across the growth plate without involving bone. A Salter-Harris II fracture courses transversely across the growth plate to exit through the metaphysis, leaving a triangular fragment of variable size attached to the epiphyseal fragment. The Salter-Harris III fracture is an intra-articular fracture that splits the epiphysis to exit through the growth plate. The Salter-Harris IV fracture is a shearing type of injury passing through the epiphysis across the growth plate and exiting through the metaphysis. The Salter-Harris V fracture is a crush injury to the growth plate that is generally a retrospective diagnosis. Any physeal injury runs the risk of premature closure, with resultant loss of growth or angular growth of the bone.

Fractures can be described in regard to their displacement (Fig. 1–45). Displacement can occur in four ways: translation, angulation, rotation, and shortening. Translation is defined as shifting of one fragment in relationship to the other. By convention, translation is described by the percent shift in relationship to the diameter of the bone, and the direction of translation is the direction in which the distal fragment has moved.

Angulation is angular malalignment. In a nonangulated fracture, the proximal and distal fragments remain parallel. The angulation is described in regard to the degrees of angulation and the apex of the deformity. If the apex of the deformity in a femur fracture points posteriorly, this is spoken of as posterior angulation.

Rotation is very difficult to judge radiographically and therefore is a clinical judgement.

Fractures may shorten due to muscle pull. The amount of shortening can be judged radiographically by measuring overlap of the fracture ends.

SUBLUXATIONS/DISLOCATIONS

The terms *subluxation* and *dislocation* are used to describe joint relationships. In a dislocation, the opposing articular surfaces of the joint are no longer in contact. In subluxation, the articular surfaces are still in contact, but the relationship is abnormal. Dislocations, like fractures, are described in regard to the relationship of the distal bone to the proximal bone. For instance, in a posterior dislocation of the knee, the tibia lies posterior to the femur.

VARUS/VALGUS

These are commonly used terms in orthopaedics. They can be applied to alignment of a joint, long bone, or fracture site. In a valgus deformity, the apex of the deformity points toward the midline of the body (see Fig. 1–3A). In a varus deformity, the apex points away from the midline (see Fig. 1–3B).

Suggested Reading

American Academy of Pediatrics, American Heart Association: Textbook of Pediatric Advanced Life Support. Dallas, American Heart Association, 1990.

American Heart Association: Guidelines for cardiopulmonary resuscitation and emergency cardiac care. JAMA 268:2171–2302, 1992.

American Orthopaedic Association: Manual of Orthopaedic Surgery, 6th ed. 1985.

Boileau-Grant JC: Grant's Atlas of Anatomy, 9th ed. Baltimore, Williams & Wilkins, 1991.

Hoppenfeld S: Orthopaedic Neurology. A Diagnostic Guide to Neurologic Levels. Philadelphia, J. B. Lippincott, 1977.

Hoppenfeld S: Physical Examination of the Spine and Extremities. New York, Appleton-Century-Crofts, 1976.

Neviaser RJ, Eisenfeld LS, Wiesel SW, Lewis RJ: Emergency Orthopaedic Radiology. New York, Churchill Livingstone, 1985.

Salter RB: Textbook of Disorders and Injuries of the Musculoskeletal System, 2nd ed. Baltimore, Williams & Wilkins, 1983.

Orthopaedic Emergencies and Infections

Kenneth Jaffe

John Greco

Jeff Wade

Orthopaedic emergencies require expeditious recognition and action, for certain orthopaedic problems may change the outcome of a patient to the extent of saving both life and limb. Although primary care physicians may not be the ones to provide the definitive treatment, their actions are quite important. It is imperative that the primary care physician maintain a high index of suspicion for orthopaedic emergencies and infections, understand the consequences, and be able to provide initial management and stabilization.

INJECTION INJURIES

High-pressure injection injuries of the hand can be disabling, resulting in loss of function. Usually, a foreign substance such as automotive grease, diesel oil, or paint is injected into the hand under force. Typically the patient is a male, who will complain initially of swelling and pain as he presents with a small puncture wound that may weep the foreign material injected.[25] Sometimes the material

may be visible radiographically. The most common injection sites are the index and long fingers, and the site may extend down to the flexor sheaths.[15]

The result of the injection of foreign material is early tissue destruction, chemical irritation, and an accompanying inflammatory reaction with possible secondary infection. Even though the puncture site initially appears innocuous, the resulting damage can be devastating (Fig. 2–1). At times, there can be immediate ischemia of a digit secondary to increased volume within a contained space. This can lead to a compartment syndrome and gangrene.

The type of material injected has a high correlation with the degree of injury.[25] In most series, it was found that paint injections resulted in the greatest number of amputations. Lubricating oils may contain impurities that cause severe inflammatory reactions. Grease injections are less irritating. Air and water injections are usually benign and require little or no treatment.[20]

The accepted treatment for these injuries starts with recognition. After a com-

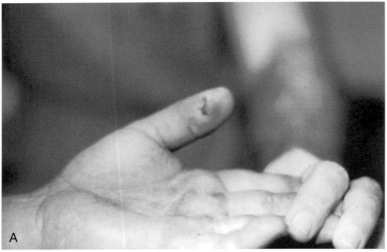

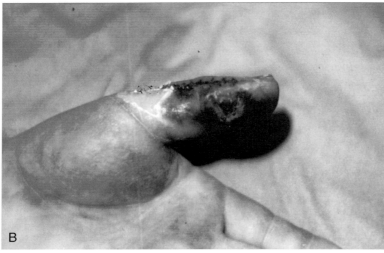

Figure 2–1. *A,* Paint gun injection injury to the thumb. *B,* Twenty-four hours postinjury, showing necrosis of the digit.

plete upper extremity and roentgenographic examination, antibiotics and anti-inflammatory medications for early use are given, sometimes including hydrocortisone.[23] Mechanical debridement and irrigation should be used to remove as much of the foreign material as possible. Wounds should be left open, with repeat irrigation and debridement as indicated. The use of paint and grease solvents has been shown to be ineffective.[26] Early surgical debridement does not guarantee a good result; some injuries progress to amputation despite early interventions. Stiffness and sensory deficits are frequent sequelae.

FAT EMBOLISM

Fat embolism is a syndrome that manifests with fever, tachycardia, acute respiratory distress with tachypnea, arterial hypoxemia, low Pco_2, and petechiae. The exact etiology remains unclear. It is fatal in 10 to 15 percent of cases. There are also mental manifestations such as restlessness, incoherency, and confusion. These usually occur 24 to 72 hours after injury.

Fat embolism occurs much more commonly in young adults than in any other age group, and it is rare in children. Its incidence correlates positively with the number of long bones fractured, open fractures, and fractures caused by vehicular accidents.[1] Embolic marrow fat from the fracture site appears to be the central pathway of the physiologic agent. Fat embolism is concentrated in the pulmonary vascular bed where it causes an inflammatory response and activates the clotting cascade, increases platelet activity, and initiates the release of vasoactive substances. The final common pathway of response of the lung is manifested by capillary leakage, inflammation and edema, and eventual fibrosis (Fig. 2–2).

The treatment of fat embolism should be designed to avoid hypoxemia and consists of the same measures used in adult respiratory distress syndrome: oxygenation and artificial ventilation whenever necessary. PEEP should be used to reach a P_{AO_2} of 60 mm Hg. Specific medications such as low molecular weight dextran, heparin, alcohol, and corticosteroids show no beneficial influence on the outcome and should not play a role in the treatment. The most important step is prevention. Early stabilization of fractures can reduce the incidence of fat embolism and its consequences.[19]

A syndrome similar to fat embolism has been reported after total hip arthroplasty. This occurs most commonly with cement fixation of the femoral prosthesis, possibly because of high intramedullary pressures that cause fats in marrow elements to be forced into the venous drainage. Another theory is related to the monomer of polymethylmethacrylate. Maintenance of normal blood volume and proper oxygenation are important in preventing the clinical manifestations. Treatment includes blood volume replacement, cardiotonic drugs, and respiratory support.

PULMONARY EMBOLISM

Pulmonary embolism is the most common cause of death immediately postoperatively in patients who have had a reconstructive operative procedure on the lower extremity.[12] Many methods of prophylaxis against deep venous thrombosis and its potential sequela of fatal embolism have been advocated, but unfortunately none have been 100 percent effective. Physical methods of prevention have included elevation of the extremity, early active motion of the hip or knee, continuous passive motion of these joints, use of compression stockings, and use of sequential-compression boots. Pharmacologic prophylaxis has included aspirin, heparin, dextran, and Coumadin (warfarin). All these measures can reduce the incidence of thromboembolism, but the extent of efficacy

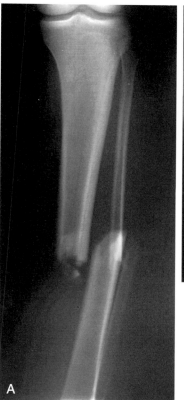

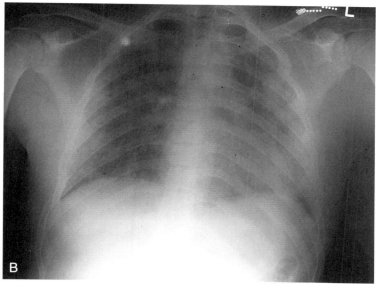

Figure 2–2. *A,* An 18-year-old man was involved in a motor vehicle accident and admitted to the hospital with a left tibia and fibula fracture. An intramedullary rod was placed. *B,* The patient developed dyspnea, and the chest radiograph was consistent with fat embolism.

has varied.[10-14,16] The patient may have a pulmonary embolism despite prophylaxis, there may be complications secondary to prophylaxis, prophylactic anticoagulation may be contraindicated, and finally, in the immediate postoperative period, therapeutic anticoagulation may compromise the healing of the wound.[28]

The diagnosis of pulmonary embolism starts with a high index of suspicion. More than 50 percent of deep venous thromboses are silent, and at least 80 percent of pulmonary embolisms are unsuspected. Physical findings include tachypnea, chest pain, hemoptysis, fever, disorientation, and tachycardia. Diagnostic procedures include ventilation perfusion lung scans, and pulmonary angiography (Fig. 2–3).

PELVIC FRACTURES

Pelvic fractures typically occur in patients who have sustained high-energy trauma. The fractures are often associated with other injuries. Priorities in the initial management are similar to those for multiple trauma. Severe pelvic fractures can be associated with a high mortality rate from significant intrapelvic bleeding and also from the associated injuries. Severe bleeding results primarily from lacerations of pelvic veins, although arterial bleeding also occurs. Injuries specifically associated with pelvic fractures include those of the neurologic, urologic, gynecologic, and gastrointestinal systems.[21]

Control of severe bleeding associated with the fractures is the primary initial concern. The severity of bleeding is highest in displaced or nonstable disruptions of the posterior pelvic ring. The first therapeutic measure for control of pelvic hemorrhage is the use of intravenous crystalloid solution or whole blood. This is sufficient in most stable pelvic fractures. Many unstable pelvic fractures may require other interventions. External fixation has been shown to decrease initial blood loss by controlling pelvic volume. The external fixation frame is typically applied to the anterior portion of both iliac crests. It is most effective in unstable fractures that increase the volume of the pelvic ring, such as injuries involving a wide separation of the symphysis pubis (Fig. 2–4). External fixation does not control vertical translation of the pelvic ring, nor does it truly immobilize the fracture site.

If fluid resuscitation and external fixation fail, the physician should proceed to selective angiography. Although most bleeding is of venous origin, often small arterial bleeders can be treated by angiographic embolization. Angiographic embolization should not be performed unless there is good evidence that the patient's condition is unstable and a significant bleeding site has been identified. If angiography shows injury to major arteries of the pelvis, direct surgical repair may be indicated.

Urologic injury in the form of injury to the bladder and urethra is common in pelvic fractures, with an overall incidence of approximately 13 percent. Most urethral injuries occur in males. The diagnosis of urethral injury is based on radiographic as well as physical findings. There may be blood at the urethral meatus, or a high-riding prostate may be found on rectal examination. An intravenous pyelogram may show an intact but elevated bladder that is compressed by a pelvic hematoma. The diagnosis is confirmed by dynamic retrograde ureterography, with radiographs taken while the contrast material is being injected.

COMPARTMENT SYNDROME

A compartment syndrome is defined as a condition in which the circulation or function of tissues within a closed space is compromised by increased pressure within that space. More than a century ago, Richard von Volkmann published the first account of a post-traumatic muscle contracture of acute onset, with increasing deformity despite splinting and passive exercises. He believed that paralysis and contraction of the limbs "too tightly bandaged" resulted from ischemic changes of the muscles. Since that time, physicians have become increasingly aware of the varied circumstances in which increased tissue pressures may compromise the microcirculation: traumatic, vascular, hematologic, neurologic, surgical, pharmacologic, renal, and iatrogenic. The most common areas for compartment syndromes to develop are the dorsal and volar forearm, the posterior and anterolateral leg, and the intrinsic muscles of the hand and foot.

The clinical presentation of compartment syndrome is often indefinite and confusing, and delays in diagnosis occur even when physicians are aware of the signs and symptoms.

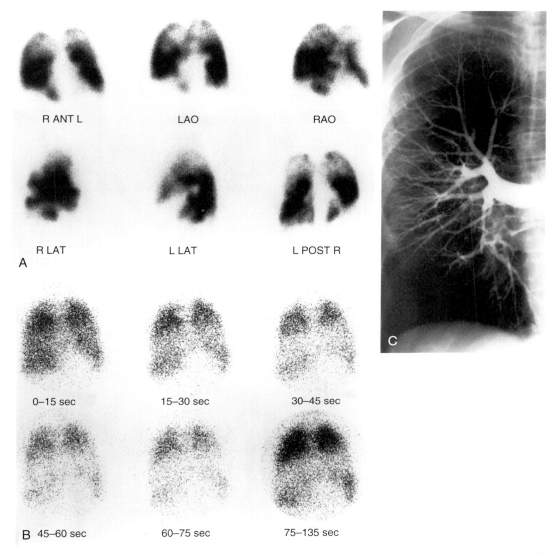

Figure 2–3. A 78-year-old man sustained a right hip fracture and developed acute shortness of breath 3 days postsurgery. His past history revealed restrictive and obstructive lung disease. *A* and *B,* V/Q scan showed a high probability of pulmonary embolus. *C,* Pulmonary angiogram showed a large filling defect in the right main and interlobal arteries.

The classic signs of impending compartment syndrome are pain, pallor, paresthesia, paralysis, and pulselessness. Pain is perhaps the earliest and most important consistent sign. Unfortunately, it is variable and not always reliable. Compartment syndromes are often associated with inherently painful conditions such as crush injuries and fractures. However, the pain of tissue ischemia is typically described as deep, unremitting, and poorly localized. It is not the type of pain usually associated with a fracture, and it is difficult to control with the usual mild anal-

gesic measures used for fractures. Passive extension of the foot or of the fingers exacerbates the pain in the extremity and is an early physical finding. Pallor may or may not be present. The extremity may appear cyanotic or mottled early in the course of events. Neither pallor nor cyanosis should be considered a sign that is necessary for the diagnosis of compartment syndrome. Paresthesia in the cutaneous distribution of the peripheral nerve coursing through the affected compartment is usually an early sign of impending, but still reversible, com-

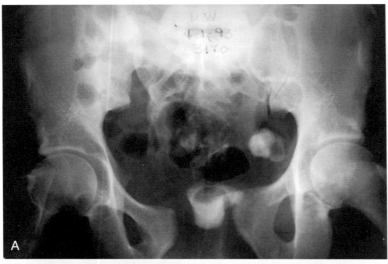

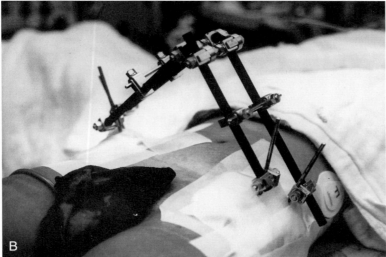

Figure 2–4. *A,* AP radiograph of a pelvic fracture. *B,* A pelvic external fixator is used to stabilize the fracture.

partment syndrome. Sensory disturbance usually precedes motor dysfunction. When a physician waits for obvious motor deficits to occur or for pulses to be obliterated, ischemia has usually been well established for some time, and there may be permanent damage.

If one suspects a developing compartment syndrome, constricting casts or circular dressings must be removed immediately. Increased intracompartmental pressure has been implicated as the primary pathogenic factor in compartment syndromes, and because the diagnosis of these syndromes is often so difficult to make on clinical grounds alone, the measurement of intracompartmental tissue pressures has been a valuable clinical tool. Several investigators recommend a measurement of intracompartmental

pressures either by infusion or with catheter technique (Fig. 2–5). Consensus is lacking on the exact tissue pressures above which a compartment syndrome occurs. Some advocate fasciotomy if the compartmental pressure is above 30 mm Hg, but others correlate pressures with the diastolic blood pressure. Compartmental pressure measurements are particularly useful when assessing an unreliable, uncooperative, or unresponsive patient.

The treatment of compartment syndromes is fasciotomy. Initially, decompression should be done by immediately splinting or removing the cast or other compromising circular dressings. The technique of fasciotomy is a matter of surgical choice. The surgical goal is salvage of a viable and functioning extremity. It is essential to decompress all tight com-

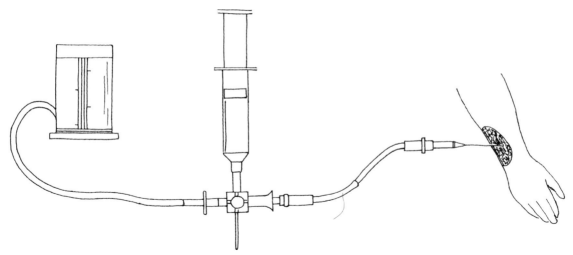

Figure 2–5. Whiteside's technique of intracompartmental pressure measurement. The catheter is introduced into a muscle belly of the compartment to be tested.

partments. The wounds are left open and may require delayed primary closing or skin grafting.

OPEN FRACTURES

An open fracture is one in which a break in the skin and underlying soft tissues leads directly into or communicates with the fracture and its hematoma. "Compound fracture" refers to the same injury, but this is an archaic and nonspecific term.[24] The prognosis in open fractures is determined primarily by the amount of devitalized bone and soft tissue caused by an injury, and by the level and type of bacterial contamination. The extent of bone and soft tissue devitalization is determined by the energy absorbed by the limb at the time of injury.

Open fractures are classified into three main groups according to the severity of the soft tissue injury.[9] Grade I fractures have a skin laceration of less than 1 cm, usually caused from a perforation of the bone from the inside out. Grade II lesions have a larger opening of less than 10 cm, with associated muscle and skin loss. Grade IIIA lesions are larger than 10 cm. A grade IIIB indicates initial soft tissue loss and periosteal stripping (Fig. 2–6). Grade IIIC fractures are associated with the disruption of a major vessel. In open fractures, antibiotic coverage should start when the patient arrives in the Emergency Department and should take into account the characteristics of the patient's

injuries and the severity of the wound contamination. For most injuries, a broad-spectrum cephalosporin should be given. For Grade III fractures, an aminoglycoside should be given as a supplement. Penicillin is added for farm-related injuries and major clostridial contamination.

When a patient with an open fracture arrives in the emergency department, general assessment of the patient should focus first on evaluating the airway, breathing, and circulation. Open fractures may have associated injuries, for they are usually a result of high-energy trauma. Once an overview of the patient is performed and the patient is stabilized, attention should then be directed toward the limbs. The area of the open fracture is splinted and assessment of the wounds made. Special attention should be paid to the neurovascular status, size of the soft tissue loss, exposure of bone, contamination, and bleeding. Wounds are cultured, a sterile dressing is applied, antibiotics and tetanus prophylaxis are administered, and radiographs are then performed. The patient will then require emergency surgical debridement.

SPINAL CORD INJURIES

Acute injuries of the spine and spinal cord are among the most common causes of feared disability and death following trauma. The diagnosis of these injuries is often delayed, and the treatment is frequently nonstan-

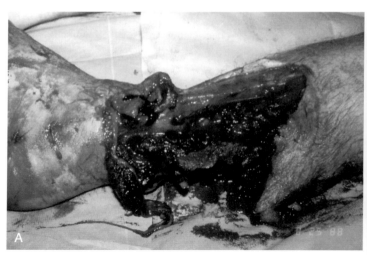
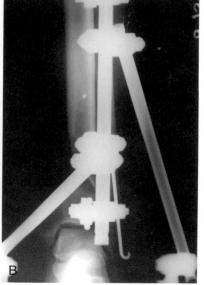

Figure 2–6. *A,* A IIIB open fracture of a lower leg with extensive soft tissue damage and exposed bone. *B,* Stabilization of the fracture with an external fixator.

dardized or inadequate, producing increasing problems with rehabilitation of the patient. Recognition of the patient with a spine or spinal cord injury is the first step toward appropriate treatment of these individuals. Ideally, these injuries should be diagnosed at the scene of the accident, and at the least any visible paralysis should be assessed and recorded. Causes of delay in the recognition of spine injuries are associated head injuries, acute alcoholic intoxication, and multiple injuries.

The evaluation of the spinal cord–injured patient should begin at the scene of the accident with trained paramedics on hand, where initial meaningful information can be gathered. The first question in obtaining a history concerns pain in the region of the neck or spine. If there is pain in the cervical region, the patient's neck should be placed in a collar or spine board; if the pain is in the lower spine, the patient should be placed on a transportation board in a neutral supine position. There should be no further movement of the spine until the patient has been completely evaluated by a physician with radiographs in the emergency department.

In the acute spinal cord injury, a predominant feature is systemic hypotension. The prime central disturbance is a sinus bradycardia due to unopposed vagal activity as a result of ablation of sympathetic activity during spinal areflexia (spinal shock). Hypotension with tachycardia should be regarded as being caused by blood loss until proved otherwise. The hypotension produces systemic shock but also reduces spinal cord blood flow. The damaged cord cannot autoregulate, and the secondary anoxic insult is applied to the cord. In isolated cord injury, hypotension is easily corrected with 500 to 1000 ml of crystalloid. Fluid replacement in the first 48 hours in an isolated spinal cord injury should be no more than 2 liters per day. Hypotension not easily corrected with IV fluids is rare. These cases may respond to pressure amines or dopamine.

In many cases, the diagnosis of an isolated spinal cord injury is obvious: there is a complete sensorimotor loss with a clear-cut sensory level and declared symptoms reproduced by a conscious patient. This diagnosis is less clear when the cord lesion is incomplete or there is a vertebral column injury in the absence of neurologic findings and yet with a capacity for spinal cord deterioration. Difficulties in diagnosis also arise when the picture is obscured by a head injury, or when multiple injuries demand precedence, with the possibility of spinal cord injury being overlooked.

A full neurologic examination of any person who has been injured in the head or trunk is mandatory. Three specific patterns of incomplete cord injury that are misdiagnosed are the Brown-Séquard lesion, the anterior cord syndrome, and the central cord lesion. The central cord lesion in particular is missed as there may be many radiologic signs, such as a widening of the anterior interbody space, or no signs at all other than a background of cervical spondylosis. The account of the injury is frequently trivial. Multiple injuries may obscure spinal cord injury, in particular head and chest injuries. Indications of the presence of a combined head and spinal cord injury include a differential level of apparent responsiveness above and below the level of the cord injury, the presence of diaphragmatic breathing, and unexplained hypotension in a patient in whom no other overt cause of shock may be found.

GAS GANGRENE

Gangrene is one of the most serious complications of traumatic wounds. It was generally regarded as a disease associated with battlefield casualties, but it is not uncommon to see this infection in civilian life. Postoperative clostridial infections are being reported with increasing frequency. It is becoming evident that many anaerobic bacteria thought to be commensals have become invasive and produce gas gangrene in the face of host changes induced by extensive surgery or therapy with corticosteroids, cytotoxic agents, or antibiotics.

Clostridium perfringens is the most important species capable of producing gas gangrene. It is a gram-positive anaerobic bacillus, regarded as an ubiquitous organism found in the human alimentary tract, in hospital corridors, and in the ground. Clostridial infections are not caused by the extra virulence of the organism, but rather by unique local conditions. The local lesion arises when the bacteria are introduced into a deep wound of muscle where, under favorable conditions, they multiply and produce toxins that diffuse into the surrounding tissues and devitalize them, allowing further colonization. Muscle ischemia and necrosis lead to a decreased oxidation reduction potential, which promotes rapid advance of the highly lethal infection. It is easy to understand how trauma from the injury itself, surgery, tight casts, and so forth can lower the oxidation reduction potential values and create the proper environment for clostridial infection. Dirty wounds, especially those closed primarily without appropriate debridement, provide an ideal setting for the onset of gas gangrene.

Different categories of traumatic wound infections need to be differentiated from clostridial myonecrosis. Anaerobic cellulitis is a clostridial infection of ischemic tissue in an inadequately debrided wound, usually occurring after several days. It may produce a rapidly spreading emphysematous infection along the fascial planes, with extensive gas formation. The onset is gradual, and the toxemia is slight. The exudate is brown and seropurulent. The gas is foul smelling and abundant, but there is no actual muscle invasion.

Infected vascular gangrene represents another specific histotoxic infection of humans in which gas-producing anaerobes are found proliferating in gangrenous but anatomically intact muscle. The organisms are saprophytes, not invaders, in a limb that is ischemic. A line of demarcation is seen, and bacterial spread is limited. A foul-smelling gas production occurs, but rarely are the signs and symptoms of acute toxemia observed. Although a relatively benign form of infection, vascular gangrene can develop into true clostridial myonecrosis if neglected.

Anaerobic myonecrosis is caused by the clostridial organism as well as a streptococcal species. Almost without exception the original wound involves injury to muscle—a deep, penetrating wound sealed off from ready access to the surface. The incubation period of clostridia is approximately 12 to 24 hours after injury. The initial symptom is pain or a sense of heaviness in the affected area, followed by local edema and exudation of a thin, dark fluid. There is dissociation between tachycardia and temperature elevation; the pulse rate is elevated, but the temperature is not high initially. The progress of the disease is rapid and spectacular, with an increase in toxemia and local spread of the infection. Profound shock may occur. The wound develops a peculiar bronze discoloration, a musty odor, and a slight amount of gas production. A symptom characteristic of gas gangrene is the mental awareness marked by terror of death in the face of a profound toxemia.

A second form of anaerobic myonecrosis is secondary to anaerobic streptococcal infection. The majority of these infections are located in the perirectal or inguinal regions. Inflammation is slight, but there is a large amount of seropurulent discharge. Toxemia is less at the outset, and marked pain and septicemia do not occur except as terminal events.

The diagnosis of clostridial myonecrosis can be made by its clinical features. The most important are severe local pain and swelling associated with severe tissue destruction and marked systemic toxemia. Gas formation is not a pathognomonic feature and in some instances may be scant. Bacteriologic demonstration of pathogenic clostridia in affected tissues is also of limited significance, since the organisms are commensal and widespread.

The successful treatment of gas gangrene depends on early diagnosis and prompt surgical decompression and debridement. Surgery remains the cornerstone of treatment for clostridial myonecrosis. Multiple incisions and fasciotomy for decompression and drainage of the fascial compartments, excision of the involved muscles, and open amputation constitute appropriate operative management. A promising adjunct in the treatment of clostridial myonecrosis is the use of hyperbaric oxygen. Large intravenous doses of penicillin should be administered. Resuscitation must include prompt replacement of fluids and electrolytes.

TRAUMATIC AMPUTATIONS/ REPLANTATION

Care for the patient as well as the amputated part is very critical to the success and survival of the replant. The overall management of the patient always takes precedence. It is important to assess the general condition of the patient with primary concern for basic life support. Once this is accomplished, attention should be directed toward the amputated part. Cooling of the amputated part helps lower the metabolic rate and thus the oxygen consumption of the tissues. The acceptable cool ischemia time is 6 hours, except for digital amputations, which have been successfully replanted after 12 to 30 hours. The amputated part should be gently irrigated with copious amounts of Ringer's lactate or saline solution. The amputated extremity then should be wrapped in Ringer's lactate with a sterile towel in order to protect the tissues from desiccation. The wrapped extremity should be placed in a sealed plastic bag, which is then placed in a container on a bed of crushed ice (Fig. 2–7). The plastic bag and the sterile towel prevent the tissues from freezing. The bag should be appropriately labeled for proper identifica-

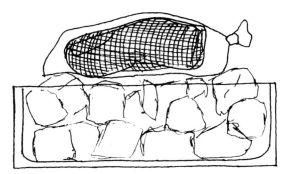

Figure 2–7. A method of storing an amputated extremity.

tion. Dry ice must not be used. The tissue must not be put directly into ice.

The stump should be irrigated and debrided and wrapped in a sterile dressing. Efforts to achieve hemostasis by the use of clamps may damage the neurovascular bundles and should be avoided. The patient is stabilized following the ABCs of trauma management. Appropriate antibiotics are given, and the tetanus immunization status is assessed. The patient is then expeditiously transported to an appropriate facility for definitive surgical treatment.

VASCULAR INJURIES ASSOCIATED WITH FRACTURES AND DISLOCATIONS

Vascular injuries associated with fractures and dislocations frequently produce complex clinical problems. These injuries are often multifactorial; therefore, a systematic as well as a team approach is necessary. Skeletal trauma can easily conceal vascular injuries because attention may be given only to obvious bone deformities. Also, the excruciating pain of arterial insufficiency may be mistaken for fracture pain. Consequently, arterial and venous defects are often recognized too late, when the likelihood of a successful repair is greatly decreased.

Three principles should govern the management of patients with vascular damage: (1) a high index of suspicion of vascular injury must prevail during the initial evaluation or treatment of any major fracture or dislocation; (2) time lost prior to the recognition of vascular injury can never be regained; and (3) prompt and appropriate definitive treatment according to established surgical principles produces the best results.

Civilian vascular trauma arises either from nonpenetrating injuries such as pelvic fractures or knee dislocations or from penetrating injuries produced by lacerations or low-velocity gunshot or stab wounds.

In vascular injuries, the vessels may be damaged by entrapment, torsion, or laceration by fracture fragments. The injury tends to occur with fractures in areas where the vessels pass close to bone or are held in a fixed position by muscles, ligaments, or adjacent bone (Fig. 2–8). The nature of the arterial injury is variable and may occur as an immediate or late complication of bone or joint injuries. Disruption of the full thickness of an artery results in a laceration or avulsion of small branches and generally is first appreciated by the presence of an expanding hematoma that may be significant enough to produce distal ischemia. Injuries of this type are almost invariably associated with comminuted fractures and are produced by bone spicules or penetrating missiles. Arterial injuries occurring as the result of sudden forces that produce traction or torsion account for the majority of civilian injuries. These injuries generally produce elevated flaps of intima or intramural hematomas. Flow past these injured areas may be present

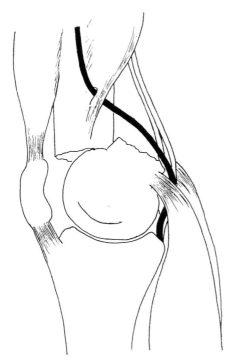

Figure 2–8. Supracondylar femur fracture. A distal fragment impinges on the popliteal artery.

initially but diminishes as the lumen narrows. Thrombosis may occur within minutes or hours of injury and depends upon such factors as the degree of underlying atherosclerosis or associated venous injuries. The major late complications include arterial venous fistulas, false aneurysms, or even true aneurysm formation. Distal ischemia may occur in the absence of arterial disruption because of extensive compression by hematoma formation or entrapment by soft tissue or bone fragments.

Restoration of normal flow is usually the rule following treatment by fasciotomies. If untreated, however, these injuries may progress to thrombosis and gangrene of the affected part. The presence of palpable pulses distal to the site of injury can in no way rule out the possibility of impending vascular compromise. Patients with major fractures and dislocations should be evaluated frequently for signs of ischemia.

DISLOCATION OF THE KNEE

Dislocation of the knee is a true surgical emergency. The vascular insult caused by such a severe injury requires immediate attention. The position of the tibia in relation to the femoral condyle is used to classify the dislocation (Fig. 2–9). A tibia that is anterior to the femur is an anterior dislocation.[17] The five major types of dislocations are anterior, posterior, lateral, medial, and rotary. The dislocation can also be described as open or closed and as a pure dislocation or a fracture-dislocation. Accidents from motor vehicles are the most common mode of injury. Sport injuries are the second most common cause of knee dislocations, but knee dislocations have been reported from lesser types of injuries such as stepping into a hole or falling down steps.

The popliteal artery is fixed both proximally and distally. It originates at the tendinous hiatus of the adductor magnus muscle, which firmly attaches it to the femoral shaft. Distally it passes beneath the tendinous arch of the soleus muscle, which also holds it firmly to the bone. Such an arrangement causes the artery to bolster across the popliteal space and allows little tolerance for skeletal distortion. Nerves of the popliteal area, the tibial and the common peroneal, do not have such a firm fixation as the popliteal artery and are therefore less likely to be

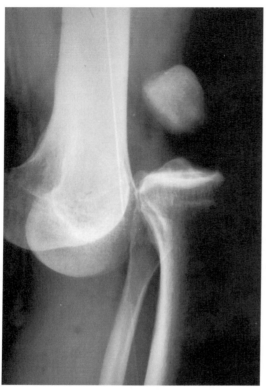

Figure 2–9. Anterior dislocation of the knee.

quite obvious, time should not be wasted obtaining radiographs, particularly if there is any question of circulatory compromise of the extremity. Even though a fracture around the knee may be suspected, if circulation is impaired, traction should be instituted to restore alignment and possibly to re-establish arterial flow. Anterior dislocations usually reduce by longitudinal traction, followed by lifting the femur into the reduced position. If closed reduction is not possible, surgical intervention is indicated.

The status of the neurovasculature must be assessed after the reduction. Lack of pulse in the dorsalis pedis or posterior tibial arteries, inability to move the toes, or the presence of tenseness in the popliteal region may be signs of developing vascular problems.[27] Such findings are indications for popliteal angiography. Controversy exists as to the indications for angiography if there is no compromise in circulation.[4]

Once the knee has been reduced and there is no apparent injury to the artery, treatment is directed toward the ligamentous damage. This will require cast immobilization or surgical repair.

injured. Nerve injuries usually are the traction type, in which the peroneal nerve is stretched across the posterior femoral condyle.

Anterior dislocation is by far the most common type.[8] It is produced by hyperextension of the knee, with tearing of the posterior capsule and cruciate ligaments. Posterior dislocations occur when there is rupture of the extensor mechanism and are usually the result of a crushing injury. Medial and lateral dislocations occur with extreme forces, usually with lateral and rotary stress. Both posterior and lateral dislocations are the type most likely to produce severe nerve damage. The dislocation may also be irreducible, with reduction prevented by the medial femoral condyle being trapped in a buttonhole rent in the medial capsule.

Because of the ease of reduction of many of these dislocations, they are often treated at the scene of an accident. High clinical suspicion must be kept in mind, and emergency medical personnel must be questioned when patients present with an unstable knee, swelling, ecchymosis, or signs of neurovascular compromise. Because the deformity is

SEPTIC ARTHRITIS

Even though septic arthritis is no longer a serious threat to life or limb, the morbidity associated with this condition if left unrecognized can be quite significant. Although any infectious agent may cause septic arthritis, bacterial or pyogenic arthritis is the most common type and is the most rapidly destructive form. Other causes include tuberculosis, mycosis, syphilis, and viruses. Most cases of bacterial arthritis are the result of a hematogenous infection that spreads to the joint. Since the synovial membrane is extremely vascular, any organism circulating in the blood may be easily trapped in the synovial space. Once inside this closed space, the bacteria rapidly multiply and are phagocytized by local synovial lining cells and inflammatory cells. Polymorphonuclear leukocytes and other circulating cells migrate to the synovium, releasing proteolytic enzymes that promote synovial hyperplasia, necrosis, and granulation tissue. Eventually cartilage is affected by the destruction of the glycosaminoglycans.

The diagnosis and treatment principles are basically similar in all types of septic arthritis. Other routes of infection of the joint may be from direct extension of osteomyelitis involving the epiphysis or an intracapsular metaphyseal infection. Direct contamination of the joint can also follow diagnostic or therapeutic interventions. Open injuries secondary to trauma may also induce an infection. The most common sites are the knee, hip, and shoulder. Basically, the condition is an acute synovitis that varies in degree, depending on the virulence of the organism and the resistance of the tissues. The affected joint is usually red, hot, swollen, and very tender. Constitutionally, there may be associated fever, glucose intolerance, and an elevated sedimentation rate.

Once a suspected diagnosis of septic arthritis is entertained, roentgenographic studies should be made. Radiographs are generally negative at the outset. However, synovial distension as well as swelling of the soft tissues may be seen. If the infection is persistent, osteoporosis as well as destruction of the cartilage with narrowing of the joint space can be seen.

Aspiration of the joint should be undertaken with sterile technique. The fluid is cultured for bacteria as well as tuberculosis, fungus, and gonococcus. A cell count as well as a Gram stain should also be ordered.

Once the diagnosis has been made, decompression of the joint is mandatory. It is controversial whether open synovectomy and debridement or repeated joint aspirations and irrigations are of the best benefit. Arthroscopic drainage and debridement have been utilized and appear to be a reasonable method of achieving the advantages of open debridement with fewer of the disadvantages. Antibiotics are given in amounts adequate to achieve therapeutic joint levels.

ACUTE HEMATOGENOUS OSTEOMYELITIS

Acute bone and bone marrow infections (osteomyelitis) usually occur via the hematogenous route.[5,18] The reported number of cases initially decreased after the introduction of penicillin but then increased with the development of antibiotic-resistant organisms.[5]

The infection occurs most commonly in the metaphyses or epiphyses of long bones. Preexisting infections, trauma, malnutrition, and compromised immune systems are all considered causative factors.[5,22]

Diagnosis can be difficult at times. A complete history, particularly noting any concurrent infection or acute onset of symptoms, is important. On thorough physical examination, any restlessness, swelling, erythema, warmth, tenderness, or limited range of motion must be documented. Initial blood work should include a complete blood count with differential, erythrocyte sedimentation rate, and blood cultures. Aspiration of the symptomatic area is helpful for bacteriologic diagnosis and subsequent antibiotic choice. A needle should be used, and separate subperiosteal and intraperiosteal aspirates are required. (Aspirates are positive approximately 60 percent of the time.[5,18]) Aspirates should be evaluated for Gram stain, acid-fast bacilli stain, culture and sensitivity, cell count, mycobacteria, fungi, viral cultures, mycoplasma isolation, and crystal analysis.

Radiographic studies can be helpful in the diagnosis of osteomyelitis. An initial set of plain radiographs is required upon presentation to the office or Emergency Department. Usually no significant bone changes are present for the first 7 to 10 days. However, deep soft tissue swelling near the metaphysis within the first 72 hours can be seen. Obliteration of deep soft tissue planes with subcutaneous edema develops between 3 and 7 days. The classic picture of sequestrum and periosteal new bone is seen approximately 10 to 14 days after onset of infection.[5,22,29]

A three-phase bone scan can be helpful in differentiating osseous versus soft tissue infection. Technetium, gallium, and indium scans are all effective in determining the activity of disease. Computed tomography scanning and magnetic resonance imaging are helpful in defining extraosseous deep soft tissue swelling and abnormal bone marrow, respectively.[5,22]

Various organisms have been identified as causing osteomyelitis. *Staphylococcus aureus* is still the predominant organism isolated from 60 to 90 percent of all reported cases. Streptococcus is the most common organism causing osteomyelitis in neonates up to 2 months of age. *Haemophilus influenzae* is a common causative agent in the 2-month to 2-year age group.[18] Other notable infectious agents include salmonella in sickle cell anemia patients, *Serratia, Pseudomonas, Brucella,* fungi, *Treponema,* and mycobacteria.[2,5,6,9,18,22]

Treatment principles are essentially based on nonoperative versus operative management. The causative organism needs to be identified as soon as possible. If no abscess is detected on aspiration or a Gram stain is negative, then broad-spectrum IV antibiotics are initiated (oxacillin/gentamicin or cefotaxime), followed by oral antibiotics once the temperature has normalized. Antibiotics should be continued until normalization of the erythrocyte sedimentation rate. If there is no response to antibiotics within 36 hours, an abscess has likely formed, and an incision and drainage procedure is necessary.[2,5,6,18]

If an abscess is present on aspiration or the Gram stain is positive, then surgical debridement is required emergently.[5,9,18,22] This is subsequently followed by intravenous antibiotics and any repeat debridements as necessary. Surgery is the only effective way of treating a proven infection.

There is considerable disagreement as to the length of time that antibiotics are required. Traditionally, 3 weeks of intravenous antibiotics followed by 3 weeks of oral therapy has been the rule. Confirmation of treatment effectiveness is seen when the erythrocyte sedimentation rate drops to less than 20 mm per hour. If there is rapid clinical improvement, oral antibiotics may be substituted for intravenous after 7 to 10 days.[5,6]

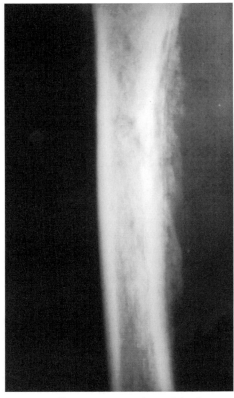

Figure 2–10. Chronic osteomyelitis of the femur, with reactive bone and soft tissue edema.

SUBACUTE/CHRONIC OSTEOMYELITIS

Chronic osteomyelitis can follow inappropriately treated acute osteomyelitis related to surgery, trauma, or soft tissue spread (Fig. 2–10). This entity is also seen in elderly patients, immunocompromised people, diabetic patients, and intravenous drug abusers. Constitutional signs and symptoms are often near normal in these patients.

Again, appropriate laboratory work, history and physical examination, plain radiographs, and nuclear medicine studies are all helpful in diagnosis. Additionally, determination of nutritional status, analysis of serum albumin, and transferrin and total lymphocyte counts are helpful in evaluating overall patient health.

The first step in treatment is debridement of necrotic, infected tissue to viable and well-perfused tissue margins. After antibiotic susceptibilities are obtained, appropriate intravenous antibiotics are instituted. Repeated debridements, bone grafting, stabilization, and soft tissue coverage are often required. Amputations are still often necessary as definitive treatment.

References

1. Baltensweiler J: Fettemboliesyndrom; Klinik und Prophylaxe. Bern, Stuttgart, Wien, Verlag Hans Huber, 1977.
2. Cierney G III: Chronic osteomyelitis: Results of treatment. Instr Course Lect 39:495–508, 1990.
3. Dennis JW, Fryberg ER, Crump JM, et al: New perspective on the management of penetrating trauma in proximity to major limb arteries. J Vasc Surg 11:84, 1990.
4. Dennis JW, Jagger C: Reassessing the role of arteriograms in the management of posterior knee dislocations. J Trauma 35:692, 1993.
5. Dorman JP: Musculoskeletal Infections in Infants and Children. Syllabus—Orthopaedic Review Course, 1993.
6. Fitzgerald RH Jr: Orthopaedic sepsis in osteomyelitis: Antimicrobial therapy for the musculoskeletal system. Instr Course Lect 31:1–9, 1982.
7. Fryberg ER, Crump JM: Nonoperative management of clinically occult arterial injuries: A prospective evaluation. Surgery 109:85, 1991.

8. Green NE, Allen BL: Vascular injuries with dislocation of the knee. J Bone Joint Surg 59A:236–239, 1977.

9. Gustilo RB: The management of open fractures. J Bone Joint Surg 72:299–303, 1990.

10. Harris WH, Salzman EW, Athanasoulis C, Waltman AC, Baum S, Des RW: Comparison of warfarin, low-molecular-weight dextran, aspirin, and subcutaneous heparin in prevention of venous thromboembolism following total hip replacement. J Bone Joint Surg 56A:1552–1562, 1974.

11. Homans J: Thrombosis of the deep veins of the lower leg, causing pulmonary embolism. N Engl J Med 211:993–997, 1934.

12. Hull RD, Raskob GE: Prophylaxis of venous thromboembolic disease following hip and knee surgery. Current Concepts Review. J Bone Joint Surg 68A:146–150, 1986.

13. Johnson R, Green JR, Charnley J: Pulmonary embolism and its prophylaxis following the Charnley total hip replacement. Clin Orthop 127:123–132, 1977.

14. Kakkar VV, Fok PJ, Murray WJG, Paes T, Merenstein D, et al: Heparin and dihydroergotamine prophylaxis after total hip replacement. N Engl J Med 309:954–958, 1983.

15. Kaufman HD: High pressure injection injuries; The problems, pathogenesis and management. Hand 2:63–73, 1970.

16. Leyvraz PF, Richard J, Bachmann F, Van Melle G, Treyvaud JM, Candardjis G: Adjusted versus fixed-dose subcutaneous heparin in the prevention of deep-vein thrombosis after total hip replacement. N Engl J Med 309:954–958, 1983.

17. Meyers MH, Harvey JP: Traumatic dislocation of the knee joint. J Bone Joint Surg 53A:16–29, 1971.

18. Miller MD: Review of Orthopaedics. Philadelphia, WB Saunders, 1992, pp 75–79.

19. Muller C, Rahn BA, Pfister U, Meinig RP: The incidence, pathogenesis, diagnosis, and treatment of fat embolism: A review paper. Orthop Rev 23(2):107–117, 1994.

20. O'Reilly RJ, Blatt G: High pressure injection injury. JAMA 233:533–534, 1975.

21. Orthopaedic Knowledge Update Home Study Syllabus I, II, and III. Chicago, American Academy of Orthopaedic Surgeons, 1984, 1987, 1990.

22. Patzakis MJ: Symposium: Current concepts in the management of osteomyelitis. Contemp Orthop 28:157–185, 1994.

23. Ramos H, Posh JL, Lie KK: High pressure injection injuries of the hand. Plast Reconstr Surg 45:221–226, 1970.

24. Rockwood CA, Green DP: Fractures in Adults, 3rd ed. Philadelphia, JB Lippincott, 1991.

25. Schoo MJ, Scott FA, Boswick JA: High pressure injection injuries of the hand. J Trauma 20(3):229–238, 1980.

26. Stark HH, Wilson JN, Boyles JH: Paint gun injuries of the hand. J Bone Joint Surg 49A:637–647, 1967.

27. Treiman GS, Yellin AE: Examination of the patient with knee dislocation. Arch Surg 127:1056, 1992.

28. Vaughn BK, Knezevich S, Lombardi AV Jr, Mallory TH: Use of the Greenfield filter to prevent fatal pulmonary embolism associated with total hip and knee arthroplasty. J Bone Joint Surg 71A(10):1542–1548, 1989.

29. Wegener WA: Diagnostic imaging of musculoskeletal infection: Roentgenography, gallium, indium-labeled white blood cell, gammaglobulin, bone scintigraphy, and MRI. Orthop Clin North Am 22:401–418, 1991.

CHAPTER 3

Injuries to the Spinal Column

John S. Kirkpatrick

Cyrus Ghavam

The evaluation and diagnosis of spine injuries elicit a broad spectrum of concerns. Injuries may involve muscle, ligament, bone, spinal cord, nerve roots, or any combination of these structures. The paramount concern during the evaluation of suspected spine injury is to prevent further injury. In acute injuries, frequently emergency medical care technicians have immobilized the patient appropriately. When trained personnel have not cared for a patient with a suspected spine injury, immobilization should be provided. This immobilization should include the application of a Philadelphia or other rigid cervical collar and placement of the patient on a back board in the supine position. Most orthoses are flexible enough for the posterior half to be passed behind the neck without moving the patient's neck or head. The anterior piece is then placed between the chest and chin and attached to the posterior piece. Alternatively, the patient may be log-rolled sufficiently (turned while holding the head, neck, shoulders, and pelvis in constant alignment) to allow placement of the posterior part of the orthosis. The patient should not have the neck flexed, extended, or rotated to place an orthosis until cervical instability has been ruled out.

The early phase of the evaluation of spine injury is performed along with the appropriate general evaluation. In the emergency department, the ABCs of emergency care must be followed. In subacute injuries, a more focused evaluation can be performed. The basic elements of any evaluation are applied to the spine. Appropriate history, physical examination, and supplemental studies lead the physician to the correct diagnosis.

HISTORY

A careful history of the injury and symptoms should be taken in any suspected spine injury. What was the nature of the injury (motor vehicle accident, fall, sports, altercation)? High-speed, high-energy trauma may cause severe spine injury. Bathtub falls in the elderly are frequent causes of upper cervical injury. Was there any head trauma, loss of consciousness, or paralysis? Trauma to the head often stresses the cervical spine to fail-

50

ure. In addition, head-injured patients may have decreased sensorium and may not complain of neck symptoms at the time of presentation. If there is paralysis, was it present initially or did it occur after the patient tried to move? Is sensation present? Answers to these questions add insight to the severity and nature of spinal cord injury.

Where is the pain? Localization of pain helps define the level of injury. Multiple levels of the spine may be injured following high-energy trauma. This is especially important in the patient with cervical paralysis, since thoracic or lumbar fractures may also be present. What is the character of the pain (sharp, burning, tingling, radiating)? Sharp pain usually occurs at the level of the injury. Burning, tingling, or radiating pain may indicate compromise of the spinal cord or nerve roots. Has there been any previous injury or previous spine condition such as degenerative changes (spondylosis)? What systemic illnesses or conditions does the patient have?

PHYSICAL EXAMINATION

The typical patient with suspected spine injury will be immobilized in a cervical collar on a back board by emergency medical technicians at the accident site. Calm assurance should be provided to the patient throughout the evaluation.

Observation of the patient's posture and position should be made, as well as of any spontaneous movement. The patient should be instructed to remain still and the front half of the cervical collar temporarily removed. The head and neck are then inspected for abrasions, contusions, lacerations, and swelling. Palpation of the head and neck is then accomplished in a systematic fashion, noting any areas of particular tenderness or bone abnormalities. The posterior neck can be palpated by the examiner without moving the head by slipping the fingers inside the posterior half of the collar. The location (upper, middle, or lower cervical spine) of any tenderness or bone abnormality should be noted. The front of the collar should then be replaced until cervical radiographs are reviewed. A lateral cervical spine radiograph is usually obtained as part of the initial survey, usually at the time a chest radiograph is obtained.

If there are no abnormalities on this cervical film, then the patient may be log-rolled to examine the rest of the back and spine. Log-rolling should be accomplished with adequate support of the head and neck so that the head, neck, and torso roll as one unit. The back is examined for evidence of trauma or deformity. The spinous processes are palpated for tenderness, malalignment, or increased spacing. The paraspinous muscles are palpated for tenderness, spasm, or defects. The patient is then placed back in the supine position.

A complete neurologic examination is critical to the evaluation of the patient with suspected spinal injury. The examination and subsequent recording of findings are based upon the segmental innervation of the body and include evaluation of motor, sensory, and reflex functions.[2]

Motor examination begins with observation of the patient's breathing mechanism. Upper cervical paralysis may result in the loss of diaphragm function (phrenic nerve C3, C4, C5) and absence of intercostal function (segmental innervation of the thoracic spine). Bilateral extremity motor function is then tested systematically, starting with shoulder abduction by the deltoid muscle (C5) and elbow flexion by the biceps (C5, C6). The wrist extensors complete the evaluation of C6. C7 is tested by elbow extension (triceps) and supplemented by wrist flexion (flexor carpi radialis and ulnaris) and finger extension (extensor digitorum). Flexion of the fingers (flexor digitorum) measures the function of C8. T1 is evaluated by abduction of the fingers (intrinsics). Lower extremity function is also tested beginning with hip flexion (L2, iliopsoas). L3 is tested by examination of knee extension (quadriceps femoris). L4 is responsible for ankle dorsiflexion and foot inversion (tibialis anterior muscle). The extensor hallucis longus (extension of the great toe) reflects L5 function. S1 is evaluated by plantar flexion of the foot (gastrocnemius-soleus muscles). Rectal sphincter tone and volitional contraction give insight to the function of lower sacral roots and should also be recorded. A summary of segmental innervation of muscle groups is contained in Table 3–1.

A grading system for motor function has been developed to help quantify motor deficits. A scale of five levels is used to describe function as follows:

Grade 0—no visible or palpable contraction;

TABLE 3–1.
Motor Segmental Innervation

Segmental Level	Function
C5	elbow flexors
C6	wrist extensors
C7	elbow extensors
C8	finger flexors (middle finger)
T1	finger abductors
L2	hip flexors
L3	knee extensors
L4	ankle dorsiflexors
L5	toe extensors (especially EHL)
S1	ankle plantar flexors

Grade 1—visible or palpable contraction without motion;
Grade 2—contraction effecting motion where gravity has been eliminated;
Grade 3—contraction effecting motion against gravity;
Grade 4—contraction effecting motion against resistance;
Grade 5—normal strength; and
NT—not testable

While this scale allows for subjective differences, it does provide a valuable clinical rating for spine-injured patients.

Sensory examination should include the evaluation of light touch and pin-prick sensation over the torso and extremities. Light touch can be evaluated with the examiner's finger or a cotton swab. A cautiously used sterile hypodermic needle works well for evaluation of pin-prick sensation. Proprioception also should be tested, particularly in patients with an incomplete neurologic deficit. The sensory distribution of segmental innervation is fairly consistent and allows for standard drawings for the recording of deficits (Fig. 3–1). It is important to note perianal sensation since it reflects the status of lower sacral roots. Sensory examination may be recorded on a three-point scale: 0—absent, 1—impaired (partial or altered perception), 2—normal, and NT—not testable. Key regions for testing sensitivity and the corresponding sensory level are listed in Tables 3–2, 3–3, and 3–4.

Reflexes should be evaluated and recorded as part of the examination. Deep tendon reflexes in the extremities aid in the evaluation of segmental innervation: biceps, C5, C6; brachioradialis, C6; triceps, C7; patellar, L3, L4; achilles, S1. Hoffman's response in the upper extremity and Babinski's response in the lower extremity are signals of upper motor neuron lesions, indicating conditions affecting neurons originating in the brain rather than the spinal cord. The bulbocavernosus reflex (anal sphincter contraction following stimulation of the glans penis, mons pubis, or traction on a Foley catheter) signifies the absence of spinal shock (see Chapter 17.)

The neurologic examination provides information that leads to the classification of spinal cord injury. The lowest normal level is used to describe the level of injury. The details of specific syndromes are contained in Chapter 17 on spinal cord injury.

ROENTGENOGRAPHIC EVALUATION

Complete roentgenographic evaluation should be performed on patients with suspected spinal injury as soon as possible within the overall evaluation. A lateral view usually will be obtained as part of the secondary survey. Once life-threatening conditions are ruled out, additional views should be obtained. The complete series includes anteroposterior, lateral, odontoid (usually an open-mouth view but may be an angled view through the foramen magnum), and oblique views. The lateral view should include the entire cervical spine to the top of the T1 vertebral body. The cervical spine cannot be radiographically "cleared" without seeing the top of the T1 vertebral body. This may require pulling the patient's arms down while obtaining the view or using a swimmer's view (raising one arm while lowering the other).

The lateral view can detect most clinically important cervical injuries (Fig. 3–2). The vertebral bodies should form a lordotic curve without subluxations. Specific signs of unstable injury include (1) subluxation of more than 3 mm, (2) more than 25 percent compression of a vertebral body, (3) widening of the interspinous distance, (4) narrowed or widened disc space, (5) facet joint widening, and (6) angulation.[1] The prevertebral soft tissue width should not exceed normal limits; if it does, bone or ligament injury is indicated. The soft tissue between the airway and the anterior inferior margin of C2 should measure less than 7 mm. The same measurement at C6 should be less than 14 mm in children and less than 21 mm in adults. The lateral

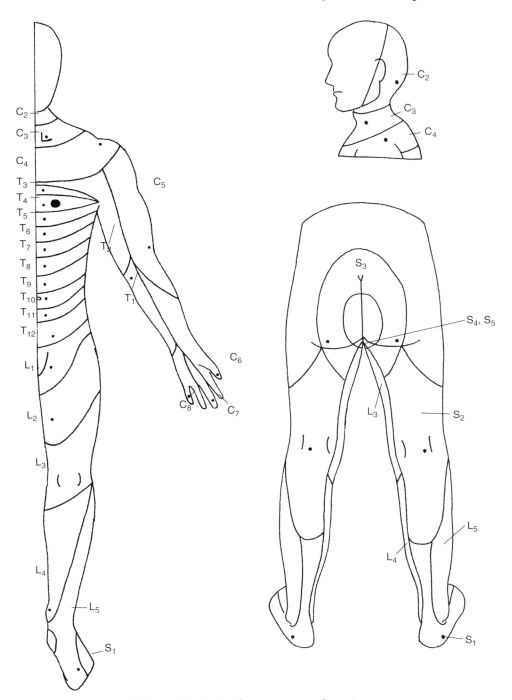

Figure 3–1. Typical human sensory dermatomes.

view will detect approximately 90 percent of cervical spine injuries.

Anteroposterior views are obtained and examined for malalignment, visible fractures, and increased spacing between spinous processes (Fig. 3–3). An open-mouth odontoid view should be obtained to visualize the odontoid process and lateral masses of C1 (Fig. 3–4). Bilateral oblique views should be obtained and reviewed for alignment and for pedicle and lateral mass fractures (Fig. 3–5). Anteroposterior and lateral views

TABLE 3–2.
Cervical Dermatomes

Segmental Level	Testing Area
C2	occipital protuberance
C3	supraclavicular fossa
C4	top of acromioclavicular joint
C5	lateral antecubital fossa
C6	thumb
C7	middle finger
C8	little finger
T1	medial antecubital fossa

TABLE 3–4.
Lumbar and Sacral Dermatomes

Segmental Level	Testing Area
L2	midanterior thigh
L3	medial femoral condyle
L4	medial malleolus
L5	dorsum of foot
S1	lateral heel
S2	midline popliteal fossa
S4, S5	perianal

alone are usually adequate for plane roentgenographic evaluation of the thoracic and lumbar spine.

Additional imaging studies may be obtained. Tomography, computed tomography, and magnetic resonance imaging (MRI) may aid in the diagnosis and treatment of spinal injuries. Appropriate use of these studies usually should be guided by those responsible for the ultimate management of the injury.

SPECIFIC INJURIES

A comprehensive review of the specific injuries of the spine and their treatment is beyond the scope of this book. Some common injuries and their appearance on radiographs will be presented. Any spinal injury noted on roentgenographic examination should be promptly evaluated by a physician familiar with the treatment of such injuries.

Upper Cervical Spine

Occipital-C1 dislocation is usually fatal at the accident scene. Patients who survive will have soft tissue swelling in the upper cervical spine and will have a widened distance between the occiput and C1.

C1-C2 subluxation may occur in the absence of an odontoid fracture. This injury is the result of a tear in the transverse and

other supporting ligaments or a rotary subluxation of the C1-C2 facets. The lateral cervical spine view should show no more than 2.5 mm between the anterior ring of C1 and the odontoid (greater than 2.5 mm would indicate injury to the transverse ligament) (see Fig. 3–2). The odontoid view should show symmetry in the space between the lateral masses of C1 and the odontoid (asymmetry indicating rotary subluxation) (see Fig. 3–4). Immobilization of the patient should be maintained, and a physician familiar with spinal injuries consulted.

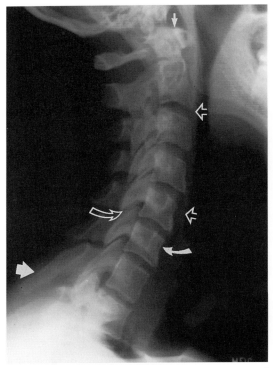

Figure 3–2. A normal lateral cervical spine radiograph illustrating the vertebral body (solid curved arrow), facet joint (open curved arrow), spinous process (solid large arrow), anterior atlantodens (C1-C2) interval (solid small arrow), and retropharyngeal soft tissue shadow (open straight arrows).

TABLE 3–3.
Thoracic Dermatomes

Segmental Level	Testing Area
T2	apex of axilla
T4	nipple line
T10	umbilicus
T12	inguinal ligament at midpoint

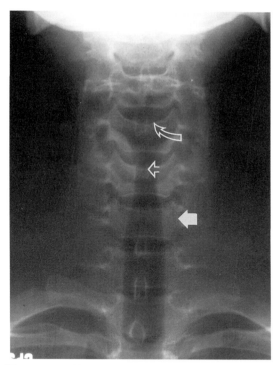

Figure 3–3. Normal anteroposterior radiograph illustrating the vertebral body (solid large arrow), spinous process (open straight arrow), and intervertebral disc space (open curved arrow).

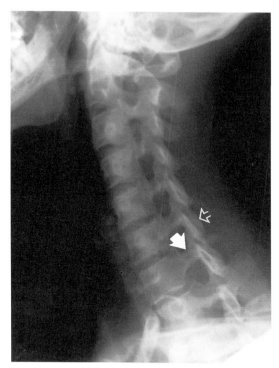

Figure 3–5. Oblique view illustrating the pedicle (solid arrow), and the lateral mass/facet complex (open arrow).

C1 fractures are usually seen on the open-mouth view. There may be asymmetry of the lateral mass–odontoid space or subluxation of the lateral masses of C1 on C2 or both.

Fractures of C2 require both open-mouth and lateral views. Odontoid fractures are classified according to the location of the fracture in the odontoid process (Fig. 3–6). Type I injuries usually require only symptomatic treatment with a rigid orthosis and analgesics, whereas Type II or Type III injuries usually require halo orthosis immobilization and

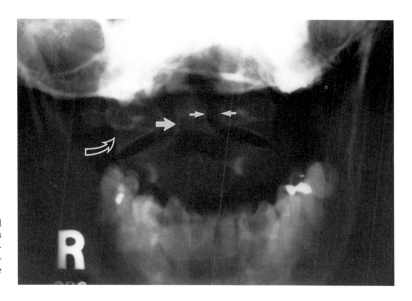

Figure 3–4. Open-mouth odontoid view illustrating the lateral mass of C1 (open curved arrow), the odontoid (solid large arrow), and the lateral mass/odontoid lateral space (solid small arrows).

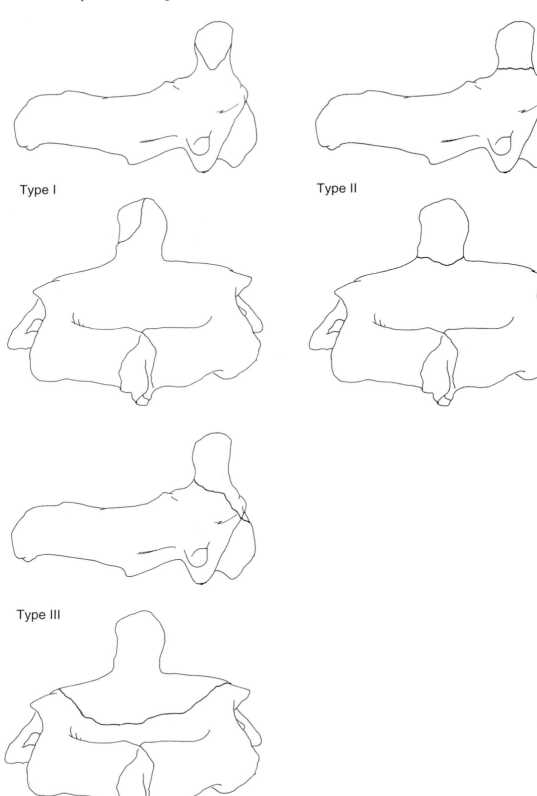

Type I

Type II

Type III

Figure 3–6. Classification of odontoid fractures and corresponding fracture locations.

occasionally surgical treatment. Fracture-subluxation of C2 may occur and is commonly known as "hangman's fracture," or traumatic spondylolisthesis. This injury is usually seen on the lateral roentgenograph as a fracture through the pedicles of C2, with forward displacement of the body of C2 on C3 (Fig. 3–7). Treatment is usually halo immobilization with fusion for late instability.

Lower Cervical Injuries

Facet dislocation is recognized by forward displacement of one vertebral body on another, angulation, widened spinous processes, and facet malalignment. Unilateral facet dislocations are associated with displacement of approximately 25 percent of the vertebral body, and bilateral with 50 percent displacement (Fig. 3–8). The anteroposterior view will usually show altered alignment of the spinous processes for unilateral disloca-

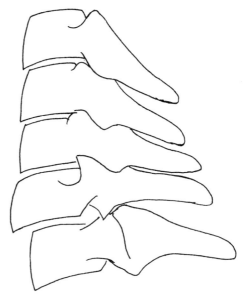

Figure 3–8. Unilateral facet subluxation with 25 percent anterolisthesis.

tions and widened processes for bilateral. These injuries, particularly the bilateral dislocations, are frequently associated with neurologic deficit. Traction for reduction followed by immobilization and occasional early surgical fusion is the typical treatment.

Vertebral body fractures may be a minor, stable injury, such as the "teardrop" fracture, or devastating and unstable, such as the burst or comminuted body fracture. The teardrop fracture is an avulsion from the anterior inferior corner of the vertebral body (Fig. 3–9). It is important to distinguish this from

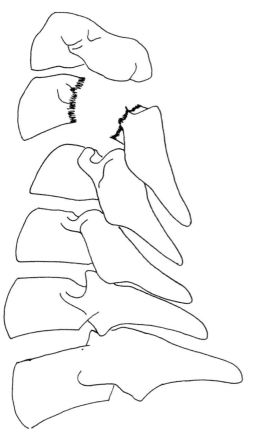

Figure 3–7. Traumatic spondylolisthesis (hangman's fracture).

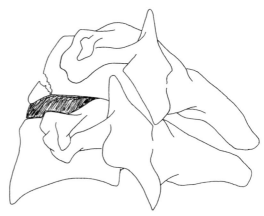

Figure 3–9. Anterior avulsion "teardrop" fracture.

a teardrop fracture-dislocation, which is unstable. The fracture dislocation will result in subluxation of the facets or vertebral bodies, or angulation of the spine at the level of injury. Burst fractures result from axial load and involve compression failure of the vertebral body. This frequently results in retropulsion of fracture fragments into the canal (Fig. 3–10). These fractures are usually identified on lateral roentgenographs by loss of vertebral body height and angulation of the spine at the injury site. The anteroposterior view may show widening of the pedicles. The initial treatment is continued immobilization and evaluation for definitive treatment by a specialist.

Spinous process fractures are known as "clayshoveler's fractures" and usually occur at C7. This injury represents an avulsion of the attachment of the ligamentum nuchae.

Dynamic (flexion and extension) radiographs may be helpful in identifying concomitant hypermobility. Treatment is symptomatic, including a rigid orthosis (Philadelphia collar or similar device) and analgesics. When symptoms improve, physical therapy incorporating active range of motion exercises and isometric strengthening exercises aids in the rehabilitation of these injuries.

Many patients will be seen in the emergency setting without roentgenographic evidence of injury, but with pain. These patients should be advised to continue to wear a cervical collar and to return if symptoms change. Follow-up dynamic radiographs should be examined 1 to 2 weeks following injury to rule out the possibility of undetected ligamentous instability. Films showing greater than 3.5-mm subluxation of the vertebral bodies or significant

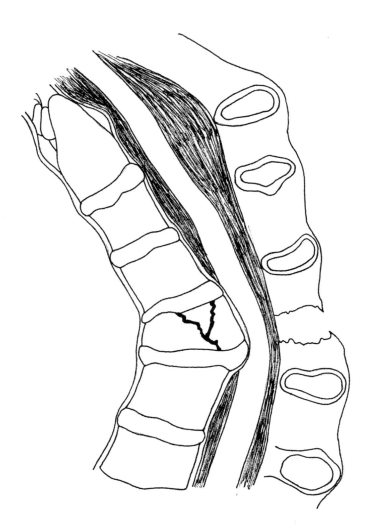

Figure 3–10. Burst fracture with retropulsion into the spinal canal and posterior ligamentous disruption.

rotational change should be evaluated by a specialist.[3]

Thoracic and Lumbar Spine

The thoracic spine is a relatively stable portion of the spine; thus, injuries in this area are usually the result of significant trauma to the torso. The cross-sectional area in the thoracic spine is relatively less than that of the lumbar spine, thus a lesser amount of displaced bone can lead to a significant neurologic injury. Anteroposterior and lateral roentgenographs are usually adequate for determining whether a fracture or dislocation is present. Any evidence of widening of the mediastinal shadow on chest roentgenographs may result from upper thoracic spine injuries.

Thoracic or lumbar compression injuries are usually seen on the lateral roentgenograph of the spine. Typically, these injuries are represented by the anterior body height being less than the posterior body height and the presence of kyphosis or angulation at the injury site (Fig. 3–11). These injuries are the result of an axial load to the spine. More severe axial load injuries may produce a "burst" fracture with displacement of bone fragments into the spinal canal. Lateral roentgenographs may reveal posterior dis-

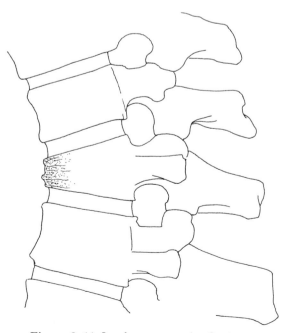

Figure 3–11. Lumbar compression fracture.

placement of the vertebral body (Fig. 3–12A). Anteroposterior roentgenographs may show that the interpedicular distance is widened (Fig. 3–12B). Differentiation between compression and burst injuries is important, since the necessary treatment will be guided by this difference. Burst fractures are more prone to neurologic deficit and instability and as such require greater attention in treatment and follow-up.

Fracture dislocations and fracture subluxations are noted as fractures with offset of the vertebral body alignment. These injuries often require both anteroposterior and lateral views for diagnosis. Flexion-distraction injuries may result in a separation of the disc space or vertebral body.

Sacral Fractures

Fractures of the sacrum are integral to the structure of the pelvis and are discussed in Chapter 4.

Neck and Low Back Pain

Clinical and roentgenographic evaluation frequently reveal no bone or ligament injury to the spine. The most common injuries without roentgenographic signs are those to the muscles of the back or neck. Although a comprehensive review of these syndromes is beyond the scope of this book, some pertinent features are discussed.

Many general issues contribute to poor outcomes in patients with neck pain or back pain, two of which are frequently identified. Compensation issues are particularly troublesome in these patients and can lead to suspicion between the physician and patient when a third party is considered "liable" by the patient. Tobacco use is another factor that contributes greatly to poor outcomes and may be one indication of an addictive personality. In the majority of patients with chronic neck or back pain, one or both of these issues affect the outcome.

Neck pain frequently is the result of strain to the paraspinal muscles or to the trapezius muscle. The whiplash type of injury may present with an associated headache. These injuries typically respond well to 48 hours of rest initially, followed by active range of motion exercises. Support in a soft cervical collar may help to relieve stress upon the

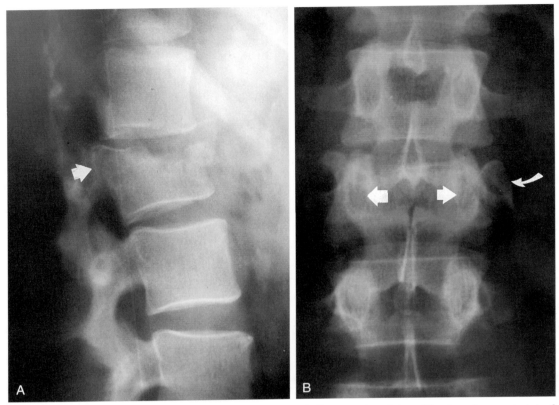

Figure 3–12. *A,* Lumbar burst fracture, lateral view. Arrow indicates retropulsion of fracture fragments into the spinal canal. *B,* Lumbar burst fracture, anteroposterior view, with pedicle widening (solid large arrows) and lateral displaced fracture fragment (curved arrow).

cervical muscles. Non-narcotic analgesics are recommended. Narcotic analgesics and muscle relaxants should be used only for very brief periods and then only in limited quantities.

Once normal range of motion is attained, isometric strengthening is begun. The services of a physical therapist experienced in treating spine patients are valuable in managing these patients. Patients who have suspected ligamentous injury but normal initial roentgenographs should have follow-up roentgenographs, including flexion and extension views, approximately 2 weeks after injury. Most patients should have obtained significant relief of their discomfort within 6 weeks.

Low back pain is second only to the common cold in causing absenteeism in the workplace. The initial evaluation of this syndrome requires differentiation of acute from chronic pain and identification of neurologic deficit and radiculopathy.

The patient with an acute episode of low back pain without neurologic signs is treated with nonoperative interventions. Reduced activity, not bedrest, should be recommended for 24 to 48 hours. Nonsteroidal anti-inflammatory agents (NSAIAs) are the mainstay of pharmacologic treatment. A physical therapist may help provide the patient with relief, using modalities such as heat, ultrasound, or traction. Flexibility exercises are begun, followed by strengthening of the abdominal muscles. Patients typically are significantly improved in 6 to 8 weeks. For patients who do not obtain relief, roentgenographs should be obtained to rule out occult injury, deformity, tumor, or infection.

Radicular Pain

Neck or back pain accompanied by radicular pain into an extremity should be evaluated with a detailed neurologic examination. Typical lumbar radiculopathy includes pain radiating distal to the knee, numbness or paresthesias in a dermatomal distribution, and complaints of muscular weakness (e.g., foot drop). Important neurologic signs include asymmetry of deep tendon reflexes, segmental motor weakness, and dermatomal sensory deficit. The initial management of these patients is the same as indicated earlier unless there is severe weakness (Grade 3 or less) or bowel or bladder incontinence. The presence of these findings or myelopathy (spasticity, impaired fine motor function, impaired vibratory and proprioception sense) indicates impairment of neurologic function; referral to a specialist should be considered.

The patient with chronic pain (longer than 6 weeks' duration) or the patient whose pain is refractory to nonoperative treatment requires a more thorough evaluation. The history of the pain should be obtained again, with particular note of any changes in the character, pattern, and associated symptoms. Review of systems may also be helpful, as weight loss may be associated with malignancy and fever and chills with infection. A social history, including type of work, retrainability, and pending litigation or compensation, will aid in determining prognosis. Physical examination, including a detailed neurologic examination, should be performed. These findings will guide the use of additional tests and imaging studies to complete the diagnostic evaluation. Some additional tests may include x-rays (deformity of the spine), myelography and CT scan (spinal stenosis, herniated disc), MRI (tumors, infections, herniated disc, stenosis), radionuclide studies (tumors, infections), complete blood count (infection, lymphoma), erythrocyte sedimentation rate (inflammatory process), protein electrophoresis (myeloma), and other blood tests as systemic markers for diseases.

Some patients warrant rigorous evaluation on inital presentation with back pain. In the pediatric population, infectious processes (osteomyelitis and discitis) must be excluded in the absence of an identifiable cause for the pain. White blood cell count, erythrocyte sedimentation rate, radiographs, and radionuclide scans may be helpful in establishing these diagnoses. The elderly patient is less likely to have typical low back pain and should be evaluated to rule out osteoporotic compression fractures or a metastatic process.

The use of MRI should be reserved for those patients whose symptoms continue to be radicular and significantly limiting following appropriate nonoperative management. The MRI scans should not be obtained until roentgenographs and nonoperative management have been attempted, usually for 4 to 6 weeks. There may be a role for MRI in patients when tumor or infection is suspected, but this should be guided by history and examination findings. In most cases, the MRI should be considered a tool for surgical planning rather than for diagnostic screening.

Spondylolysis and Spondylolisthesis

Spondylolysis may be associated with low back pain in patients, particularly in the young and active patient. The typical patients are adolescent female gymnasts or football linemen who have frequent forced hyperextension of the spine. This disorder consists of a stress fracture or fibrous defect in the pars interarticularis region of the vertebrae. Frequent symptoms include low back pain with radiation into the buttocks or thighs and hamstring spasm or tightness that may limit forward flexion at the hips. Oblique radiographs of the lumbosacral spine may display the pars defect. A bone scan is often required to make the diagnosis when the defect is not seen on roentgenographs. Relief is often obtained with decreased activity. There may be an increased risk for spondylolisthesis, and this should be discussed with the patient.

Spondylolisthesis refers to the anterolisthesis (sliding forward) of one vertebral body on another. Two frequently seen types of spondylolisthesis are isthmic and degenerative.

The isthmic type frequently occurs in adolescents and may be associated with nerve root compression signs. Management is first nonoperative, with activity modification and lumbar spine–strengthening exercise. If pain is unremitting in the adolescent with spondylolisthesis, or if the deformity is progressive, surgical fusion may be indicated.

Degenerative spondylolisthesis is rarely seen in people under age 40 years. Symptoms are usually of insidious onset and consist of low back, buttock, and thigh pain. Spinal stenosis frequently develops in degenerative spondylolisthesis. The patients may develop neurogenic claudication in addition to other symptoms. The effectiveness of nonoperative measures in this patient group is somewhat limited, and surgical decompression and fusion are frequently indicated.

References

1. Brown ML, Berquist TH: Imaging of the musculoskeletal system. *In* Fitzgerald RH Jr (ed): Orthopaedic Knowledge Update 2. Park Ridge, Illinois, American Academy of Orthopaedic Surgeons, 1987.

2. Ditunno JF Jr (ed): Standard for Neurological and Functional Classification of Spinal Cord Injury. Chicago, American Spinal Injury Association, revised 1992.

3. White AA, Panjabi MM: Update on the evaluation of instability of the lower cervical spine. Instr Course Lect 36:513–520, 1987.

Additional Reading

Hoppenfeld S: Physical Examination of the Spine and Extremities. New York, Appleton-Century-Crofts, 1976.

Rothman R, and Simeone F (eds): The Spine, 3rd ed. Philadelphia, WB Saunders, 1992.

Frymoyer J (ed): The Adult Spine. New York, Raven Press, 1991.

Pelvic and Acetabulum Fractures

Jorge E. Alonso

In the past decade, fractures of the pelvis and acetabulum have been on the rise, owing to the high-energy trauma so prevalent in our society today. Massive force is necessary to disrupt a pelvic ring in a young individual; therefore, injury to other organs is common and often life threatening.[7,14]

Connolly and Hedberg noted that fractures of the pelvis are secondary only to those of the skull in terms of mortality, morbidity, and other complications.[3] With aggressive methods of treatment, the mortality rate for pelvic injury patients has decreased significantly. The mortality ranges from 5 to 50 percent. Forty percent of patients die within 5 hours of hospital admission, and an additional 18 percent die within 2 days of hospitalization.[3]

Approximately two thirds of all pelvic fractures occur as a result of traffic accidents, with pedestrians being injured more frequently than occupants of vehicles. Representative figures show that 40 percent of pelvic injuries were secondary to motor vehicle accidents, 28 percent secondary to a fall, 17 percent were pedestrians run over by an automobile, 9 percent were motorcycle accidents, and 6 percent were from other causes.[1,13,14,17]

In a study of the probability of sustaining a pelvic fracture while in a car, McCoy and associates reported that at 20 miles per hour, there is a 9 percent chance of sustaining a pelvic fracture. At 30 miles per hour, there is a 50 percent chance.[10] Perry and McClelland, in an autopsy study of 127 patients following fatal traffic accidents, concluded that the second most common cause of death was injury to the pelvis and lower extremities.[13] These statistics support the need for early diagnosis and early emergency treatment by the initial physician, thereby improving the survival of patients with these difficult fractures.

ANATOMY

The pelvis has two functions: structural support and soft tissue protection. The pelvis represents the link between the axial skeleton and the major weight-bearing structures, the lower extremities. With this in mind, it is easy to see that any fractures or dislocations that alter the structural support will affect the locomotive function of the lower extremities. The forces of sitting and weight-bearing are transferred through the pelvis and through the major structures that it protects: the vascular, neurologic, genitourinary and gastrointestinal systems that pass through its arches and are thus injured.[1,7]

The pelvic ring is made up of three bones: the sacrum and two innominate bones. The innominate bone is formed from three ossification centers: the ilium, the ischium, and the pubis. These centers fuse at the triradiate cartilage of the acetabulum, forming the complete innominate bone (Fig. 4–1).

These three bones are joined posteriorly at the sacroiliac joint and anteriorly at the pubic symphysis. These three joints and three bones have no structural stability. The ligamentous structures provide vital stability to the pelvis. The ligaments can be divided into three areas, in order of importance: anterior ligaments, ligaments of the floor of the pelvis, and posterior ligaments (Fig. 4–2).

The symphysis is composed of fibrocartilage and a band of fibrous tissue. It is reinforced anteriorly by the arcuate ligament. Sectioning of the symphysis will show a diastasis of about 2 to 2.5 cm, with no instability of the pelvis.

The ligaments of the floor of the pelvis are those that span from the sacrum to the innominate bone. The sacrotuberous ligament is a strong band that runs from the posterolateral aspect of the sacrum to the ischial tuberosity. It is especially important in maintaining both rotational and vertical

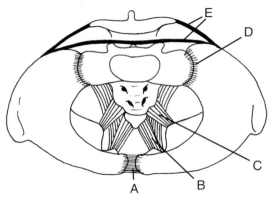

Figure 4–2. Ligamentous structures. Anterior ligaments: Symphysis pubis (*A*). Ligaments of the floor of the pelvis: Sacrotuberous ligaments (*B*); sacrospinous ligaments (*C*). Posterior ligaments: Anterior sacroiliac ligaments (*D*); posterior sacroiliac ligaments (long and short) (*E*).

stability of the pelvis. The sacrospinous ligament is triangular and runs from the lateral margins of the sacrum and coccyx to the ischial spine. It is important in maintaining rotational stability and, to a lesser degree, vertical stability.[7]

The strongest and most important ligamentous structures are in the posterior aspect, connecting the pelvis with the sacrum. These are divided into anterior and posterior sacroiliac ligaments. With these ligaments sectioned, a pelvis goes from being rotationally unstable to vertically unstable.[1,7]

Other posterior ligamentous structures are the iliolumbar ligaments, which run from the transverse processes of L4 and L5 to the posterior iliac crest. A fracture of the transverse process of L5 is a sign of vertical instability of the pelvis.

Force Patterns of Pelvic Fractures

Anteroposterior Force Pattern

Injury to the ligaments depends upon the amount of anteriorly applied force. Tile, in testing the pelvis, found that sectioning only the symphysis resulted in a pubic diastasis of no more than 2.5 cm. Further opening will injure the sacrospinous ligament. As long as the posterior sacroiliac ligaments are intact, only an anteroposterior rotatory instability is present with no component of vertical instability[15] (Fig. 4–3).

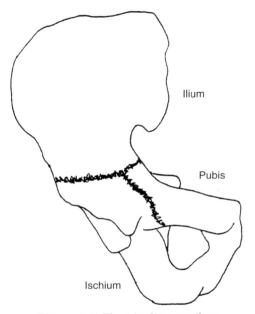

Figure 4–1. The triradiate cartilage.

Ilium

Pubis

Ischium

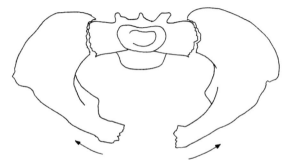

Figure 4–3. Anteroposterior force pattern.

Lateral Compression Force Pattern

The second and most common force pattern of pelvic fractures is lateral compression. Depending on the area of impact and magnitude of the force, different types of injury will be seen. Usually, there will be a very minimal soft tissue injury and a stable fracture configuration.

External Rotation/Abduction Force Pattern

This type of force is common in motorcycle accidents. The leg is caught and externally rotated and abducted, sectioning or fracturing all the structures in the posterior hemipelvis or sacrum. An unstable vertical pattern is created.

Shear Force Pattern

The last force pattern is the vertical shear. This will lead to a completely unstable fracture with a triplanar displacement. It indicates a complete disruption of the posterior osseous and ligamentous structures (Fig. 4–4).

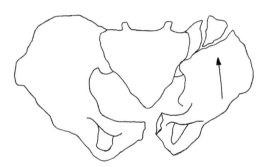

Figure 4–4. Shear force pattern.

Classification

The classification of a pelvic ring disruption is important to establish a diagnosis and treatment option and to aid in determining prognosis. The classification by Young and associates is based on the mechanism of injury and alerts the surgeon to potential resuscitation problems associated with these fractures.[18] This classification follows the different force patterns.

Letournel and Judet suggested a classification based on the site of injury.[8] This classification seems more straightforward and is easier to understand and to communicate. It is depicted in Figure 4–5. A combination of these fractures can occur.

EVALUATION AND EMERGENCY MANAGEMENT

A history of the injury can give a clue as to the type of fracture. A fall from a short height, or tripping, is usually a low-energy injury and is generally seen in elderly, osteoporotic patients. Pathologic fractures are usually nondisplaced or minimally displaced fractures. High-energy injuries are usually secondary to an automobile or motorcycle accident. These patients are usually multi-traumatized, and the initial evaluation must include assessment of immediate life-threatening problems of head, chest, abdominal, and, most importantly, retroperitoneal vascular injuries caused by the fracture. Sixty to eighty percent of high-energy pelvic fractures have associated musculoskeletal injuries.[7,12,17]

The initial standard resuscitation priorities need to be established to make sure the patient is stabilized. Of paramount importance is the airway and breathing, and then care of the circulatory system. High-energy pelvic fractures are associated with significant hemorrhage in 75 percent of patients,[3] urogenital injuries in 12 percent, and lumbosacral nerve injuries in 8 percent.[3,7,10]

Once the airways and breathing are stabilized, care of the hypovolemic shock is mandatory. First, two 14- to 16-gauge intravenous cannulas are inserted in the upper extremity, and crystalloid solution is given with type-specific or noncross-matched universal donor O group negative blood, if type-specific blood is not available. The patient's

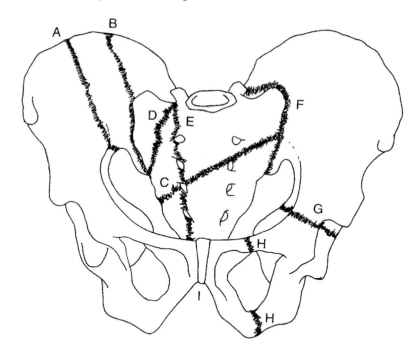

Figure 4–5. Pelvic fracture classification (modification of Judet and Letournel). *A*, Iliac wing fracture. *B*, Wedge fracture. *C*, Transverse sacral fracture. *D*, Fracture of the sacral wing. *E*, Transforaminal sacral fracture. *F*, Diastasis of sacroiliac joint. *G*, Fracture of the acetabulum. *H*, Superior and/or inferior pubic ramus fracture. *I*, Diastasis of the symphysis.

response is monitored by urinary output and body temperature.

If there is no improvement of the hypovolemic shock, antishock trousers should be used.[5] The antishock trousers are a pneumatic compression device that will produce increased systemic vascular resuscitation and promote autotransfusion of blood by applying circumferential pneumatic compression. These trousers are inflated to pressures of from 20 to 50 mm Hg at increments of 5 mm Hg. Once the serial hematocrit and hemodynamic parameters are stable, the patient can be transferred to a trauma center.

Another method of diminishing the pelvic volume includes the application of an anterior external fixation device. This external fixation frame stabilizes the pelvis and immobilizes the jagged bone edges that contribute to vascular damage[6,11] (Fig. 4–6).

In addition to fluid replacement and external fixation or antishock trousers in the patient with massive, continuous bleeding, angiography is useful as a means of locating the site of bleeding and embolizing to control arterial bleeding. The embolization can be done with clotted autologous blood, gel foam, or coils.[7]

Once the patient is stable and a thorough physical examination is performed, radiographic evaluation of the pelvis is done.[4]

Young and associates showed that the majority of cases can be diagnosed correctly by using an anteroposterior projection alone.[18] Ninety-four percent of their series had a correct diagnosis, although it is always recommended that three views be taken: anteroposterior, inlet, and outlet views (Fig. 4–7).

The use of the CT scan has revolutionized the evaluation of the posterior ligaments of the pelvis, and it is mandatory in assessing the exact injury to the posterior ligaments or bone.

If there is any indication of an unstable fracture, urethrography should be done. This is performed by placing a small catheter into the urethral meatus, inflating the balloon, and injecting 25 to 30 ml of radiopaque dye. Once the urethra is visualized, the balloon is deflated, the catheter is advanced to the bladder, and another 400 ml of dye is injected and a radiograph taken. If there is still no pathology but hematuria is noted, an intravenous pyelogram should be ordered[2] (Fig. 4–8).

In the past few years, a more aggressive course to stabilize these unstable fractures, usually with internal fixation using plates and screws, has proved to be the best method of achieving an intact pelvic ring and assuring the best possible result. Not all pelvic fractures require stabilization, but with

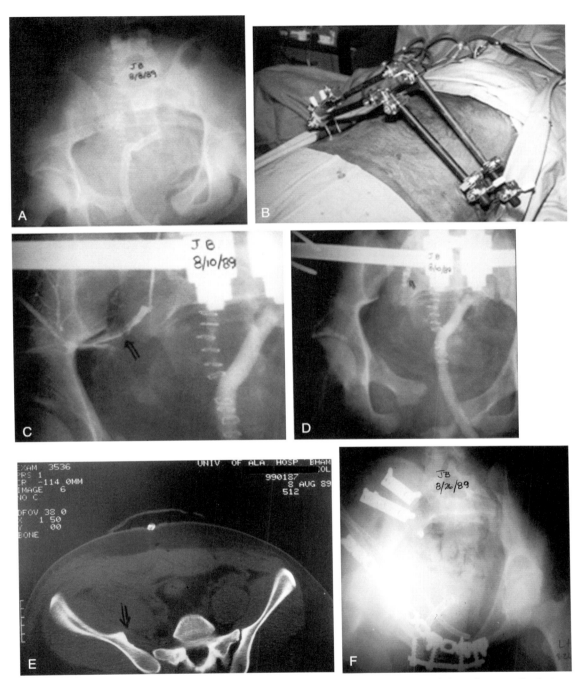

Figure 4–6. Diastasis of the sacroiliac joint. *A,* Anteroposterior radiograph of a vertical shear fracture. Patient was hemodynamically unstable. *B,* An external fixator was applied. *C,* Anteroposterior arteriogram showing bleeding from the internal iliac artery. *D,* Anteroposterior arteriogram showing embolization with coils. *E,* Computed tomography scan showing the posterior pathology. *F,* Anteroposterior radiograph showing open reduction and internal fixation of the pelvic fracture.

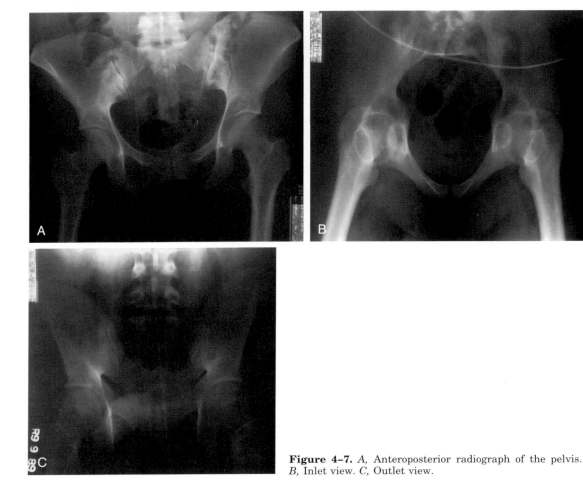

Figure 4–7. *A,* Anteroposterior radiograph of the pelvis. *B,* Inlet view. *C,* Outlet view.

appropriate early evaluation we can improve the management of these injuries[16] (see Fig. 4–6).

ACETABULAR FRACTURES

It is important to remember that most acetabular fractures are the result of high-energy forces, and multiple organ systems may be injured. Long bone fractures are the most frequently associated musculoskeletal injuries and should be stabilized early. Careful evaluation of the neurovascular status is important. It is particularly important to document sciatic nerve injuries, which are often associated with posterior and central dislocations.[7,9,15] After the patient has been fully evaluated and stabilized, evaluation of the acetabular fracture is continued.

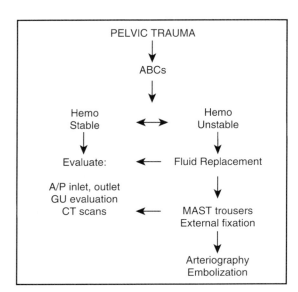

Figure 4–8. Stabilizing pelvic fractures.

Radiographic Evaluation

Because of the anatomy, three views are mandatory for the evaluation of acetabular fractures.[8,9,15] (1) The anteroposterior view usually demonstrates the fundamental landmarks of the acetabulum. (2) The obturator oblique view is taken at a 45-degree tilt, with the normal side closer to the x-ray tube; this will give information about the anterior column and the posterior lip. (3) The iliac oblique view is taken at a 45-degree tilt, with the normal side closer to the x-ray tube; this gives information regarding the posterior column and the anterior lip (Fig. 4–9). Proper positioning is essential to ensure that these views give accurate information.

Computed tomography scanning of the acetabulum is an accepted adjunct in the diagnosis of these fractures. It is particularly helpful in demonstrating incarcerated loose bodies, marginal impaction, the size of the wall fragment, and femoral head fractures. It should be ordered to aid in planning definitive treatment (Fig. 4–10).

Three-dimensional scans can produce striking images and also help in the classification of these difficult fractures and in planning definitive treatment (Fig. 4–11).

Classification

There are different types of classifications for acetabular fractures, but not until Judet and Letournel[8] integrated pelvic anatomy and fracture biomechanics did a clinically useful form arise. The five elemental fractures encompass single lesions of the respective walls and columns and an additional transverse fracture (Fig. 4–12):

(1) posterior wall fracture,
(2) posterior column fracture,
(3) anterior wall fracture,
(4) anterior column fracture, and
(5) transverse fracture.

The five associated or complex acetabular fractures combine at least two of the elemental forms (Fig. 4–13):

(1) T-shaped fractures,
(2) posterior wall–posterior column fracture,
(3) transverse posterior wall fracture,
(4) anterior with posterior hemitransverse, and
(5) both column fractures.

These classifications will guide the surgeon in the type of approach and fixation of these fractures.

Fractures of the acetabulum may produce an incongruity between the cartilage of the femoral head and the acetabulum. Thus, fractures in this area are intra-articular fractures. If these fractures are allowed to heal in a displaced position, weight-bearing forces applied to the small areas of contact lead to rapid cartilage breakdown and result in posttraumatic arthritis. Surgical treatment and anatomic reduction can restore the normal

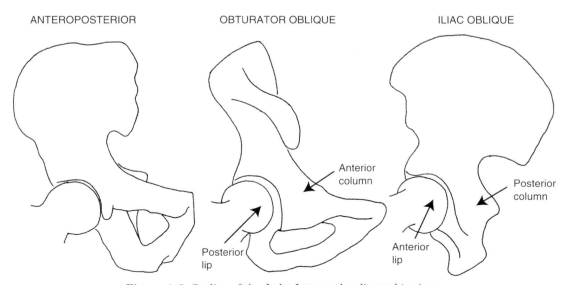

ANTEROPOSTERIOR   OBTURATOR OBLIQUE   ILIAC OBLIQUE

Anterior column

Posterior column

Posterior lip

Anterior lip

Figure 4–9. Outline of the Judet-Letournel radiographic views.

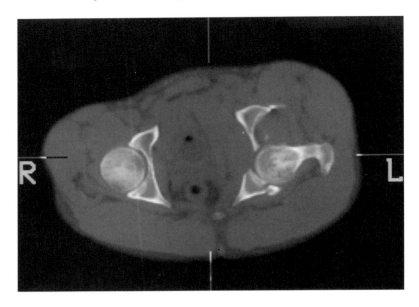

Figure 4–10. Computed tomography view of a posterior wall/posterior column fracture with fragments in the joint.

shape of the acetabulum and decrease the risk of early post-traumatic arthritis. The combined Judet-Letournel operative experience of over 1000 cases provides validation for their contention that operative restoration of joint anatomy is the treatment of choice for nearly all displaced fractures.[8]

Management

A nondisplaced acetabular fracture can be treated by traction for 4 to 6 weeks and then crutch-walking with toe touch to the affected side for 6 to 8 weeks.

Any fracture that is displaced more than 4 mm can produce joint incongruity and post-traumatic arthritis. In the last few years, an

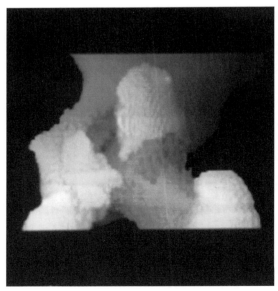

Figure 4–11. Three-dimensional reconstruction of a computed tomogram showing comminution of the posterior wall.

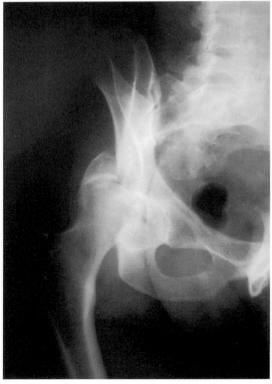

Figure 4–12. Iliac oblique radiograph showing a posterior wall fracture (elemental fracture).

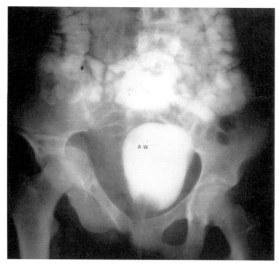

Figure 4–13. Iliac oblique radiograph of an anterior with posterior hemitransverse fracture (associated fracture).

aggressive approach to these fractures has given excellent results in more than 80 percent of patients.[7,12]

References

1. Burgess AR, Tile M: Fractures of the pelvis. Rockwood CA, Green DP (eds): Fractures in the Adult. Philadelphia, JB Lippincott, 1991.
2. Colapinto V: Trauma to the pelvis: Urethral injuries. Clin Orthop 151:46–55, 1980.
3. Connolly WB, Hedberg EA: Observations on fractures of the pelvis. J Trauma 9:150–169, 1969.
4. Edeiken-Monroe BS, Browner BD, Jackson H: The role of standard radiographs. Radiology, 129–139, 1986.
5. Kaplan BC, Civetta J, Nagel E, et al: Military anti-shock trousers in civilian pre-hospital emergency care. J Trauma 13:843–848, 1973.
6. Kellam JF: The role of external fixation in pelvic disruptions. Clin Orthop 241:66–82, 1989.
7. Kellam JF, Browner BD: Fractures of the pelvic ring. *In* Browner BD, Jupiter JB, Levine AM, Trafton PG, (eds): Skeletal Trauma. Philadelphia, WB Saunders, 1992.
8. Letournel E, Judet R (eds): Fractures of the Acetabulum. New York, Springer Verlag, 1993.
9. Matta J: Surgical treatment of acetabular fractures. *In* Browner BD, Jupiter JB, Levine AM, Trafton PG (eds): *Skeletal Trauma.* Philadelphia, WB Saunders, 1992.
10. McCoy GF, Johnstone RA, Kenwright K: Biomechanical aspects of pelvic and hip injuries in road traffic accidents. J Orthop Trauma 3(2):118–128, 1989.
11. Mears DC, Fu FH: Modern concepts of external fixation of the pelvis. Clin Orthop 151:65–70, 1980.
12. Mears DC, Rubash H: Pelvic and Acetabular Fractures. Thorofare, New Jersey, Charles B. Slack, 1986.
13. Perry JF, McClelland FR: Autopsy findings in 127 patients following fatal traffic accidents. Surg Gynecol Obstet 119:586–590, 1964.
14. Peter NK: Care of patients with traumatic pelvic fractures. Crit Care Nurse 8:62–76, 1980.
15. Tile M: Fractures of the Pelvis and Acetabulum. Baltimore, Williams & Wilkins, 1984.
16. Tile M: Pelvic fractures: Operative vs. nonoperative treatment. Orthop Clin North Am 11:423–464, 1980.
17. Trunkey PD, Chapman M, Lim R, et al: Management of pelvic fractures in blunt trauma injury. J Trauma 14:912–923, 1974.
18. Young JWR, Burgess AR, Brumback RJ, Poka A: Pelvic fractures: Value of plain radiography and early assessment and management. Radiology 160:445–451, 1986.

CHAPTER 5

Hip Fractures and Dislocations

Kenneth Jaffe

John T. Killian

Scott Morris

The hip is a ball and socket joint that includes both the acetabulum of the pelvis and the proximal femur. Fractures of the hip are generally divided into acetabular, femoral head, femoral neck, intertrochanteric, and subtrochanteric, or a combination of these. Patients usually present from either low-energy trauma, such as a slip or fall, or high-energy trauma, such as a motor vehicle accident or fall from a height. Generally, patients complain of severe pain in the hip or an inability to walk and loss of control of their leg.

FEMORAL HEAD FRACTURES

Femoral head fractures in adults and children are usually the result of a hip dislocation. The thigh is axially loaded with the femur in neutral or in the adducted position. Most fractures occur as the result of a posterior dislocation of the femoral head. A shear or cleavage injury to the femoral head occurs as the head impinges on the rim of the acetabulum (Fig. 5–1). However, femoral head

fractures also may result from a ligamentum teres avulsion or direct blow causing an indentation or crush fracture. Acetabular fractures, patellar fractures, femoral fractures, and knee ligament injuries may be associated with femoral head fractures.

ANTERIOR HIP DISLOCATIONS

Anterior hip dislocations occur in approximately 10 to 15 percent of all traumatic hip dislocations.[3,11] They have been subdivided into superior (iliac) and inferior (obturator) types. Superior dislocations result from extension, abduction, and external rotation forces. The femoral head is displaced anteriorly and may compress the femoral neurovascular bundle. Inferior dislocations, which are more common, result from flexion, abduction, and external rotation forces (Fig. 5–2). Closed reduction can be accomplished by traction, followed by extension and internal rotation (Fig. 5–3). Femoral head fractures can occur and are either transcondylar or indentation fractures. These may be difficult

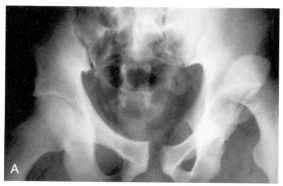

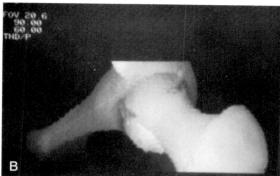

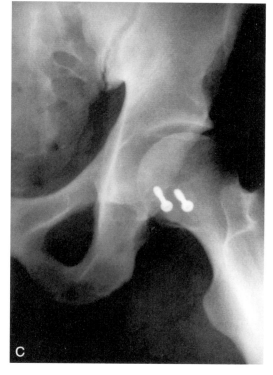

Figure 5–1. *A,* Posterior dislocation of the hip with a femoral head fracture. *B,* Three-dimensional CT scan imaging showing the fracture after the hip was relocated. *C,* Open reduction and internal fixation of the femoral head fracture/dislocation.

to identify without tomograms or computed tomographic scans. Transcondylar fractures that result in nonconcentric reduction require open reduction and either excision or internal fixation of the fragment, depending on its size and location.

POSTERIOR HIP DISLOCATIONS

Posterior hip dislocations account for the majority of all hip dislocations.[3,11] They may be associated with a femoral head or acetabular fracture or both. Posterior dislocations occur as a result of a force applied to the flexed knee along the axis of the femur. If the hip is in neutral or adduction, a simple

dislocation occurs. If the hip is in abduction, an associated posterior acetabular fracture occurs.

The reduction of a dislocated hip with or without a femoral head fracture should be undertaken as soon as the diagnosis has been made. The patient must be fully evaluated by a physical examination and radiography. Associated fractures of the femoral neck, femoral shaft, patella, and tibia should be ruled out. Cruciate ligament injuries of the knee may be sustained as well. The presence of any one of these associated injuries may alter the method of reduction as well as treatment of the dislocation. The neurovascular status of the lower extremity should also be examined and documented. Good quality

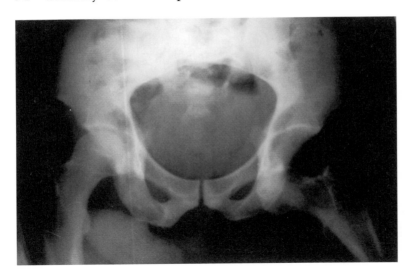

Figure 5–2. Inferior anterior hip dislocation secondary to a motor vehicle accident. The hip is abducted, externally rotated, and flexed.

radiographs (AP and lateral views) of the hip should be carefully evaluated for the presence of femoral neck fractures prior to treatment. AP radiographs of the pelvis should be obtained following reduction. Oblique views at 45 degrees (Judet) are used to evaluate the anterior and posterior acetabular walls.

Once the initial work-up has been completed, a gentle closed reduction should be attempted using the Bigelow, Allis, or Stinson techniques (Fig. 5–4). If this is successful, the patient should be placed in traction and should be scheduled for a complete radiographic analysis, including a computed tomographic scan. A CT scan is the best method for visualizing incarcerated intra-articular fragments as well as for demonstrating the presence of femoral head and acetabular fractures.[3] Following successful closed reduction, surgery may be indicated for removal of the osteochondral fragments or repair of the acetabular fragments.

If a concentric stable reduction is attained, treatment should include a brief period of bedrest until symptoms subside. In adults, this is followed by protective weight-bearing ambulation for 4 to 6 weeks until soft tissue healing occurs. The patient can then progress to full weight-bearing. In pediatric

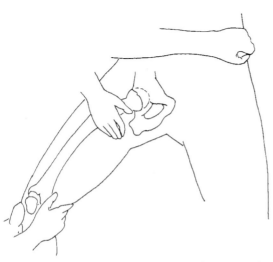

Figure 5–3. Allis's reduction maneuver for an anterior dislocation of the hip.

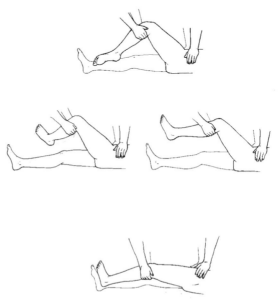

Figure 5–4. Bigelow's reduction maneuver for a posterior dislocation of the hip.

patients, a spica cast is frequently used for several weeks. If the reduction is concentric but unstable and there are no associated fractures, the patient should be placed in traction until soft tissue healing occurs. This is followed by progressive weight-bearing ambulation. A nonconcentric reduction can result from intra-articular osteochondral fragments, interposed soft tissue, or malreduction of associated femoral head fractures. This is an indication for open reduction, joint exploration, and removal of osteochondral fragments. Treatment of associated femoral head or acetabular fractures depends on the location and size of the fragments and the stability of the reduction.

In children under 18 months of age who appear clinically to have a dislocated hip, care must be taken to ensure that a displaced femoral neck fracture through the unossified proximal femoral epiphysis has not occurred.[10] Arthrography, ultrasound, or magnetic resonance imaging may be needed for visualizing the unossified femoral head.

Complications of hip dislocations can be immediate or late. Femoral artery and femoral nerve injuries are rare and are associated with anterior dislocations. Sciatic nerve injuries are associated with approximately 10 percent of posterior dislocations. Osteonecrosis of the femoral head may occur after dislocation, the risk ranging from 10 to 15 percent in adults and 15 to 35 percent in children.[15] It can occur several years after injury. The risk of osteonecrosis depends on the severity of injury, delay in reduction, and repeated closed reduction attempts. The presence of a posterior acetabular fracture significantly increases the risk of osteonecrosis. A delay of reduction for more than 6 to 12 hours after injury also increases the risk. Degenerative post-traumatic arthritis depends on the severity of the hip injury and is a more frequent sequela in adults than in children. Contusion to the articular cartilage or the presence of an osteocartilaginous fragment may be the etiologic factor. The incidence is documented to be 33 percent at 10 years and up to 75 percent at 30 years. Posterior dislocations may go unrecognized, particularly in multiple trauma patients when there is an ipsilateral femoral shaft fracture.

FEMORAL NECK FRACTURES

Fractures of the femoral neck are intracapsular and can be classified as either nondis-

placed or displaced (Fig. 5–5). The most significant complications of femoral neck fractures are nonunion and osteonecrosis. These fractures are primarily a disease of patients older than 50 years. In younger patients, they may be associated with motor vehicle accidents. Stress fractures may also occur in this region in athletes. In the child under 3 years of age presenting with a proximal femur fracture, child abuse should be suspected (Fig. 5–6). Femoral neck fractures disrupt the vasculature of the femoral head and neck; the degree of displacement determines the severity of damage.[9] A study by Catto shows that if the femoral neck is displaced greater than 50 percent, it will disrupt the posterior hip capsule.[5] In addition, an intracapsular hematoma will increase the pressure, decreasing the venous outflow and decreasing the arterial inflow.

Nonunion and osteonecrosis are the usual complications;[1] the incidence of nonunion ranges from 10 to 30 percent and that of osteonecrosis from 15 to 33 percent. Primary replacement with a prosthesis is advocated in displaced fractures to avoid the problems with nonunion and osteonecrosis and to allow immediate weight-bearing after surgery[2,6] (Fig. 5–7). In all pediatric patients and young adults, anatomic reduction and internal fixation are required for all displaced fractures (Fig. 5–8).

INTERTROCHANTERIC FRACTURES

Intertrochanteric fractures of the hip occur along the line between the greater and lesser trochanters. This fracture is totally extracapsular. These fractures usually occur as a result of a fall, involving both direct and indirect forces. The bone is usually osteoporotic in elderly people. Patients present with the involved limb usually markedly shortened, with a deformity as much as 90 degrees of external rotation. The external rotation deformity is usually greater than that seen in patients with intracapsular fractures. There may be swelling in the hip region and ecchymosis over the greater trochanter.

Attempts to move the fractured limb are painful and should be avoided. Immediate immobilization of the fractured limb with Buck's traction or sandbags may be necessary to prevent further soft tissue damage in addition to bone comminution. After the limb is immobilized, AP roentgenograms in inter-

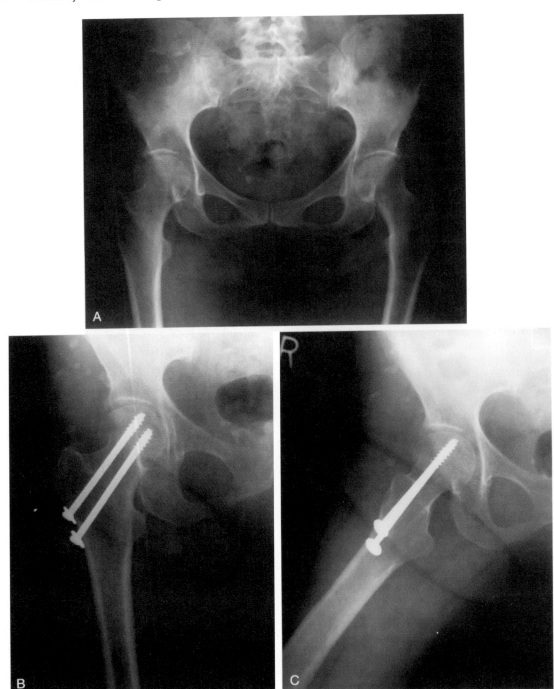

Figure 5–5. *A*, AP view of the pelvis with a right subcapital femoral neck fracture, minimally displaced. *B* and *C*, AP/lateral hip radiograph, showing internal fixation of a hip fracture with multiple cannulated screws.

nal rotation and lateral roentgenograms are taken to confirm the diagnosis and delineate the fracture pattern.

The goal of treatment of an intertrochanteric fracture must be restoration of the patient to his or her preoperative status at the earliest possible time. If the patient was confined to bed and chair before injury, the goal of treatment is pain relief. If prior to injury the patient was active and vigorous,

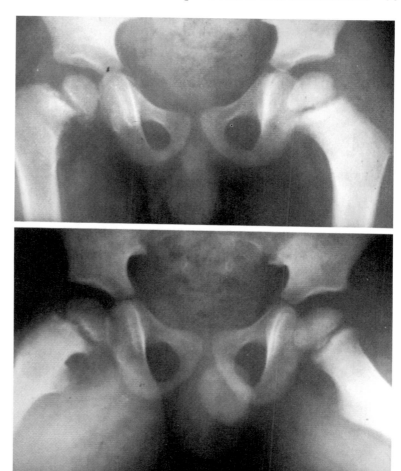

Figure 5–6. Radiographs of a child with a transepiphyseal femoral neck fracture due to nonaccidental trauma.

the treatment should return him or her to the preoperative status. Both these goals can best be achieved through reduction and internal fixation in a stable fashion that allows early mobilization of the patient (Fig. 5–9). The overwhelming majority of intertrochanteric fractures, therefore, should be treated operatively to afford ease of nursing care, rapid mobilization, decreased mortality, decreased hospital stays, and restoration of function. However, nonoperative treatment may be considered in debilitated nonambulatory patients.

Nonoperative treatment includes simple support with pillows or splinting to the opposite limb, Buck's traction, well-leg traction or external fixation, plaster spica or immobilization, balanced traction, and skeletal traction. Nonoperative treatment of intertrochanteric fractures may follow one or two fundamentally different approaches. One approach is toward early mobilization. The

patient is given analgesics and placed in a chair daily. If after chair mobilization the physical condition improves, the patient then begins nonweight-bearing crutch training. The second approach to conservative treatment is traction to maintain the alignment of the fracture so that varus, shortening, and external rotation do not ensue. Great care must be taken to avoid the secondary complications of pneumonia, urinary tract infections, pressure sores over the sacrum and heels, equinus contractures of the foot, and thromboembolic disease. Because of the high cost of health care, this method of treatment is rarely used.

If operative treatment is selected, the goal is to achieve stable fixation internally.[4] For significantly comminuted unstable fractures in elderly osteopenic patients, a prosthetic replacement may be indicated. Studies have shown that by cementing the prosthesis in place, patients are permitted to ambulate

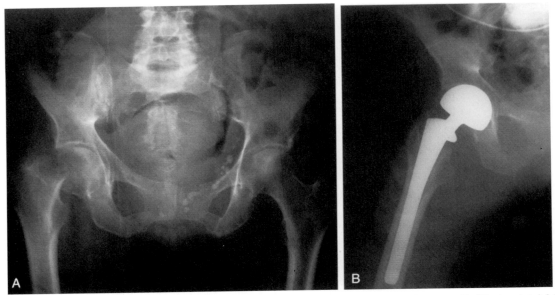

Figure 5–7. *A,* AP radiograph of the pelvis, showing a displaced femoral neck fracture. *B,* Bipolar total hip arthroplasty for reconstruction.

sooner without the increased risk for thrombophlebitis, decubitus ulcers, malunion, and nonunion seen after use of other internal fixation devices.

SUBTROCHANTERIC FRACTURES

Subtrochanteric fractures are those fractures of the hip that extend below the lesser trochanter. Anatomically, the greater tro-

chanteric fragment is abducted by the gluteus medius and minimus, and the iliopsoas flexes and externally rotates to the proximal fragment via the lesser trochanter to which it is attached. Adductors and hamstrings cause shortening and adduction of the shaft fragment.

In younger patients, these fractures are most commonly caused by high-energy trauma, such as motor vehicle accidents, penetrating injuries, or falls from heights.

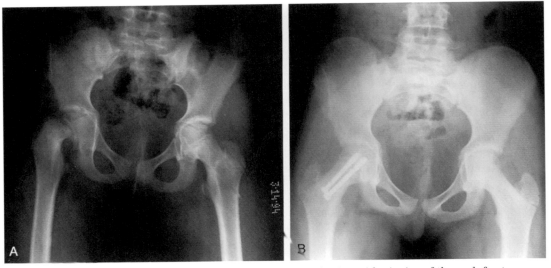

Figure 5–8. *A,* Femoral neck fracture. *B,* Femoral open reduction with pinning of the neck fracture.

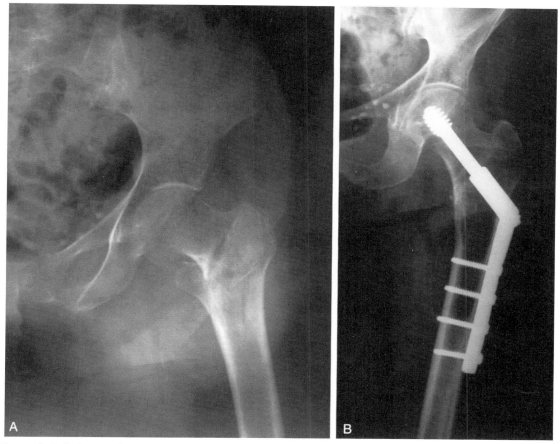

Figure 5-9. *A,* Intertrochanteric hip fracture. *B,* Open reduction and internal fixation of an intertrochanteric hip fracture treated with a sliding compression screw.

In the older age group, fractures are most commonly caused by simple falls. Pertinent history usually includes the mechanism of injury and ability to bear weight after the incident. Also important is the past medical history, social history, pulmonary status, and pharmacologic history. Physical examination usually reveals pain with any hip motion, and the leg is shortened and internally or externally rotated with swelling and deformity. After initial overall assessment, the limb is evaluated for pulses, capillary refill, skin temperature, neurovascular compromise, and muscle strength.

The pertinent x-ray views are an AP pelvis, an AP and lateral of the affected hip, and an AP and lateral of the ipsilateral femur, including the knee. Adults are usually treated with open reduction and internal fixation.[12] In pediatric patients under 12 years of age, subtrochanteric fractures are treated with skeletal traction and a hip spica cast.

References

1. Beaty JH, Calandruccio JH, Canale ST, Carnesale PG, Crenshaw AH, Crenshaw AH Jr, et al.: Campbell's Operative Orthopaedics, 8th ed. St. Louis, Mosby Year Book, 1991.
2. Bochner RM, Pellicci PM, Lyden JP: Bipolar hemiarthroplasty for fracture of the femoral neck. J Bone Joint Surg 70A:1001–1010, 1988.
3. Browner BD, Jupiter JB, Levine AM, Trafton PG: Skeletal Trauma. Vol 2. Philadelphia, WB Saunders, 1992.
4. Canale ST, Bourland WI: Fracture of the neck and intertrochanteric region of the femur in children. J Bone Joint Surg 59A:431–443, 1977.
5. Catto M: Histological study of avascular necrosis of the femoral head after transcervical fracture. J Bone Joint Surg 47B:749–776, 1965.
6. Delamarter R, Moreland JR: Treatment of acute femoral neck fractures with total hip arthroplasty. Clin Orthop 218:68–74, 1987.

7. Greenough CG, Jones JR: Primary total hip replacement for displaced subcapital fracture of the femur. J Bone Joint Surg 70B:639–643, 1988.

8. Morrissy R: Hip fractures in children. Clin Orthop 152:202–210, 1980.

9. Ratliff AHC: Fractures of the neck of the femur in children. Orthop Clin North Am 5:903–921, 1974.

10. Ratliff AHC: Traumatic separation of the upper femoral epiphysis in young children. J Bone Joint Surg 50B:757–770, 1968.

11. Rockwood CA, Green DP: Fractures in Adults, 3rd ed. Philadelphia, JB Lippincott, 1991.

12. Ruff ME, Lubbers LM: Treatment of subtrochanteric fractures with a sliding screw-plate device. J Trauma 26:75–80, 1986.

13. Steinberg GG, Desai SS, Kornwitz NA, et al.: The intertrochanteric hip fracture: A retrospective analysis. Orthopaedics 11:265–273, 1988.

14. Swiontkowski MF, Winquist RA: Displaced hip fractures in children and adolescents. J Trauma 26:384–388, 1986.

15. Trueta J: The normal vascular anatomy of the femoral head during growth. J Bone Joint Surg 39B:359–393, 1957.

Fractures of the Femur

Femoral Shaft Fractures in Adults

Stuart Stephenson

In the adult, fracturing of the femoral shaft almost without exception requires major and quite violent trauma. The leading causes of femoral shaft fractures are motor vehicle or motorcycle accidents, gunshot wounds, and falls from heights. Lesser degrees of trauma in the elderly osteoporotic patient or the patient with a metastatic neoplasm may result in a fracture; however, some degree of trauma even in these individuals is usually required.

Invariably, these patients will present with significant pain, and the mechanism of injury usually will be quite evident. As in any patient presenting with extreme trauma, a full and complete history and physical examination are always indicated. Careful examination should always be given to the hip and knee as it is not uncommon for these areas to be injured as well.

Examination of the upper thigh should include inspection for penetrating wounds and any related lacerations. Swelling and bruising of the thigh should be noted since compartment syndromes can develop because of the massive bleeding into the soft tissues surrounding the shaft of the femur. A neurovascular examination should be documented; however, it is quite rare in the case of a closed femoral shaft fracture to alter significantly the distal perfusion of the extremity or the distal sensation and motor function.[1] Because of the associated muscle spasm involving the quadriceps and ham-string musculature, muscle strength may be diminished but should be present nonetheless.

Careful monitoring of the patient's blood pressure and vital signs always should be maintained, since the hemorrhage from the bone following a femoral shaft fracture can be life threatening. Loss of 2 to 4 units of blood volume, even in the most simple fractures, is common. Therefore, maintaining an assessment of vital signs is critical.

RADIOGRAPHIC ASSESSMENT

Once stabilized, the patient should have standard anteroposterior and lateral radiographs of the femur. The x-rays should always include the entire femoral shaft, hip, and knee. Ideally, this is done once the patient has been stabilized in a splint or temporary traction device, available in most emergency departments. Not only should the fracture pattern itself be evaluated, but more subtle findings that could indicate more extensive bone involvement (such as pathologic or infectious processes), or other osseous lesions that would contribute to the degree of fracture, should be sought.

CLASSIFICATIONS OF FRACTURES

The majority of classifications for fractures of the femoral shaft in adults are based largely on the degree of comminution, the length of the fracture, or some description of the geometry of the fracture. These classification schemes are mainly geared toward decision making for the best form of surgical approach, fixation, and long-term prognosis. Regardless of which fracture classification a physician chooses to use, the degree of comminution is the best indicator for treatment and long-term outcome.

TREATMENT

In the isolated femoral shaft fracture, it is generally felt that the earlier treatment is instituted, the better the anticipated long-term outcome.[2]

In the isolated closed femoral shaft fracture, intramedullary nailing has become virtually universal. Although a technically demanding procedure, it is now widely accepted and practiced. Most fracture patterns are amenable to intramedullary fixation.[3] The continued availability of more specialized devices means that such fixation can be used in virtually all shaft fractures (Fig. 6–1). Other surgical alternatives include plate and screw fixation, multiple small rod fixation, external fixation, or a variety of these. In the very special or unusual case, long-term traction can still be employed; however, this is now rarely indicated or used in the adult.

LONG-TERM PROGNOSIS

The majority of patients whose isolated femoral shaft fracture is treated with early intramedullary fixation can expect a good long-term outcome. Although the time to union directly depends upon the degree of fracture comminution and concomitant soft tissue injury, most patients can expect good ambulatory function within 4 to 6 weeks. The femoral shaft fracture, once treated with intramedullary fixation, should be healed within 6 months. Factors that may delay healing include soft tissue damage, open

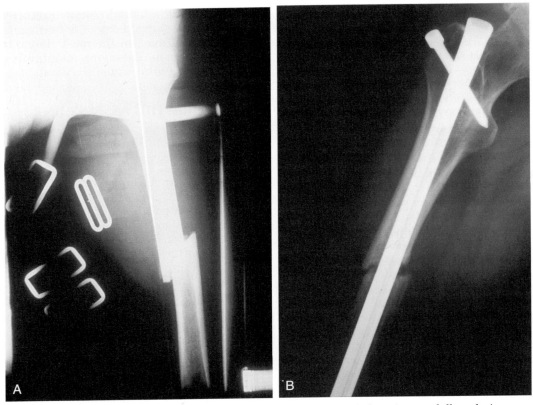

Figure 6–1. *A,* Simple fracture of the femoral shaft. *B,* Fixation with an intramedullary device.

fractures, inadequate fracture stabilization, poor surgical technique, and infection.[4]

CONCLUSION

Patients presenting with an isolated femoral shaft fracture usually will have an impressive presentation and invariably will have been involved in some form of violent trauma. However, with good trauma management, patient stabilization, attention to other injuries if present, and early surgical intervention for the femoral fracture, the majority of these patients can expect excel-lent early mobilization and a good long-term prognosis.

References

1. Barr H, Santex G, Stephenson I: Occult femoral artery injury in relation to fracture of the femoral shaft. J. Cardiovasc Surg 28:193–195, 1987.
2. Clawson DK, Smith RF, Hanse ST: Closed intramedullary nailing of the femur. J Bone Joint Surg 53A:681–692, 1971.
3. Eriksson E, Wallin C: Immediate or delayed Küntscher-rodding of femoral shaft fractures. Orthopedics 9:201–204, 1986.
4. Webb LX, Winquist RA, Hansen ST: Intramedullary nailing and reaming for delayed union or nonunion of the femoral shaft; A report of 105 consecutive cases. Clin Orthop 212:133–141, 1986.

PART II

Femoral Shaft Fractures in Children

Michael J. Conklin

Fractures of the femoral shaft occurring before closure of the proximal or distal physis should be treated with special pediatric considerations in mind. The proximal and distal femoral growth plates are closed somewhere between the ages of 14 and 16 years, earlier in females than males. Femoral fractures are relatively common in children and should be considered serious injuries because of the potential blood loss and the amount of force involved.

ANATOMY

The femur can be divided into a proximal epiphysis or femoral head, the proximal metaphysis including the femoral neck and intertrochanteric region, the diaphysis or shaft, a distal metaphysis, and the distal epiphysis (Fig. 6–2). Fractures occurring between the subtrochanteric region and the beginning of the flare of the distal metaphysis are considered femoral shaft fractures. The femoral shaft has a slight anterolateral bow, with the apex in the middle one third. This is the most common location for fractures of the femoral shaft. Fracture patterns can be either greenstick, transverse, oblique, spiral, or comminuted. Transverse fractures are the result of direct trauma. Oblique fractures are generally the result of indirect trauma, such as torsional or angular forces. Comminuted fractures are the result of more severe direct trauma. The displacement of the fracture fragments can be described in regard to angulation, translation, and rotation (Fig. 6–3). Displacement depends upon the initial force causing the injury, the action of muscles attached to the fragments, and the force of gravity acting upon the limb.

Fractures of the upper third of the femur show flexion, abduction, and external rotation proximal to the fracture site secondary to the action of the iliopsoas, abductors, and short external rotators, respectively. Middle one third fractures do not show any specific displacement pattern because of muscle pull but rather depend on the initial force and the forces acting upon the limb by gravity or external splinting. Fractures of the distal third tend to be posteriorly translated by the action of the gastrocnemius origin.

There is always a component of soft tissue injury with any femoral shaft fracture. This may range from minimal tearing of the periosteum on the tension side of a greenstick injury to complete disruption of the perios-

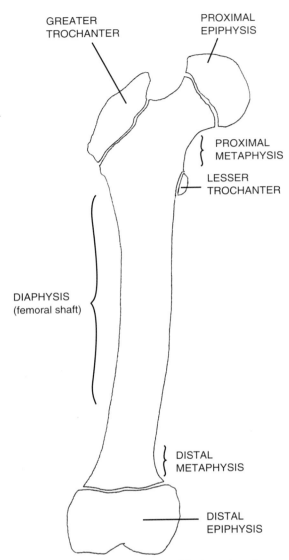

GREATER TROCHANTER

PROXIMAL EPIPHYSIS

PROXIMAL METAPHYSIS

LESSER TROCHANTER

DIAPHYSIS (femoral shaft)

DISTAL METAPHYSIS

DISTAL EPIPHYSIS

Figure 6–2. Ossification centers of the immature femur.

teum and muscular sleeve, as well as soft tissue defects seen in open fractures. The severity of the soft tissue injury depends upon the fracturing force. Blood loss can occur from injury to branches of the profunda femoris artery, the surrounding muscles, or the intramedullary vessels. The femoral artery is rarely injured.

MECHANISM OF INJURY

Femoral fractures can be secondary to direct or indirect trauma. Trauma can be either blunt or penetrating (e.g., gunshot wounds).

Indirect trauma involves angular or rotational forces applied to the lower leg with the body in a fixed position or forces applied to the body with the foot planted. Common mechanisms of injury in children involve playground accidents such as falls from swings or monkey bars, auto/pedestrian, auto/bicycle, and auto passenger accidents. In children without a history of significant trauma, the diagnosis of child abuse or osteogenesis imperfecta or other pathologic bone lesions should be entertained.

DIAGNOSIS

History

An adequate history is indispensable in the evaluation of pediatric femoral fractures. Possible sources include the patient, parent, witness of the event, or emergency medical technician present at the scene. In cases of motor vehicle accident or other high-energy trauma, it is imperative to ask about loss of consciousness, the presence of neck, back, or abdominal pain, and other possible injuries.

In cases of suspected abuse, the child should be interviewed separately from the parents or caretakers and histories compared to assess for discrepancies. The history of previous multiple fractures may be a clue to possible metabolic bone disease or osteogenesis imperfecta.

Physical Examination

A thorough examination is likewise indispensable in the evaluation. In cases of high-energy trauma, the examination is divided into two phases: (1) the primary rescuscitative, and (2) the secondary, definitive injury-specific examination. The initial rescuscitative effort involves assessment of airway, breathing, and circulation.[5,11] The secondary examination is injury-specific and is directed at not only the obviously injured extremity but also other possible sources of injury, such as the head, cervical spine, back, abdomen, or other extremities.

Specific examination of the injured extremity should be very gentle, as all but the greenstick fractures of the femur are grossly unstable and very painful. The skin should be inspected for evidence of soft tissue injury. An open fracture may be so subtle that it

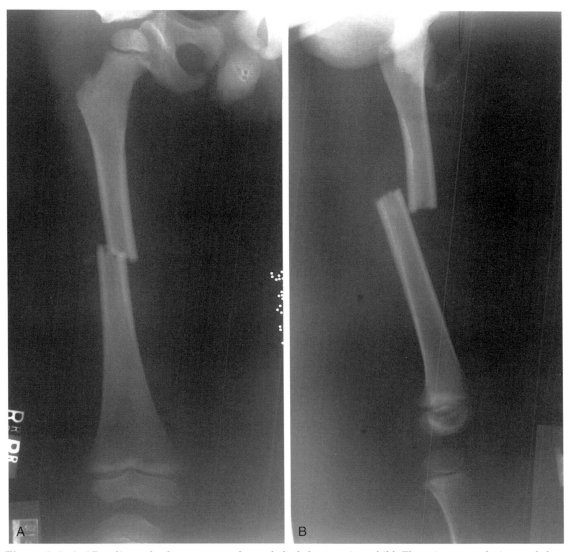

Figure 6–3. *A,* AP radiograph of a transverse femoral shaft fracture in a child. There is no angulation, and there is 40 percent lateral displacement. *B,* The lateral radiograph shows 20 degrees of posterior angulation, 100 percent posterior displacement, and 1 to 2 cm of shortening.

presents only as a pin-point laceration with minimal bloody drainage. The circumference and consistency of the thigh should be assessed, as this may give some indication of the amount of blood loss and the state of the muscular compartments. Compartment syndrome is rare in femoral fractures but does occur. The alignment of the limb should be judged in regard to both angulation and rotation. Generally the distal fragment, including the lower leg, will be externally rotated from the force of gravity. The neuro-vascular status should be assessed with pal-pation of the popliteal, dorsalis pedis, and posterior tibial pulses. Popliteal artery

injury can occur in the more distal fractures. Careful motor and sensory examination of both the peroneal and tibial branches of the sciatic nerve is imperative. Because of pain, it is difficult to evaluate femoral nerve func-tion (quadriceps muscle function) in a patient with a grossly unstable femoral fracture.

The remainder of the examination involves assessment of the pelvis proximally and the lower leg to rule out ipsilateral fractures.

Radiologic Evaluation

It is imperative when evaluating pediatric femoral fractures that the AP and lateral radiographs of the femur include both the hip and knee joints. If the entire femur, including the hip and knee joints is not visualized, other fractures or dislocations may be missed. The remainder of the x-ray examination is tailored to the patient's history and physical examination but frequently may include an AP pelvic view and a view of the ipsilateral tibia.

TREATMENT

The initial management of any femoral fracture involves immobilization. This is best accomplished with a Thomas splint. If none is available, a splint may be improvised from boards. The splint should extend on the lateral side from just under the axilla to the foot and on the medial side from the groin to the foot. Usually the patient has been splinted by the emergency medical technician before presentation to the physician. If the extremity is unsplinted, splinting should be accomplished after the initial survey, before the patient is transported for further studies. This is particularly applicable in the multiple trauma patient.

Treatment of pediatric femoral shaft fractures may involve spica casting,[1,4,8] skin traction, skeletal traction,[3] external fixation,[2] intramedullary nailing,[13] or open reduction and internal fixation (ORIF). In deciding on treatment, age is a major factor. Three age groups are considered.[10,12]

Infancy to 2 Years of Age

Most isolated femoral fractures in this age group can be treated adequately with immediate spica casting either in the emergency department or under general anesthesia in the operating room.[1] The patient is observed overnight to monitor circulatory status, the parents are instructed in spica cast care, and the patient generally is discharged the day after injury. Patients with multiple trauma or those being observed to rule out abdominal trauma may need to undergo delayed spica casting. In this case, either splinting or skin traction can be used to stabilize the fracture until definitive care can be rendered. If child abuse is suspected, the patient should be admitted to the hospital for appropriate evaluation.

3 to 10 Years of Age

In this age group, the treatment of choice is spica cast application. Generally the patient is hung in 90/90 skeletal traction through a distal femoral pin until she or he can safely be taken to the operating room for spica cast application under general anesthesia. The pin may be incorporated in the cast to give extra stability and control of length.[4] Time in the cast averages 8 weeks. Alternatively, the patient can be treated for 2 to 3 weeks in traction until the fracture becomes stable and then placed in a spica cast. This prolongs hospitalization and is relatively labor intensive; also, frequent radiographs are needed to check the fracture position.

11 to 15 Years of Age

Historically, adolescent femoral fractures have been treated with 90/90 skeletal traction until the fracture is relatively stable at 3 weeks postinjury.[3] The patients can then be placed in a one half hip spica cast or a cast brace.[6] In recent years there has been a push to proceed with intramedullary nailing in this age group.[7] This offers the advantage of early mobilization and short hospital stay. This must be balanced against the increased risks from operative intervention.

Special Considerations

Open Fractures

All open fractures require formal irrigation and debridement in the operating room, prophylactic antibiotic therapy, and stabilization of the fracture to decrease the incidence of infection. Stabilization usually will take the form of external fixation.

Polytraumatized Patients

Patients with polytrauma may require more aggressive treatment of the femoral shaft fracture.[9] This applies to patients with multiple long bone fractures, patients with ipsilateral femoral and tibial fractures ("floating knee"), and patients with a closed head injury and spasticity.[14] These fractures may require external fixation or ORIF and plating in the younger age group and external fixation versus intramedullary rodding for those 11 years of age or older.

References

1. Allen BL, Kant AP, Emery FE: Displaced fractures of the femoral diaphysis in children: Definitive

treatment in a double spica cast. J Trauma 17:8–19, 1977.

2. Alonso JE, Geissler W, Hughes JL: External fixation of femoral fractures; Indications and limitations. Clin Orthop 241:83–88, 1989.

3. Aronson DD, Singer RM, Higgins RF: Skeletal traction for fractures of the femoral shaft in children. J Bone Joint Surg 69A:1435–1439, 1987.

4. Curtis JF, Killian JT, Alonso JE: Improved treatment of femoral shaft fractures in children utilizing the pontoon spica cast. A long term follow-up. J Pediatr Orthop, 15:36–40, 1995.

5. Emergency Cardiac Care Committee and Subcommittees: Guidelines for Cardiopulmonary Resuscitation and Emergency Cardiac Care Recommendations of the 1992 National Conference. JAMA 268:2251–2281, 1992.

6. Gross RH, Davidson R, Sullivan JA: Cast brace management of the femoral shaft fracture in children and young adults. J Pediatr Orthop 29–32, 1983.

7. Herndon WA, Mahnken RF, Yngve DA: Management of femoral shaft fractures in the adolescent. J Pediatr Orthop 9:29–32, 1989.

8. Irani RN, Nicholson JT, Chung SM: Long-term results in the treatment of femoral-shaft fractures in young children by immediate spica immobilization. J Bone Joint Surg 58A:945–951, 1976.

9. Routt MLC: Fractures of the femoral shaft. *In* Green NE, Swiontkowski MF (eds): Skeletal Trauma in Children. Philadelphia, WB Saunders, 1994, pp 345–368.

10. Staheli LT: Fractures of the shaft of the femur. *In* Rockwood CA, Wilkins KE, King RE: Fractures in Children, 3rd ed. Philadelphia, JB Lippincott, 1991, pp 1121–1164.

11. Subcommittee on Pediatric Resuscitation: Chameides L (ed): Textbook of Pediatric Advanced Life Support, Dallas, TX, 1990.

12. Tachdjian MO: Fractures of the femoral shaft. In Tachdjian O: Pediatric Orthopaedics, 2nd ed. Vol. 4. Philadelphia, WB Saunders, 1990, pp 3248–3282.

13. Ziv I, Blackburn N, Rang M: Femoral intramedullary nailing in the growing child. J Trauma 24:432–434, 1984.

14. Ziv I, Rang M: Treatment of femoral fracture in the child with head injury. J Bone Joint Surg 65A:276–278, 1983.

CHAPTER 7

Fractures and Ligamentous Injuries of the Knee

• PART I

Knee Injuries in Sports

William P. Garth, Jr.
Kimberly Morris Fagan

Much progress has been made in the surgical treatment and rehabilitation of knee injuries; however, they remain among the most frequent and feared injuries in athletes. Some progress in prevention of knee injuries has been made by rule changes in various sports. For example, in football, rules against crack back blocking and blocking below the waist when downfield from the line of scrimmage are aimed at protecting the knee. However, the location of the knee at the center of the lower extremity leaves it very vulnerable to injury in sports. Prophylactic knee bracing has not been proven to be practical or effective in preventing these injuries.[3,4,11,19,20,23,38,39,43,46] In the foreseeable future, it is unlikely that we will see a significant decrease in the incidence of knee injuries among athletes. It will remain important for those people associated with athletic endeavors to maintain a basic level of knowledge about knee injuries.

KNEE ANATOMY

The term *knee* actually refers to three different joints: the tibiofemoral, the patellofemoral, and the tibiofibular (Figs. 7–1 and 7–2). Both the tibiofemoral and patellofemoral joints are commonly involved in athletic injuries. Occasionally, the proximal tibiofibular joint is involved in sprains and dislocations, but this is relatively insignificant in the discussion of athletic injuries to the knee.

The intra-articular surfaces of the tibiofemoral and the patellofemoral joints are covered with an articular cartilage that is analogous to the treads on a tire. Articular cartilage provides a smooth surface, allowing efficient motion between the bones and dampening forces transmitted through the bones to the joints. When considering response to injury, it is important to keep in mind that articular cartilage lacks nerves, blood vessels, and a lymphatic system.

A second type of cartilage within the tibiofemoral joint is that found in the medial and lateral menisci. These soft, pliable cartilages are held between the articular cartilaginous surfaces of the tibia and femur by coronary ligaments attached peripherally to the margin of the tibia and femur (Fig. 7–3). The menisci function to reduce stress in the tibiofemoral joint by distributing forces over a greater surface area.[29,50] They also assist in providing some degree of joint stability.[30,46]

Intra-articular and extra-articular ligaments serve as static stabilizers of the tibiofemoral joint. During motion, these

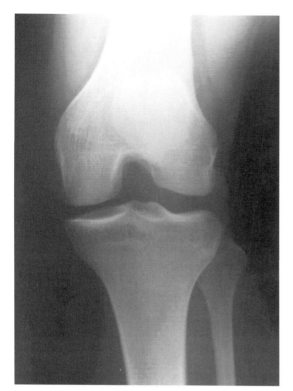

Figure 7–1. Anterior posterior view of the knee reveals the tibiofemoral joint and the tibiofibular articulation.

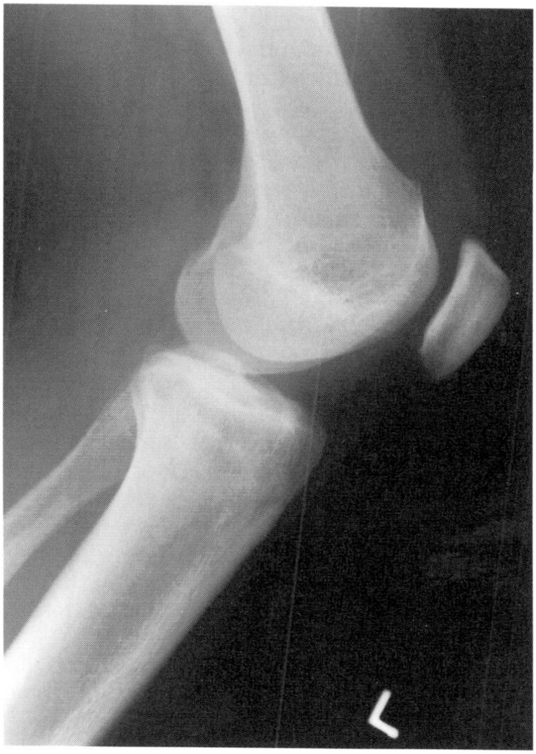

Figure 7–2. Lateral view of the knee reveals the patello-femoral joint.

ligaments force the tibia to follow the articular surface of the femur. The intra-articular ligaments of the knee are the anterior cruciate ligament (ACL) and posterior cruciate ligament (PCL). The ACL functions as the primary restraint to anterior tibial translation and as a secondary restraint to tibial rotation.[13,33] The PCL functions as the primary restraint to posterior translation of the tibia on the femur.[6]

The extra-articular ligaments aid in maintaining varus and valgus stability of the knee. These consist of the medial collateral ligament, the primary restraint preventing valgus instability, and the lateral collateral ligament. The lateral collateral ligament, in association with the popliteus tendon, the iliotibial band, and a complex of ligaments in the posterolateral knee known as the arcuate complex, helps prevent varus instability of the knee. Muscle and tendon units crossing the tibiofemoral joint provide additional dynamic stability and aid the ligaments in maintaining efficient motion and good stability.

The patellofemoral joint is stabilized statically by soft tissue restraints collectively known as the patellar retinaculum. The patellar retinaculum fans out from the patella medially and laterally. The functional portions of the medial retinaculum consist of the medial patellofemoral ligament (MPFL), the medial patellomeniscal ligament (MPML), and the less significant medial patellotibial ligament (MPTL). The MPFL extends from the adductor tubercle of the femur to the superomedial margin of the patella, with additional attachment to the deep surface of

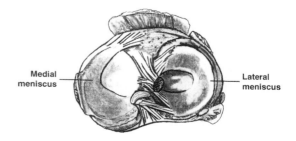

Medial meniscus

Lateral meniscus

Figure 7–3. The shape of the menisci ensures the maximal area of force transmission from the femur to the tibia. Loss of a meniscus reduces the contact area of force transmission and results in wear of the articular cartilage.

the vastus medialis obliquus (VMO) portion of the quadriceps muscles.[7,50] The MPML arises from the distal half of the medial border of the patella and inserts on the periphery of the anterior horn of the medial meniscus.[7,27,37] The MPTL originates on the inferomedial border of the patella and inserts below the joint line on the anterior medial portion of the tibia.[48,49] The MPTL provides little structural support. The MPFL and the MPML account for approximately 75 percent of the static strength preventing dislocation of the patella.[7]

The lateral patellar retinaculum tethers the patella laterally. It consists of the lateral patellofemoral ligament, the lateral patellomeniscal ligament, and the iliopatellar ligament that runs from the iliotibial band to the lateral patella.[14,40,48] If these structures become abnormally taut, they can contribute to patellar instability, resulting in lateral patellar subluxation or lateral patellofemoral compression syndrome.

The quadriceps muscle consists of the vastus medialis, the rectus femoris, the vastus intermedius, and the vastus lateralis (Fig. 7–4). Proper balance and strength within the quadriceps muscles are extremely important in preventing painful conditions in the patellofemoral joint and in maintaining patellofemoral stability. Perhaps the most im-

portant portion of the quadriceps muscle in maintaining patellofemoral stability is the vastus medialis obliquus (VMO). It originates on the distal adductor magnus tendon and the medial intermuscular septum and inserts by way of its tendon onto the superomedial patella, with additional attachment to the medial patellofemoral ligament.[5,7] The VMO's primary function is to give dynamic support in preventing lateral subluxation or dislocation of the patella.[31,32,42]

REHABILITATION OF THE KNEE

Prior to discussing the various soft tissue injuries found in the knee, it is important to understand current concepts of rehabilitation that are true for all these injuries, with only minor modifications for certain specific injuries.

Immobilization, as has been so frequently used for injured or postoperative knees in the past, is rarely if ever indicated following soft tissue injuries to the knee. Protective bracing of the injured structure, e.g., a valgus-stabilizing knee brace for medial collateral ligament sprain or a lateral buttress knee sleeve following patellar dislocation, should be used while a physical therapist works with the patient to regain motion and functional strength. An exercise bicycle is very useful. Full active knee extension is most important to gain full weight-bearing ambulation. Crutches or other walking aids should be utilized until the patient can demonstrate sufficient strength to maintain knee extension while weight-bearing. Quadriceps exercises progress from isometric contraction at full extension and knee extension with light ankle weights to knee extension against progressive resistance (in the absence of patellofemoral pain). Flexibility of the quadriceps, hamstrings, and gastrocnemius, and soleus muscles should be obtained, with stretching maneuvers performed following strength-building exercises.

INJURIES TO THE TIBIOFEMORAL JOINT

Articular Cartilage Injuries

Purely cartilaginous injuries involving the knee are common. They may be described as chondral fractures when a traumatic fissure

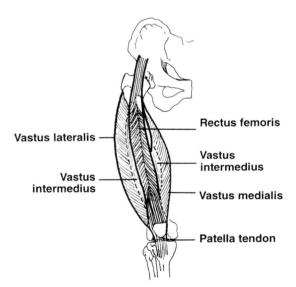

Figure 7–4. The quadriceps femoris is comprised of the rectus femoris, the vastus lateralis, and the vastus medialis. The fourth component, the vastus intermedius, lies deep to these. All insert on the patella and on the tibial tubercle via the patellar tendon. Collectively, they serve as an extensor mechanism for the leg.

Vastus lateralis

Vastus intermedius

Rectus femoris

Vastus intermedius

Vastus medialis

Patella tendon

is present in the articular cartilage surface, or as chondromalacia when softening and degenerative cracking of the articular cartilage occur. These injuries can occur with repetitive use over a period of years, resulting in degeneration of the articular cartilage, or they can occur with an acute impact-loading injury, resulting in a chondral fracture. Occasionally, chondral fractures can dissociate and become fragments that move as loose bodies within the knee. It is important to remember that ligamentous injuries can also occur in association with cartilaginous lesions.

Initially, symptoms associated with articular cartilaginous lesions may be vague and intermittent. The patient may complain of a popping sensation within the knee joint. In the case of chondromalacia, the patient may have a sensation of grinding or grating, and these conditions may be both audible and palpable. Occasionally, the patient will feel that something is moving within the knee, which would suggest a loose body. Clinical manifestations can include an effusion, a yellow-tinged clear fluid within the knee. With a pure cartilaginous lesion, the development of effusion generally requires 24 to 48 hours. Immediate onset is more suggestive of a hemarthrosis, which is more typically associated with an intra-articular ligamentous injury or osteochondral fracture. Other suggestive findings on physical examination are tenderness to palpation of the patella or the involved femoral condyle when the knee is in flexion and occasionally the presence of a palpable loose body or chondral defect.

Radiographic evaluation should include the standard anterior/posterior, lateral, and sunrise or Merchant views of the knee. It is important to remember that a normal x-ray series of the knee does not exclude an articular cartilage lesion. Further diagnostic measures have been reported to be capable of identifying these lesions. Arthrograms of the knee that can show irregular joint surfaces or separated fragments have been routinely recommended by some in the past but are now seldom performed.[1] More recently, noninvasive studies are commonly utilized. However, our experience has been that these imaging studies frequently fail to demonstrate chondral lesions or to make a significant difference in their management. Although we have little experience with contrast-enhanced magnetic resonance imaging, focal articular cartilage defects as small as 2 mm have been reported to be detectable using MRI in conjunction with an enhancing agent such as gadolinium.[17]

Arthroscopy may be used as the primary diagnostic tool for evaluating the knee for articular cartilage damage. The advantage of this method is that treatment can be rendered at the same time without the additional expense of other diagnostic tests. This technique allows one to visualize directly the damaged area, determine the degree of articular cartilage separation, and, if necessary, remove any loose bodies. In addition, drilling and reattachment of separated osteochondral fragments can be performed, if necessary, using this single procedure. If symptoms of effusion and crepitus, suggestive of cartilaginous derangement, have not responded to noninvasive treatment, it is more cost effective to proceed directly to arthroscopic examination and treatment than to spend further time and money on other diagnostic studies.

Acute osteochondral fracture will present routinely with hemarthrosis, and fat droplets from exposed bone marrow will be identified in the bloody aspirate. Nondisplaced osteochondral fractures as identified by routine radiographs may be treated by protection against activities that may produce displacement of the fracture. A cast may be required. When the fracture does not appear to be significantly unstable, range of motion of the knee should be maintained while protecting against displacement of the fracture with nonweight-bearing. Displaced fractures must be treated by surgical reduction and fixation of intra-articular fragments or excision of smaller fragments.

Osteochondritis dissecans will present more subtly. In early cases, the young patient presents with complaints only of vague pain with activity. Effusion and popping will be present only in advanced cases when complete or partial detachment of osteochondral fragments has occurred. Osteochondritis dissecans typically occurs in late childhood or preadolescence. It is believed due to segmental loss of subchondral blood supply. The cause of this avascularity is unknown. The most common location is on the medial femoral condyle adjacent to the intercondylar notch. The lesion at that location is best identified by the tunnel radiographic view, which demonstrates the intercondylar notch of the femur.

Osteochondritis dissecans has the capacity to heal in the growing child. Treatment consists of avoidance of aggravating activity. If a fragment persists ununited to the femoral condyle after growth is complete, then surgical fixation of the lesion while it remains in situ will promote union and prevent eventual detachment. Should detachment occur, treatment consists either of surgical replacement in the crater with fixation or excision of the fragment (Fig. 7–5).

The prognosis for recovery following an articular cartilage injury largely depends upon the size of the lesion. As will be recalled, articular cartilage has no blood vessels and no innate healing capabilities. Surgical shaving of the articular cartilage surface may decrease joint symptoms and effusion but does not appear to stimulate significant repair.[36,44] More aggressive abrasion down to bleeding subchondral bone can result in the appearance of a weaker fibrocartilaginous repair tissue, but there is no evidence for normal articular cartilage regeneration.[24–26]

Reconstructive surgery for replacing the entire surface of the articular cartilage is per-formed when extensive involvement is present. That surgery, known as total knee replacement, covers the end of the bone with metal and polyethylene surfaces. Joint replacement is not suggested for athletic individuals since it tends to break down over a period of years in response to the stresses applied to it.

Meniscal Injuries

Meniscal injuries related to sports such as football, basketball, and wrestling are common. The mechanism of injury is usually a twisting maneuver or a move that requires a rapid change in direction. Isolated injuries of the menisci can occur with improper squatting with or without weights or hyperflexion while weight bearing. These injuries may occur particularly if the hyperflexion under a load occurs in combination with a twisting motion of the tibia on the femur.

A careful history is of utmost importance in making the diagnosis of meniscal injury. The patient often complains of a sudden onset of pain with the initial injury. Swelling within 1 to 2 days is commonly noted (again, the more immediate onset of swelling would suggest intra-articular ligamentous injury or osteochondral fracture). Both pain and swelling may resolve spontaneously only to recur with repeated activity. True knee locking or lack of full extension of the knee is also an important diagnostic clue. On examination, joint line tenderness is felt to be most important, and it is found in 77 to 86 percent of cases.[2,45] This is especially true if the posterior medial or posterior lateral corners of the knee are involved.[12] Provocative tests are useful in identifying the torn meniscus. McMurray's test is one of the most commonly used (Fig. 7–6). This is performed by placing the knee in full flexion with the leg externally rotated for lateral meniscus and internally rotated for medial meniscus evaluations. The knee is then taken from full flexion to full extension with rotation maintained. Pain or a click or both along the joint line is suggestive of a meniscal tear. The location of the click at the joint line is important, because patellofemoral problems can also cause a click. It is also important during the physical examination to rule out any associated ligamentous instability.

Roentgenograms of the knee are recommended to rule out bone lesions in any acute

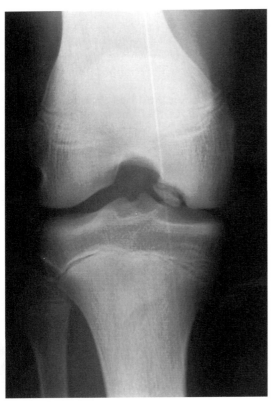

Figure 7–5. Loose osteochrondral fragment noted on the medial femoral condyle.

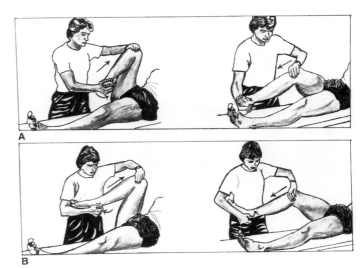

Figure 7–6. McMurray's test is used to detect meniscal pathology. The hip and then the knee are brought into full flexion. The tibia is then internally rotated and the leg extended to apply a compressive force to the medial meniscus (*A*). For lateral meniscus testing, the tibia is externally rotated and the leg extended (*B*). The examiner's hand should be placed along the joint lines in order to palpate a possible click associated with a meniscal tear.

injury. However, these will not demonstrate meniscal pathology.

In most patients, unless the knee is locked, i.e., lacking full extension secondary to a displaced meniscal flap, an initial rehabilitation approach is desirable. Relative rest, that is, avoiding any offending activity, and measures to decrease pain and swelling are the first steps. Increasing activities are then gradually instituted as rehabilitation restores the normal strength of the quadriceps and hamstrings. If these measures fail and the patient has persistent pain, recurring effusion, or continued episodes of locking, then surgical intervention may be required. If the examination is equivocal, an MRI scan may confirm or rule out the diagnosis. Accuracy rates of 93 to 98 percent for medial meniscal tears and 90 to 96 percent for lateral meniscal tears have been reported using MRI.[22,40] However, when the history and physical examination both support an intra-articular lesion, arthroscopy is likely the most cost-effective diagnostic tool. As in the case of articular cartilage lesions, it allows direct visualization and the opportunity for definitive treatment in one procedure.

The type of surgical procedure for a torn meniscus depends upon the location of the tear. A tear of the meniscus along the inner two thirds of its rim generally will not heal due to the lack of blood supply to this area. Therefore, that type of tear requires an operation known as an arthroscopic partial meniscectomy. On the other hand, a tear of the meniscus along its outer periphery, which is generally well vascularized, is treated with a procedure known as an arthroscopic meniscus repair.

Partial meniscectomies require little protection following the surgical procedure, and athletes are generally back to full activity as early as 2 to 3 weeks following the operation. Meniscus repairs, however, must be protected by limited weight-bearing for at least 3 weeks while waiting for the meniscus to heal. Rehabilitation otherwise does not differ from the general knee rehabilitation discussed earlier. Generally, after a meniscus repair the athlete should wait approximately 12 weeks before returning to full activity.

Meniscal tears are commonly associated with tears of the anterior cruciate ligament. In those instances, the meniscal tears are managed as discussed, along with definitive management for the anterior cruciate ligament tear, which generally requires a more extensive surgical procedure.

Medial and Lateral Collateral Ligament Injuries

Injuries of the extra-articular ligaments, the medial and lateral collateral ligaments, also occur in sports. In the past, these ligament sprains (tears) were routinely treated surgically by repairing the torn ligaments. However, in the last decade, it has been recognized that isolated extra-articular ligament sprains can be treated nonsurgically with rehabilitation and bracing and result in good healing and prognosis.[21]

The medial collateral ligament (MCL) is the most commonly injured ligament of the knee.[9,21] MCL injury results from a valgus stress, i.e., the knee being displaced into a knock-kneed position, generally from a blow on the lateral side of the knee. Less severe injuries can occur via a noncontact twisting mechanism, as is seen in cutting and pivoting activities.

Clinical findings depend upon the severity of the injury. A grading system based on physical findings is helpful in planning treatment and predicting the outcome of MCL injuries. First-degree MCL sprains (mild injuries) show tenderness with possibly some minimal swelling along the MCL. In addition to localized swelling and edema, second-degree sprains, which are considered moderate in nature, are noted to have some signs of instability. The MCL is stable to valgus stress when the knee is in full extension; however, at 30 degrees of flexion, some degree of opening is noted. A firm endpoint is felt in cases of moderate sprains. In contrast, a third-degree or severe sprain of the MCL shows instability to valgus stress both in flexion and extension, with no definite endpoint noted (Fig. 7–7A). Associated cruciate ligament or meniscal lesions should be sought on examination.

Diagnostic studies should begin with AP, lateral, and patellofemoral roentgenograms. Ligamentous avulsions, fractures, and loose bodies should be ruled out. In the skeletally immature, a valgus stress radiograph of the

knee is important in differentiating a physeal injury from a MCL injury.

Treatment for acute isolated MCL injuries, regardless of grade, is generally nonoperative. Bracing and rehabilitation are the mainstays of treatment. The time frame for return to activity ranges anywhere from 2 to 8 weeks and generally depends on the degree of initial injury. In essentially all cases, strength evaluation following MCL sprain will demonstrate weakness of the hamstring on leg curl exercise. This corresponds with tenderness of the semimembranosus at its insertion inferior and parallel to the medial joint line. Knee rehabilitation follows the general prescription, but care should be taken to ensure that full knee flexion strength has been restored prior to resumption of full activities. Generally hamstring strength and the patient's subjective confidence in the knee will improve as the semimembranosus tenderness resolves with time. Occasionally, corticosteroid injections of the semimembranosus tendon sheath are necessary to get full resolution of symptoms.

If the MCL is injured in conjunction with the ACL or menisci, then treatment varies accordingly. An acute MCL sprain in the presence of a significant effusion should be considered to have a concomitant ACL injury unless aspiration fails to confirm hemarthrosis. Medial meniscal injuries rarely if ever occur with MCL sprains. In our experience, lateral meniscus tears occur in approximately 5 percent of Grade II or III MCL sprains.

Isolated injury to the lateral collateral ligament is rare. If it is injured, the mechanism is generally a blow to the inside of the knee, resulting in a "bow-leg" or varus force. Examination should reveal tenderness along the ligament and possibly a mild opening on varus stress with the knee at 30 degrees of flexion (Fig. 7–7B). Treatment is nonoperative and similar to that for an isolated MCL injury.

Unfortunately, injury to the lateral collateral ligament is often associated with tearing of the arcuate complex and possibly the popliteus tendon, resulting in posterolateral rotary instability. In this case, the tibia may rotate abnormally posteriorly and laterally on the femur with resulting functional instability. Also, concomitant cruciate ligament injuries are not uncommon. Both situations require more complex diagnostic and treatment plans.

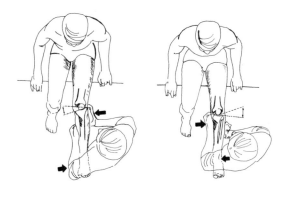

A　　　　　　　**B**

Figure 7–7. Valgus and varus stress tests are used to assess medial and lateral stability. A, Valgus stress is applied by stabilizing the femur and moving the lower leg laterally. This is performed with the knee at 0° and 30° of flexion. B, Varus stress is applied by stabilizing the femur and moving the lower leg medially. This too is performed at 0° and 30° of flexion.

Cruciate Ligament Injuries

The ACL is located inside the knee joint and acts as the primary stabilizer preventing forward displacement of the tibia upon the femur.[13,34] Much to the surprise of many patients, this important structure may be torn without a contact injury. It may occur simply with a sudden stop, hyperextension, or twisting injury of the knee.

The patient may relate a sensation of shifting or hyperextension of the knee at the time of injury. A pop may be felt or heard. Rapid swelling is characteristic of the injury and is a result of bleeding within the knee joint (hemarthrosis). The athlete usually is unable to continue play at the time of the injury but in many cases can walk off the field unassisted. Swelling and soreness may subside in a few days or weeks, and the significance of the injury may not be recognized until recurrent giving way occurs upon return to sports. Chronic recurrent symptoms that may occur as a result of the tearing of the ligament include a sudden "giving way" of the knee, much as occurs at the time of initial injury.

The physical examination may reveal an effusion, with aspiration proving it to be bloody. However, if the injury is not acute, neither swelling nor tenderness may be present. The diagnosis in either case depends on abnormal anterior displacement of the tibia. The anterior drawer test (Fig. 7–8A) can be used in making the diagnosis of an anterior cruciate ligament tear. However, Lachman's test, if positive, is considered to be a much more sensitive test for anterior cruciate instability (Fig. 7–8B). It is performed with the patient in a supine position with the examiner standing on the side of the affected knee. The patient's femur is then stabilized by grasping the distal thigh. The proximal tibia is then drawn forward while maintaining approximately 30 degrees of knee flexion. Increased tibial translation or the lack of a definite endpoint in comparison with the unaffected knee is considered a positive test for ACL instability. The pivot shift test (Fig. 7–9) also is used in making the diagnosis of an anterior cruciate rupture. Regardless of the test used, the degree of patient relaxation and the skill of the examiner are important variables in making an accurate diagnosis.

Standard radiographic views of the knee are routinely obtained. Occasionally an avulsion fracture of the ACL or an avulsion from the lateral tibial plateau (Segond's fracture) may be present and are considered pathognomonic of ACL tears (Fig. 7–10). If there is a question concerning the diagnosis of an ACL tear or if there is concern over associated lesions such as a meniscal tear or bone lesion, an MRI scan may confirm the diagnosis. With complete tears of the ACL, MRI, when performed under the supervision of and read by an experienced radiologist, has a proved accuracy rate of 95 percent.[35] However, a skilled examination should diagnose the

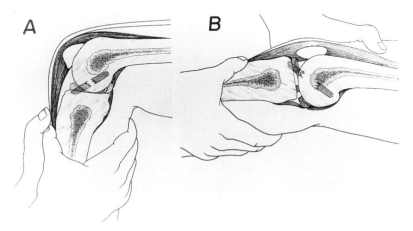

Figure 7–8. *A,* Anterior translation of the tibia in the knee with intact extra-articular ligaments tested in the 70° to 90° flexed position may be restrained to the point that anterior laxity may not be appreciated even in the absence of the anterior cruciate ligament (ACL). *B,* ACL incompetence can be more easily identified because greater anterior excursion occurs at 10° to 30° of knee flexion. As shown in this specimen, anterior translation of a portion of the menisci may still be obstructed by the femoral condyles.

(Used with permission from Garth WP: Current concepts regarding the anterior cruciate ligament. Orthop Rev 21:568, 1992.)

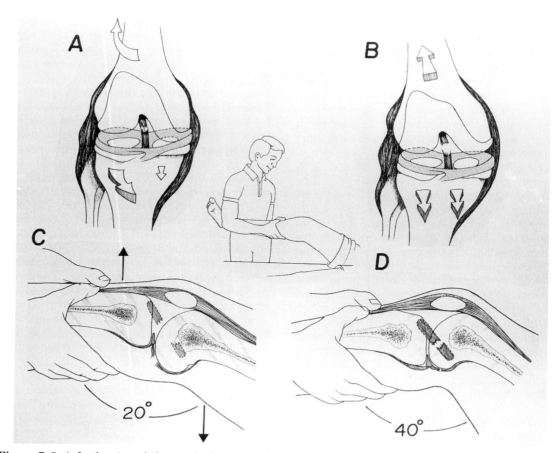

Figure 7–9. *A,* In the pivot shift test, the knee is held near full extension, and anterior displacement of the tibia occurs as a result of holding the leg while gravity acts on the thigh. Subtle internal rotation occurs with anterior translation of the tibia as the lateral femoral condyle sags posteriorly. *B,* Valgus and anterior translating force is then placed on the tibia by the examiner. *C,* Further anterior displacement of the tibia on the femur occurs as the valgus-loaded knee is gradually flexed to 30°. In this specimen, the posterior capsule, which is one of the extra-articular secondary restraints, is shown also to be torn, which would result in even more anterior translation of the tibia than an isolated tear of the ACL. *D,* When flexion proceeds beyond 30°, the acute change in shape of the femoral condyles lessens resistance to reduction of anterior subluxation and results in instantaneous reduction of the anterior subluxation with a sudden acceleration of knee flexion. This instantaneous reduction is recognized by the physician and patient as a sudden shift.

(Used with permission from Garth WP: Current concepts regarding the anterior cruciate ligament. Orthop Rev 21:567, 1992.)

great majority of ligament tears without the need for MRI.

It is generally well accepted to consider surgical repair or reconstruction of the ACL in young individuals who are physically active and intend to remain in sports that involve sudden stopping, jumping, and cutting. In more sedentary individuals who are perhaps older and willing to restrict their activities, nonoperative management consisting of rehabilitation and possible arthroscopic surgery with trimming of torn cartilage is considered. Exceptions may be made. If repair or reconstruction of a torn ACL would prohibit an athlete from partici-

pating in an important season, then delay is reasonable if there is minimally detectable instability on examination and functional testing. Adequate rehabilitation and appropriate bracing are essential. An arthroscopic surgery that requires only a short rehabilitation period may be necessary to trim torn cartilage when the athlete elects not to proceed with the more extensive ligament repair or reconstruction until after the season.

Rehabilitation for nonoperatively treated ACL injuries follows the general outline for rehabilitation described for soft tissue injuries about the knee. However, special empha-

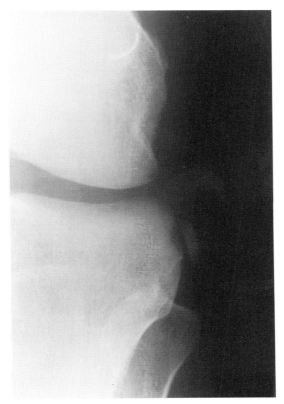

Figure 7–10. Segond's fracture.

sis is placed on regaining and maintaining hamstring strength, since these knee flexors direct the posterior displacing force on the tibia, giving dynamic resistance to the pathologic anterior laxity. Also, special braces in ACL-deficient knees are useful, though expensive.

It is important to keep in mind that the recurrence of pivot shifts during sports not only results in impaired ability to compete but also predisposes the knee to other significant injuries, including the tearing of menisci and damaging of articular cartilage. It is the damage to the menisci or joint cartilage that may result in irreparable damage to the knee and subsequent post-traumatic degenerative arthritis.[15]

The posterior cruciate ligament (PCL) is the primary restraint preventing backward displacement of the leg upon the thigh.[6,18] The mechanism of injury to the posterior cruciate ligament is commonly a direct blow to the anterior portion of the proximal tibia. For the athlete, this would mean falling directly onto the anterior aspect of the distal portion of the flexed knee or taking a direct blow to

the proximal tibia with the leg in extension, thus forcing the tibia posteriorly on the femur. Hyperflexion of the knee without a direct blow is also felt to be a mechanism of injury. Compared with anterior cruciate ligament tears, PCL tears are relatively rare.

There is often a delay in diagnosis, and posterior cruciate ligament injuries are often missed. There may be little swelling and only minimal soreness or stiffness of the knee. On examination, one should look for the posterior sag sign of Godfrey (Fig. 7–11). This is observed with the patient in a supine position with the knee flexed 90 degrees. From the side view, the examiner is able to detect posterior subluxation of the tibia on the femur. Radiographs are usually negative unless there is an associated avulsion fracture of the PCL. Magnetic resonance imaging, if necessary, can be used to confirm the presence of posterior cruciate ligament injury.

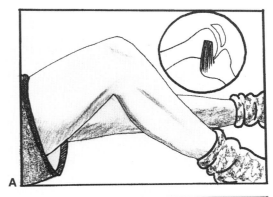

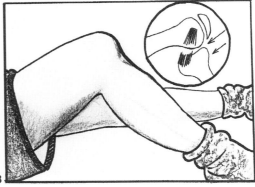

Figure 7–11. *A,* The sag sign of Godfrey is an observation noted when the posterior cruciate ligament is torn. When the ligament is intact, a normal knee profile is observed. *B,* When the ligament is torn and the patient is supine with the leg flexed at 90°, a "drop off" is noted just distal to the patella. This signifies posterior translation of the tibia on the femur resulting from a torn posterior cruciate ligament.

Unlike injury to the ACL, posterior cruciate injuries are commonly treated nonsurgically. Patients who work diligently at knee extension exercises to regain and maintain quadriceps strength tolerate PCL tears best, since the quadriceps muscles provide dynamic resistance to posterior sagging of the tibia. Braces are usually not necessary or beneficial. Reconstruction of the PCL is generally done only if the patient fails to obtain a good result with nonoperative management. More recent studies, however, may change this way of thinking. Independent follow-up studies by Dejour and associates and Keller and colleagues have noted significant morbidity in cases of conservatively managed PCL injuries.[8,28] The degenerative changes and functional deficits noted may lead to earlier surgical intervention in the future. When patellofemoral injury and pain occur concomitantly with significant posterior laxity, cases are generally doomed to failure with nonoperative management.

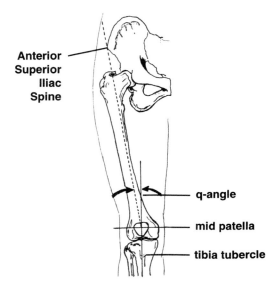

Figure 7–12. The Q-angle (quadriceps angle) is formed by the intersection of the line from the anterior superior iliac spine to the midpoint of the patella and the line from the tibial tubercle to the midpoint of the patella. An excessive Q-angle predisposes the patella to abnormal lateral stresses.

INJURIES TO THE PATELLOFEMORAL JOINT

Aside from direct trauma, most patellofemoral disorders are related to an anatomic predisposition. Predisposing factors include an increased quadriceps angle (Q-angle) (Fig. 7–12). The Q-angle is determined by measuring the angle formed by a line through the center of the patella and femur extending up to the anterior superior iliac spine and a line from the center of the patella through the tibial tubercle. This typically does not exceed 15 degrees in the normal patient. With more acute angles, the contraction of the quadriceps muscles that pulls the patella proximally will also tend to displace the patella laterally. In addition, a congenital laxity of the medial soft tissue restraints will allow deviation of the patella laterally. It is felt, however, that the most common anatomic predisposition to patellofemoral instability occurs when the groove or sulcus of the femur in which the patella glides is abnormal. A relative flattening of this sulcus, as noted on roentgenographic studies, is present in approximately 70 percent of knees with a history of patellar dislocation.[16] Flattening of the sulcus results in an inadequate lateral buttress, which allows for lateral displacement of the patella. Additionally, an abnormally long patellar tendon will result in the

patella riding high (patella alta) in the femoral sulcus, which causes the patellofemoral joint to act in a similar fashion as the flat sulcus. This condition of patella alta is found in approximately 50 percent of individuals who experience patellar dislocations.[16] These anatomic predispositions can lead to various "malalignment syndromes" of instability or pain or both.

The most obvious patellar instability problem is that of dislocation. For a patellofemoral dislocation to occur, however, there must be more than the predispositions just noted. Failure of the medial retinaculum must occur. Tearing or disruption of the medial patellar retinaculum results in loss of the medial tethering of the patella in the femoral sulcus, allowing lateral displacement to occur.

The mechanism of injury in the case of patellar dislocation is typically a twisting injury associated with a strong contraction of the quadriceps. A direct blow to the knee is not necessarily present. Athletes will often report that they felt a shifting sensation and heard or felt a pop. Often the patella will relocate by simply straightening the knee and, therefore, will not be displaced on initial physical examination. Significant swelling, which occurs fairly rapidly, is expected.

On examination, the patella may or may not be in a laterally dislocated position. However, there will be swelling and tenderness over the medial retinaculum. A positive apprehension sign, which is solicited by flexing the knee to approximately 30 degrees and attempting to displace the patella laterally, should be present. Plain radiographs of the knee should be obtained in all cases of patellar dislocation. This is important to rule out avulsion or osteochondral fractures.

If a large hemarthrosis is present, aspiration is appropriate in order to relieve pain and evaluate for the possibility of fat globules in the aspirate, which would suggest an occult osteochondral fracture. Control of pain and swelling is then the primary concern. Appropriate bracing with a lateral patellar buttressing felt pad and knee sleeve should be prescribed.

An aggressive rehabilitation program follows, with particular attention placed on strengthening the vastus medialis obliquus (VMO) portion of the quadriceps muscle. The strengthening program should be supervised under care by a physical therapist and generally consists of terminal knee extension exercises and strengthening of the medial thigh muscles with adduction exercises. Bicycling and other low-impact exercises are excellent forms of rehabilitation to be utilized until soreness is reduced and function is restored. Adequate rehabilitation should be gauged by demonstrating normal quadriceps strength compared with the uninvolved leg, with absence of any significant atrophy and complete restoration of muscle tone. When adequate rehabilitation has been tried and failed or in the case of recurrent patellar dislocations with the threat of more significant damage, then surgical intervention should be considered.

Patellar subluxation, although more subtle in its presentation, can be the cause of persistent knee pain, functional disability, and chondral pathology secondary to recurrent episodes of subluxation. The mechanism of injury is similar to that for dislocations. The patient will usually complain of a slipping sensation in the knee cap upon twisting, cutting, or pivoting. Usually, only mild swelling is associated with the subluxation. If the subluxation is recent, examination should reveal a positive apprehension sign as seen with a dislocated patella. Treatment options are similar to those for patellar dislocations.

Aside from the instability problems demonstrated by patellar dislocations or subluxations, there are malalignment syndromes in which pain rather than instability predominates. An example of this is the lateral patellofemoral compression syndrome or excessive lateral compression syndrome.[10] In this case, the patella tends to ride laterally, causing increased compressive forces of the lateral facet of the patella against the lateral femoral condyle. Generally a tightness of the lateral patellar retinaculum tethers the patella against the lateral femoral condyle.

The patient with lateral patellofemoral compression syndrome will usually give a history of a spontaneous onset of knee pain without any preceding trauma. Activities such as going up and down stairs, kneeling or squatting, or turning or twisting may aggravate the problem. Also, the patient may complain of pain following prolonged periods of sitting with the knee in the flexed position (the "movie theater" sign). There is usually no history of swelling; however, the patient may complain of a sensation of puffiness around the knee. Crepitation may also be present. On examination, special attention should be given to the alignment of the lower extremity. The Q-angle is usually exaggerated. Also, typically there is tenderness over the lateral facet of the patella, which is demonstrated by displacing the patella laterally and palpating under the lateral edge of the patella. Vastus medialis oblique atrophy also may be noted. Patellofemoral radiographs, such as the Merchant's view, may reveal a lateral tilt to the patella.

Treatment, if at all possible, is nonsurgical. Aggressive rehabilitation, especially focusing on strengthening the vastus medialis oblique portion of the quadriceps muscles, is undertaken. Hamstring and gastrocnemius flexibility is addressed. Hamstring flexibility is addressed by performing passive and active assistive hamstring stretching by flexing the hip while maintaining knee extension. The gastroc-soleus muscles are stretched with typical Achilles stretching exercises: passive and active assistive dorsiflexion of the ankle, both with the knee extended and with the knee flexed. When there is hypermobility of the patella and lateral patellofemoral compression, a lateral buttressing patellofemoral knee sleeve or McConnel taping is routinely used,[34] as well as patellofemoral bracing or taping. Occasionally, activity modification is recommended. If all these measures fail, then surgical options are considered.

Acknowledgment

A special thanks to Lee Ann Manasco for drawing the illustrations in this section.

References

1. Almgard LE, Wikstad I: Late results of surgery for osteochondritis dissecans of the knee joint. Acta Chir Scand 127:588, 1964.
2. Anderson AF, Lipscomb AB: Clinical diagnosis of meniscal tears; Description of a new manipulative test. Am J Sports Med 14:291–293, 1986.
3. Baker BE, VanHanswyk E, Bogosian SP, et al: A biomechanical study of the static stabilizing effect of knee braces on medial stability. Am J Sports Med 15:566–570, 1987.
4. Baker BE, VanHanswyk E, Bogosian SP, et al: The effect of knee braces on lateral impact loading of the knee. Am J Sports Med 17:182–186, 1989.
5. Bose K, Kanagasuntheram P, et al: Vastus medialis oblique: An anatomic and physiologic study. Orthopedics 3:880–883, 1980.
6. Butler DL, Noyes FR, Grood ES: Ligamentous restraints to anterior-posterior drawer in the human knee. A biomechanical study. J Bone Joint Surg 62A:259–270, 1980.
7. Conlan T, Garth WP, Lemons JE: Evaluation of the medial soft tissue restraints of the knee extensor mechanism. J Bone Joint Surg 75A:682–693, 1993.
8. Dejour H, Walch G, Peyrot J, Eberhard PH: The natural history of rupture of posterior cruciate ligament. French J Orthop Surg 2:112–120, 1988.
9. Fetts JF, Marshall JL: Medial collateral ligament injuries of the knee: A rationale for treatment. Clin Orthop 132:206–217, 1978.
10. Ficat RP, Hungerford DS: *Disorders of the Patellofemoral Joint.* Baltimore, Williams & Wilkins, 1977.
11. France EP, Paulos LE, Jayaraman G, Rosenberg TD: The biomechanics of lateral knee bracing. Part II: Impact response of the braced knee. Am J Sports Med 15:430–438, 1987.
12. Fu FH, Baratz M: Meniscal injuries. In DeLee JC, Drez D Jr (eds): *Orthopaedic Sports Medicine.* Philadelphia, WB Saunders, 1994, pp 1146–1162.
13. Fukubayashi T, Torzilli PA, Sherman MF, Warren, RF: An in vitro biomechanical evaluation of anterior-posterior motion of the knee; Tibial displacement, rotation, and torque. J Bone Joint Surg 64A:258–264, 1982.
14. Fulkerson JP, Gossling HR: Anatomy of the knee joint lateral retinaculum. Clin Orthop 153:183–188, 1980.
15. Garth WP: Current concepts regarding the anterior cruciate ligament. Orthop Rev 21:565–575, 1992.
16. Garth WP, Pomphrey M, Merrill K: Functional treatment of patellofemoral instability in an athletic population. Presented at Alabama Orthopaedic Society, Pt. Clear, Alabama, May, 1990.
17. Glys-Morin VM, Hajek PC, Sartoris BJ, Resnick D: Articular cartilage defects: Detectability in cadaver knee with MR. AJR 148:6, 1987.
18. Gollehon DL, Torzilli PA, Warren RJ: The role of the posterolateral and cruciate ligaments in the sta-
19. Grace TG, Skipper BJ, Newberry JC, Nelson MA, Sweetser ER, Rothman ML: Prophylactic knee braces and injury to the lower extremity. J Bone Joint Surg 70A:422–427, 1988.
20. Hewson GF, Mendini RA, Wang JB: Prophylactic knee bracing in college football. Am J Sports Med 14:262–266, 1986.
21. Indelicato PA: Non-operative treatment of complete tears of the medial collateral ligament of the knee. J Bone Joint Surg 65A:323–329, 1983.
22. Jackson DW, Jennings LD, Maywood RM, Berger PE: Magnetic resonance imaging of the knee. Am J Sports Med 16:29–47, 1988.
23. Jackson RW, Reed RC, Dunbar F: An evaluation of knee injuries in a professional football team—risk factors, type of injuries and the value of prophylactic knee bracing. Clin J Sports Med 1:1–7, 1991.
24. Johnson LL: Diagnostic and Surgical Arthroscopy. St. Louis, CV Mosby, 1980.
25. Johnson LL: Arthroscopic abrasion arthroplasty. Historical and pathologic perspective: Present status. Arthroscopy 2:54–59, 1986.
26. Johnson LL: The sclerotic lesion: Pathology and the clinical response to arthroscopic abrasion arthroplasty. *In* Ewing JW (ed): *Articular Cartilage and Knee Joint Function; Basic Science and Arthroscopy.* New York, Raven Press, 1990, pp 319–334.
27. Kaplan EB: Factors responsible for the stability of the knee joint. Bull Hosp Joint Dis 17:51–59, 1956.
28. Keller PM, Shelborne KD, McCarroll JR, Rettig AC: Nonoperatively treatment for isolated posterior cruciate ligament injury. Am J Sports Med 21(1):132–136, 1993.
29. Krause WR, Pope MH, Johnson RJ, Wilder DG: Mechanical changes in the knee after meniscectomy. J Bone Joint Surg 58A:599–604, 1976.
30. Levy IM, Torzilli PA, Warren RF: The effect of medial meniscectomy on anterior-posterior motion of the knee. J Bone Joint Surg 64A:883–888, 1982.
31. Lieb FF, Perry J: Quadriceps function; An anatomical and mechanical study using amputated limbs. J Bone Joint Surg 50A:1535, 1968.
32. Mariani PP, Caruso I: An electromyographic investigation of subluxation of the patella. J Bone Joint Surg 61B:169–171, 1979.
33. Markolf KL, Mensch JS, Amstutz HC: Stiffness and laxity of the knee—the contributions of the supporting structures. A quantitative in vitro study. J Bone Joint Surg 58A:583–594, 1976.
34. McConnell J: The management of chondromalacia patella: A long-term solution. Aust J Physiother 32(4):215–223, 1986.
35. Mink JH, Levy T, Crues JH: Tears of the anterior cruciate ligament and menisci of the knee: MR evaluation. Radiology 167:769–774, 1988.
36. Mitchell N, Shepard N: Effects of patellar shaving on the rabbit. J Orthop Res 5:388–392, 1987.
37. Paulos LE, et al: Infrapatellar contracture syndrome. An unrecognized cause of stiffness with patella entrapment and patella infera. Am J Sports Med 15:331–341, 1987.
38. Paulos LE, Cawley PW, France EP: Impact biomechanics of lateral knee bracing: The anterior cruciate ligament. Am J Sports Med 19:337–342, 1991.
39. Paulos LE, France EP, Rosenberg TD, Jayaraman G, Abbott PJ, Jaen J: The biomechanics of lateral knee bracing. Part I: Response of the valgus

restraints to loading. Am J Sports Med 15:419–429, 1987.

40. Polly DW, Callaghan DD, Sikes RA, McCabe JM, McMahon K, Savory CG: The accuracy of selective magnetic resonance imaging compared with the findings of arthroscopy of the knee. J Bone Joint Surg 70A:192–198, 1988.

41. Reider B, Marshall JL, Koslin B, Ring B, Girgis FG: The anterior aspect of the knee joint: An anatomical study. J Bone Joint Surg 63A:351–356, 1981.

42. Reynolds L, Levin TA, Mederios JM, Adler NS, Hallum A: EMG activity of the vastus medialis oblique and vastus lateralis muscles in their role of patellar alignment. Am J Phys Med 62:61–70, 1983.

43. Rovere GD, Haupt HA, Yates CS: Prophylactic knee bracing in college football. Am J Sports Med 15:111–116, 1987.

44. Schmid A, Schmid F: Results after cartilage shaving studied by electron microscopy. Am J Sports Med 15:386–387, 1987.

45. Shakespeare DT, Rigby HS: The bucket-handle tear of the meniscus. A clinical and arthrographic study. J Bone Joint Surg 65B:383–387, 1983.

46. Shoemaker SC, Karkolf KL: The role of the meniscus in the anterior-posterior stability of the loaded anterior cruciate deficient knee. J Bone Joint Surg 68A:71–79, 1986.

47. Sitler M, Ryan J, Hopkinson W, et al: The efficacy of a prophylactic knee brace to reduce knee injuries in football. Am J Sports Med 18:310–315, 1990.

48. Slocum DB, Larson RL, James SL: Later reconstruction of ligamentous injuries of the medial compartment of the knee. Clin Orthop 100:23–45, 1974.

49. Terry GC: The anatomy of the extensor mechanism. Clin Sports Med 8:163–177, 1989.

50. Voloshin AS, Wosk, J: Shock absorption of meniscectomised and painful knees. A comparative in vivo study. J Biomed Eng 5:157–161, 1983.

51. Warren LF, Marshall JL: The supporting structure and layers on the medial side of the knee. J Bone Joint Surg 61A:56–62, 1979.

- PART II

Fractures About the Pediatric Knee

John Killian

The increase in bone injuries of the immature knee is a direct result of increased participation of children in athletic programs and increased vehicular accidents. Because of the presence of the epiphysis, physeal plates, and secondary ossification centers, the bone injuries that result can be classified into growth plate injuries or bone avulsion injuries.

KNEE ANATOMY

The pediatric knee function is unique in the presence of large cartilaginous epiphyses articulating in the form of a modified hinged joint. The distal femoral physeal plate and proximal tibial physeal plate contribute substantially to the overall length of the limb and development of the knee. The distal femoral physeal plate has an undulating nature designed to resist shear forces generated by injuries or the extensor mechanism. The distal femoral physeal plate closes between 16 and 20 years of age. The proximal tibial physeal plate is flatter in nature but extends distally on the anterior surface beneath the insertion of the patellar tendon. This physeal plate typically closes between 14 and 17 years of age. The medial and lateral collateral ligaments attach to the epiphyses of the distal femur and the proximal tibia. The anterior cruciate and posterior cruciate ligaments originate from the epiphyses of the distal femur. The anterior cruciate ligament inserts onto the proximal tibial epiphysis at the tibial eminence. The posterior cruciate ligament inserts on the posterior aspect of the proximal tibial epiphysis.

The distal femoral epiphyses and physeal plate contribute approximately three eighths inch of growth per year to the overall stature of an individual, while the proximal tibial physeal plate contributes approximately one fourth inch of growth per year. Combined, they are responsible for more than 60 percent of the overall length of the limb, with the femur contributing approximately 60 percent of that total growth.

DISTAL FEMORAL AND METAPHYSEAL FRACTURES

Fractures of the distal femoral area can be characterized according to the Salter-Harris

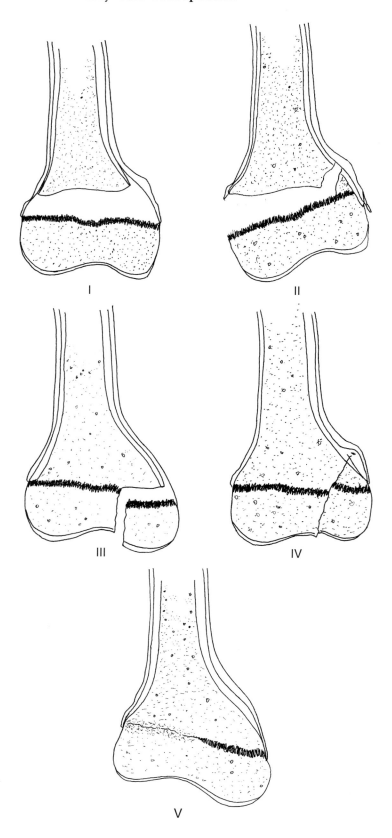

Figure 7–13. Fractures of the distal femur are classified according to the amount of involvement of the physeal plate, metaphysis, and epiphysis.

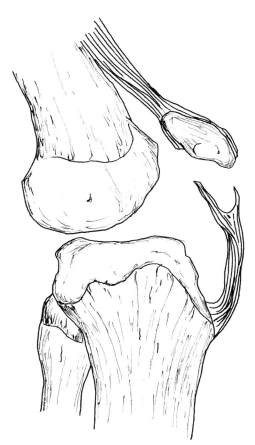

Figure 7–14. The patellar ligament and its bone attachment are avulsed in this injury.

classification (see Chapter 1) (Fig. 7–13). Most are the result of a direct injury to the extremity or a fall. In children under 3 years of age, suspected child abuse should be part of the differential diagnosis, and associated injuries should be ruled out.

The Salter-Harris classification attempts to group injuries in this area based on the propagation of the fracture relative to the epiphysis and the physeal plate. Salter-Harris Type I fractures represent a transverse separation of the distal femoral physeal plate from the metaphysis. These may occur at any age and, if nondisplaced on the initial radiograph, may require a diagnostic varus or valgus stress film to demonstrate displacement or widening through the growth plate. These are typically managed with a closed reduction and long leg cast. After 4 to 6 weeks of partial weight-bearing, the cast may be removed.

Salter-Harris Type II fractures represent the largest group of injuries to the distal femur. The typical fracture line extends transversely across the physeal plate and then extends proximally into the metaphysis, where it exits. The triangular piece of metaphyseal bone left attached to the epiphysis, thus separating it from a Salter I type of injury, is referred to as the "Thurston-Holland" fragment. Treatment, again, is usually with a closed reduction and long leg cast. Occasionally internal fixation and cast immobilization are required for fractures in which an anatomic reduction cannot be obtained.[11]

Salter-Harris Type III fractures typically involve a medial or lateral epiphysis. The fracture line extends transversely across the physeal plate and then exits distally through

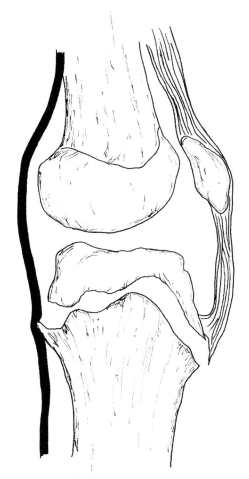

Figure 7–15. With displacement of the proximal tibial epiphysis, the neurovascular bundle may be compressed or injured.

the epiphysis, typically through the intercondylar notch. This fracture requires an anatomic reduction to optimize healing and minimize further growth problems. Internal fixation will be required more frequently with Type III fractures.[3]

Salter-Harris Type IV fractures are relatively rare and are characteristically described as an oblique fracture from the epiphysis transversely across the physeal plate, then exiting through the proximal metaphysis of the distal femur. Anatomic reduction of this injury is required as well.

Salter-Harris Type V fractures are often referred to as the "overlooked" fracture. Unless there is frank impaction of the distal femoral metaphysis into or through the physeal plate, this diagnosis is often made only retrospectively. It is characterized as a crush injury to the distal femoral physeal plate, resulting in aberrant growth.

Occasionally, growth disturbances from a physeal fracture may not be evident for up to 2 years.[4] Genu varum, genu valgum, recurvatum, and leg length inequality may occur owing to a growth arrest or asymmetric growth of the physeal plate.[10] Parents and patients should be advised of these potential complications, and extremity radiographs or scanograms should be obtained as necessary.

PATELLAR FRACTURES

Patellar fractures represent a group of bone avulsion fractures involving the immature knee. These fractures usually occur in the adolescent group as the immature patella appears to be protected from fracture. Typically the adolescent will present with the history of a direct blow to the area, or of attempting to jump or leap. The patellar fractures are referred to as a bone avulsion injury in that the two most common fractures involve either a displacement of the inferior pole of the patella with its attached patellar ligament (Fig. 7–14), or an avulsion of the medial aspect of the patella associated with patellar subluxation or dislocation. Anatomic reduction of large displaced fractures of the patella is required to minimize problems of diminished knee motion, extensor lag, or chondromalacia.[6] Virtually always this will require an open reduction and internal fixation.

PROXIMAL TIBIAL FRACTURES

Fractures to the proximal tibial growth plate are relatively uncommon. Salter-Harris Type I and Type II fractures predominate and are generally the result of direct trauma. Occasionally with a Type II injury and significant displacement or with an open injury, there may be an altered neurovascular examination of the distal limb (Fig. 7–15). Fractures that have a suspected vascular insult or associated neurologic deficit distally should be referred for further assessment and possible internal fixation of the fracture. Undisplaced fractures may be treated with

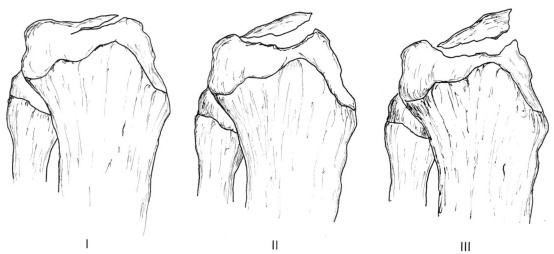

I   II   III

Figure 7–16. Type I and Type II tibial eminence fractures are minimally elevated from the surface. Type III fractures are completely displaced and rotated.

a long leg cast for 4 to 6 weeks. Displaced and open fractures require surgery.[1]

The majority of Salter-Harris Type III and Type IV fractures are nondisplaced and can be managed with long leg cast immobilization. Osseous healing occurs in 4 to 6 weeks. If there is displacement, then an anatomic reduction is required. This may necessitate surgical fixation.

TIBIAL EMINENCE FRACTURES

Tibial eminence fractures represent a group of bone avulsion injuries to the immature knee. The child or adolescent typically presents with a tense hemarthrosis after a fall or athletic injury. Valgus, external rotation, and hyperextension forces result in the subsequent injury. A portion of the tibial eminence is avulsed by the intact anterior cruciate ligament. The Meyer and McKeever classification of the injury is based on the amount of displacement and associated rotation of the fracture fragment[9] (Fig. 7–16). Type I and Type II fractures are best managed by evacuation of the hematoma and casting in full extension. Type III injuries occasionally are converted to a Type I or Type II injury with a gentle manipulation of the knee into full extension and then casting in extension in a long leg cast.[8] The majority of Type III fractures, however, require open reduction and internal fixation in order to restore the anterior cruciate ligament to its normal tension.[7]

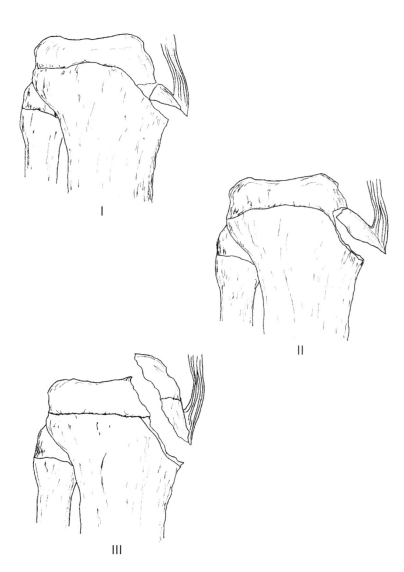

Figure 7–17. Type I and Type II fractures of the tibial tubercle are incomplete and may reduce with extension casting. The Type III fracture is intra-articular and requires open reduction and internal fixation.

TIBIAL TUBEROSITY FRACTURES

Injuries to the proximal tibial tuberosity represent a group of bone avulsion injuries that characteristically occur during a well-defined period of growth. Between 13 and 16 years of age, the proximal tibial physeal plate is completing its growth. Typically, the cessation of growth proceeds asymmetrically from the center of the physeal plate peripherally.

The usual history is of an attempted leap or pushing off during which there is a forced contraction of the quadriceps muscle against a fixed leg.[2]

The Watson-Jones classification is still used, and although these injuries represent a Salter-Harris III fracture, they are treated based on the relative amount of displacement[12] (Fig. 7–17). Type I and Type II fractures can be successfully treated with immobilization in full extension for 6 weeks. Serial radiographs are taken to document adequacy of the reduction. Displaced Type II and all Type III injuries require anatomic reduction and stabilization with internal fixation. Problems with excessive swelling with Type III fractures have been reported; if there is evidence of a compartment syndrome primarily involving the anterior compartment, then immediate referral is recommended.

CONCLUSIONS

Injuries to the pediatric knee usually take the form of a bone injury. The relative weakness of the physeal plate and epiphyses compared with the ligaments about the knee results in forces that tend to fracture bone rather than strain or disrupt ligaments. Fractures that extend into the joint or part of the articular surface of the joint require an anatomic reduction, but fortunately the majority of injuries are nondisplaced. Displaced Salter II injuries of the distal femur or proximal tibia and Watson-Jones Type III fractures of the proximal tibial tuberosity have been associated with vascular injuries or compartment syndromes.[5]

References

1. Burkhardt SS, Peterson HA: Fractures of the proximal tibial epiphyses. J Bone Joint Surg 61A: 996–1002, 1979.
2. Christie MJ, Devonch VM: Tibial tuberosity avulsion fractures in adolescents. J Pediatr Orthop 1:391–394, 1981.
3. Crawford AH: Fractures about the knee in children. Orthop Clin North Am 7:639, 1976.
4. Graham JM, Gross RH: Distal femoral physeal problem fractures. Clin Orthop 225:51–53, 1990.
5. Green NE, Allen BL: Vascular injuries associated with dislocation of the knee. J Bone Joint Surg 59A:236–239, 1977.
6. Griswold AS: Fractures of the patella. Clin Orthop 4:44, 1954.
7. Groenkvist H, Hirsch G, Johansson L: Fracture of the anterior tibial spine in children. J Pediatr Orthop 4:465–468, 1984.
8. Meyer MH, McKeever FM: Fracture of the intercondylar eminence of the tibia. J Bone Joint Surg 41A:209–222, 1959.
9. Meyer MH, McKeever FM: Fractures of the intercondylar eminence of the tibia. J Bone Joint Surg 52A:1677–1684, 1970.
10. Risborough EJ, Barrett IR, Shapiro F: Growth disturbances following distal femoral physeal fracture separation. J Bone Joint Surg 65A:885–893, 1983.
11. Roberts JM: Operative treatment of fractures about the knee. Orthop Clin North Am 21:365–379, 1990.
12. Watson-Jones R: *Fractures and Joint Injuries,* 4th ed. Edinburgh, E&S Livingstone, 1955–1956.

* P A R T   I I I

Fractures About the Adult Knee

Stuart Stephenson

In the adult patient presenting to the physician with a knee effusion following trauma, one should not only carefully search for ligamentous or intra-articular injury but should also pay very careful attention to the bone structures because fractures in and about the knee are very common and sometimes overlooked. Although probably not as common as hip or femoral shaft fractures, fractures involving the most distal aspect of the femur, patella, and proximal tibial plateau are very challenging treatment problems; if improperly handled, they may create significant functional disability.

In any patient with a history of trauma and knee effusion, a careful history and physical examination should be performed. Significant trauma has occurred in the majority of cases, resulting in the aforementioned physical findings. However, in elderly patients even minor falls can result in occult fractures that are commonly missed if not diligently sought. Usually multiple radiographic views, including AP, lateral, and oblique films, are necessary. Careful inspection of the contours of the patella, distal femur, and tibia should be done. Even subtle changes in the appearance of any articular surfaces in the patient presenting with a history of knee trauma should be considered abnormal, and a full explanation for these changes should be sought.

FRACTURES OF THE DISTAL FEMUR

The distal 9 to 10 cm of the femoral shaft are considered the supracondylar region of the femur. Fractures in this area often extend into the knee joint, thereby causing a large intra-articular hemarthrosis. With an intra-articular hemarthrosis, the knee will lose its normal bone landmarks. Often one will not be able to distinguish the patellar prominence or the characteristic medial and lateral appearance of the quadriceps mechanism. Unlike other joint effusions, an intraarticular hemarthrosis often will be very tense to palpation and often very painful to the patient.

Fractures with significant displacement in this area may involve the femoral artery as it enters the adductor canal. The distal vascular and neurologic function should be documented and monitored. If there is any question of the presence or absence of distal pulses, a vascular surgeon should be consulted and an arteriogram strongly considered (Fig. 7–18).

FRACTURES OF THE PATELLA

The majority of patellar fractures will occur with direct trauma to the patella itself. Invariably, there is some separation or splitting of the patella, and the patient will be unable to fully extend the knee joint. A palpable defect may be felt or seen in a patellar fracture. However, because of related injury or extreme patient anxiety, deep palpation in this area is often difficult and unadvisable. Fractures of the patella are usually more evident on the lateral radiograph (Fig. 7–19).

FRACTURES OF THE TIBIAL PLATEAU

The majority of fractures of the proximal portion of the tibial plateau are related to violent trauma. However, patient falls with torsion on the proximal tibia and varus or valgus ligamentous stress can result in a displaced tibial plateau fracture.[2] The elderly osteoporotic patient is more likely to sustain a fracture of the tibial plateau versus a ligamentous or meniscal injury with seemingly minor twisting trauma (Fig. 7–20).

After careful radiographic and neurovascular assessment, the majority of tibial plateau fractures can be treated temporarily by

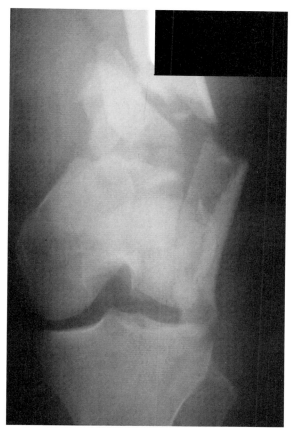

Figure 7–18. A comminuted supracondylar femur fracture.

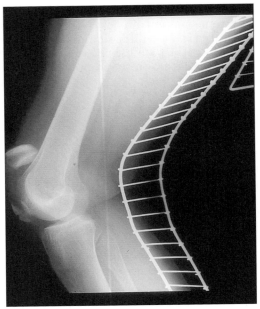

Figure 7–19. Lateral radiograph showing a displaced patella fracture.

splinting, with the knee in extension or slight flexion. Aspiration of the joint to evacuate a large hemarthrosis may provide temporary pain relief; however, great care should be given to rigid aseptic techniques, for conver-

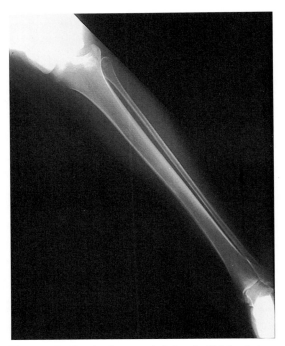

Figure 7–20. A depressed lateral tibial plateau fracture.

sion of a closed intraarticular knee fracture to an open one by aspiration and bacterial contamination could be devastating. As with any fracture, examination should be done to evaluate for any open lacerations into the fracture site. If found, local debridement can be done and the wound covered with a sterile bandage. Tetanus prophylaxis should be given when appropriate. Intravenous antibiotics, usually a first-generation cephalosporin, should be started.

Definitive surgical treatment for these fractures should be well planned and meticulously executed, with careful rehabilitation. Many of these fractures are best treated surgically within the first 24 hours of injury, if possible. Therefore, prompt recognition of the fracture, early attention to other subsystem involvement, and early referral are indicated.

CLASSIFICATION

As with any fracture, many classifications exist for fractures of the distal femur, patella, and proximal tibia. The important factors are the degree of comminution, displacement, and concomitant soft tissue injury.

TREATMENT

Critical to any surgical procedure for fractures involving the knee is restoration of normal anatomic alignment, congruent intraarticular surfaces, and rigid fixation. Fractures of the distal femur often will require specialized plates with screws applied to the lateral surface of the femur to maintain this normal anatomic alignment.

Fractures of the patella require exploration for concomitant laceration of the extensor mechanism. Bone reconstruction is usually done with pins and wires as well as screw fixation.

As with fractures of the distal femur, fractures of the proximal tibia often require buttress plates with multiple screws. Supplemental bone graft is not uncommon.

Postoperatively, most of these fractures are splinted in a brace or functional device to provide further fracture stabilization, yet allow early rehabilitation.

Fractures of the distal femur, patella, or tibial plateau often do not require surgical intervention.[1] However, this depends largely upon the degree of comminution and displacement, as well as consideration of the patient's age and functional status. Fractures involving the tibial plateau with minimal displacement or severely osteoporotic bone or both can do quite well if treated with appropriate casting or splinting. If treated nonoperatively, careful and frequent follow-up should be maintained to avoid any further fracture displacement and subsequent development of fracture malunion.

CONCLUSIONS

Fractures involving the knee should always be considered in a patient presenting with a history of trauma and knee joint effusion. The distinction between soft tissue injury, ligamentous injury, and bone fracture should be made. One should remember that elderly patients with osteoporotic bone and seemingly minor trauma often will have a fracture involving the knee that may not be evident on routine radiographic analysis.

Once a fracture involving the knee is documented, it is imperative that early fracture management be instituted. Fracture management varies from those patients requiring early surgical intervention to those meeting the criteria for functional casting or bracing. The ultimate goal for these patients is to provide fracture stabilization such that early resumption of joint motion can be reestablished. Delay in the appropriate management of these injuries may lead to long-term and possibly permanent restriction of joint motion and, ultimately, long-term disability.

References

1. Hohl M, Johnson EE, Wiss DA: Fractures of the knee. *In* Rockwood CA, Green DP (eds): *Fractures in Adults.* 3rd ed. Philadelphia, JB Lippincott, 1991, p 1756.
2. Weis E Jr, Pritz H, Hassler C: Experimental automobile-pedestrian injuries. J Trauma 17:823–828, 1977.

CHAPTER 8

Tibial Shaft Fractures

Jorge E. Alonso

The tibia and fibula are the most common bones to fracture. The estimated incidence is 185,000 per year in the United States,[13] with an estimated 2,472,000 days lost from work or school annually. Nicoll stated that "fractures of the tibial shaft are important for two reasons. The first is that they are common; the second is that they are controversial, and anything that is common and controversial must be important."[11]

An accurate diagnosis and disposition of these fractures is mandatory. To achieve this goal, one should keep in mind the following 12 commandments.[6]

(1) Most fracture patterns can be predicted by knowing the chief complaint, the age of the patient, and the mechanism of injury.

(2) A careful history and physical examination will predict radiographic findings with a high degree of accuracy. (Remember that the majority of fractures were described before the advent of radiology.)

(3) Splint all extremities, including the joint above and the joint below, before sending the patient to radiology.

(4) Do a thorough neurovascular examination initially before sending the patient to radiology.

(5) Be familiar with the proper radiographic views. At least two views 90 degrees from each other and including the joint above and the joint below are necessary.

(6) If the radiographs are negative but a fracture is suspected clinically, treat for a fracture.

(7) Obtain the radiographs before reduction of the fracture.

(8) Circumferential casts can cause many complications if the physician is unaccustomed to their application. They are usually not mandated in the acute setting and should be applied later when swelling has diminished.

(9) Patients should be checked for the ability to ambulate with crutches and should receive explicit aftercare instructions before leaving, including a warning to watch for signs of neurovascular compromise.

(10) In the multiple trauma patient, noncritical injuries take second place to airway, head, and intracavitary injuries.

(11) All orthopaedic injuries should be described precisely.

(12) The injury should not be overtreated.

Competency in the treatment of tibial shaft fractures requires fluency in the language of orthopaedics. Because the general practitioner or the emergency physician frequently describes fractures to consultants over the telephone, the ability to give a precise description according to established minimal guidelines is important.[14]

A *fracture* is a break in the continuity of bone or cartilage (Fig. 8–1). If the fracture line involves one cortex, it is termed *incomplete,* and if it involves both cortices, it is termed *complete.* A fracture is either closed or open. *A closed fracture* is a fracture in which the skin overlying the fracture is intact. In an *open fracture* the fracture communicates with the environment (Fig. 8–2). Open fractures are considered orthopaedic emergencies because of the risk of infection. Gustillo and Anderson have classified open tibial fractures according to injuries of the soft tissues (Table 8–1). Therefore, no time should be wasted. The emergency physician should apply a sterile dressing, provide appropriate tetanus prophylaxis and antibiotic coverage, and transfer the patient or call the orthopaedic surgeon.

The exact anatomic location must be described. The tibia can be divided into thirds: proximal, middle, and distal. Describe the direction of the fracture line in relation to the long axis of the tibia (Fig. 8–3). A *transverse fracture* occurs at a right angle to the long axis of the tibia. A *spiral fracture* results from a rotational force and encircles the bone. A fracture in which more than two fragments are present is termed *comminuted*[6] (Table 8–2) (see Fig. 8–1).

CLOSED TIBIAL FRACTURES

Tibial fractures have many causes, ranging from simple falls with a twisting force to severe injuries such as those sustained in motorcycle accidents or bumper injuries. It is essential to distinguish between low- and high-energy injuries.[1-4]

The history, physical examination, and radiographs provide a guide to the type of fracture. The history provides significant information concerning the type of fracture. Much more kinetic energy is produced by a skiing injury than by a simple fall. The amount of comminution shown in the radiograph is proportionate to the amount of energy that produced the fracture.

Once a physical examination with neurovascular evaluation is performed, the extremity is splinted, and the patient is sent to radiology for an AP and lateral radiograph, including the knee and ankle. The splint is applied to include the joint above and the joint below. The purpose of splinting the leg is twofold: to immobilize the bone fragments, thus decreasing the pain, and to decrease the damage to the soft tissues.

After the patient has returned from the radiology suite, a second physical examination should be performed. When a conscious patient is developing a compartment syndrome, pain can be produced by passively stretching the muscles in the involved compartments. (Anterior compartment pain is produced by plantar flexing the patient's toes passively.[3,9,13,14]) Compartment syndromes are covered in more detail in Chapter 2.

In the treatment of these fractures, a long leg splint should be applied, including the proximal and distal joints. The patient should be referred to an orthopaedic surgeon, since definitive treatment often requires sur-

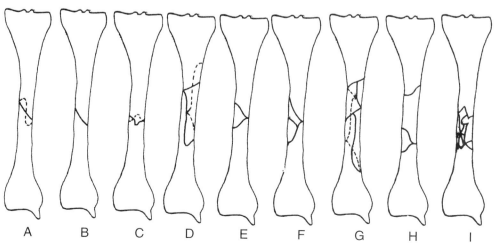

Figure 8–1. Fracture patterns. *Spiral fractures: A,* spiral fracture; *B,* oblique fracture; *C,* transverse fracture. *Butterfly fractures: D,* butterfly by torsion; *E,* butterfly by bending (one); *F,* butterfly by bending (several). *Comminuted fractures: G,* comminuted by torsion; *H,* segmental fracture; *I,* crush.

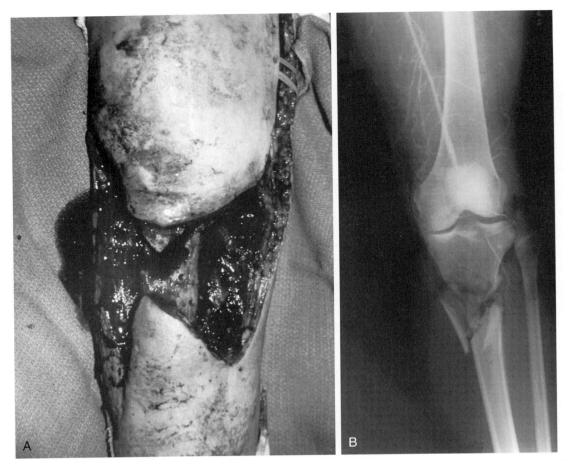

Figure 8–2. *A,* Clinical photograph of a Grade IIIC proximal tibial fracture. *B,* Anteroposterior radiograph with an arteriograph showing a comminuted proximal metaphyseal fracture of the tibia with vascular injury.

gical fixation. Circumferential casting is best left for the physician providing definitive care and follow-up examinations. The patient should be given explicit instructions, including watching for signs of neurovascular compromise (numbness, excessive swelling, or loss of normal color in the toes), and

should also be checked for the ability to ambulate safely with crutches or a walker before being discharged from the clinic or emergency department.

Although the average tibial fracture heals in approximately 17 weeks, with more time added for complete rehabilitation, some patients are disabled for a year or more.[5] Tibial fractures in themselves are rarely lethal injuries now, but their prolonged recovery period and their potential for permanent disability are of great significance.[7]

OPEN TIBIAL FRACTURES

Open fractures are a serious surgical emergency. They demand urgent yet thoughtful intervention by the surgeon. The steps taken during the first few hours after fracture can make the difference between complete recovery and a lifetime of disability.

TABLE 8–1.
Gustillo-Anderson Classification of
Open Fractures

Grade I		Wound less than 1 cm long, punctured from within
Grade II		Laceration up to 5 cm long, no contamination or crush, frequently a segmental fracture
Grade III		Large laceration associated with contamination or crush. A segmental or comminuted fracture
	IIIA	Soft tissue stripping of bone
	IIIB	Periosteal stripping
	IIIC	Major vascular injury present

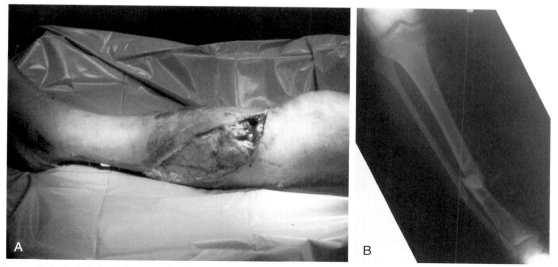

Figure 8–3. *A,* Clinical photograph of a Grade IIIA midshaft tibial fracture. *B,* Anteroposterior radiograph of a midshaft spiral fracture of the tibia.

In 1866, Theodor Billroth said, "I can state from my own experience that the most remarkable operative case has never given me such satisfaction as the successful treatment of a severe open fracture." In his series of 93 patients with open tibial fractures, there were 36 deaths and 28 amputations. Since then we have advanced to the era of "functional preservation." Today, higher priority is given to the functional integrity of the injured extremity. Even with a severe open fracture, the patient not only expects that the bone will heal but also insists upon a complete return to normal function of the extremity.[3,9,13,14]

With this in mind, early care of an open tibial fracture begins at the accident scene.[15]

TABLE 8–2.
Describing a Fracture

Is the fracture open or closed?
Location of the fracture: right or left tibia?
proximal third
middle third
distal third
Type of fracture
transverse
oblique
spiral
comminuted
segmental
Does it extend to the joint?
tibial plateau
to the ankle joint

The main objective in the prehospital care of an open tibial fracture is to avoid further soft tissue injury. The fractures should be gently straightened and splinted on the scene, as this will relieve pressure on the injured, ischemic soft tissues. Swelling and the spread of hematoma are controlled by placing a sterile dressing over the wound and immobilizing the extremity in a pneumatic splint, including the joint above and below. External bleeding is controlled with a sterile compression dressing. In rare instances, a tourniquet is indicated. It is used only in the face of unmanageable hemorrhage or traumatic amputation, and never should be left in place longer than 1 hour.[9,13,14]

The benefit of this early care is substantial. The infection rate in open tibial fractures can decrease from 22.2 percent in patients who reached their final destination by way of another hospital within 10 hours postinjury, to 3.5 percent when the primary care was administered and the patient transferred to the final destination within an hour.[15] As we can see, the time factor has a significant bearing on the end result, regardless of the quality of primary care.

Usually these high-energy fractures are the result of extreme violence, and many patients may present with multiple injuries. As many as 30 percent of tibial fractures occur in patients with multiple injuries.[10,14,15] Once life-threatening problems have been corrected and the patient is in stable condition, a more definitive diagnostic evaluation may be made, with emphasis placed upon speed, accuracy, and thoroughness.

The initial sterile dressing and the splint should not be disturbed until the orthopaedic surgeon examines the extremity. In a study by Tscherne and Gotzen, dressings that were removed by the emergency physician or initial physician had an infection rate of 19.2 percent; when the sterile dressing was left intact from the accident scene and removed by the orthopaedic surgeon under sterile conditions, the infection rate was 4.3 percent.[15]

Often it is impossible to obtain a complete history. Nevertheless, every effort should be made to establish at least the time, cause, and mechanism of the accident. Remember that the "golden time" for repair of these injuries is within 6 hours from injury to surgical debridement and stabilization. Therefore, an expedient history and physical examination are mandatory.

In the physical examination, the joints adjacent to the open fractures are carefully examined so that coexisting injuries will not be overlooked. Vascular evaluation should be thorough, especially in open fractures, as vessels are injured either from the initial trauma or from the fracture fragments. In tibial fractures, large amounts of blood loss (500 to 700 ml) can occur just from the fracture, even without vascular injury.[6]

Nerve injuries can occur by both blunt and penetrating trauma. In tibial fractures, the peroneal nerve is the nerve most frequently injured. The injury can manifest as a neuropraxia (contusion of the nerve in which normal function usually returns in weeks to months), an axonotmesis (severe crush injury to the nerve), or a neurotmesis (severance of a nerve, usually necessitating surgical repair).

Evaluation of compartment syndrome should be considered even in open fractures. Pain is usually out of proportion to the injury and is increased with passive stretching of the involved muscles. Compartment syndrome is a surgical emergency, and it is covered in Chapter 2.

Once the extremity has been examined, radiographs are essential. At least two views are obtained 90 degrees to each other, conventionally in the frontal (AP) and sagittal (lateral) planes. It may be difficult to position the injured limb precisely. It should be rotated as a unit and not twisted through the fracture site. The unstable fracture should

be aligned and splinted prior to obtaining radiographs. Then the entire splint is rotated for x-ray positioning. Insufficient radiographs should not be accepted, and it is essential that all bone injuries be well documented before taking the patient to the operating room.

In communicating with the orthopaedic surgeon, it is important that appropriate terminology be used to describe the radiographic appearance of a tibial shaft fracture. Its location, pattern, degree of comminution, and extent and direction of displacement and alignment are all essential information in assuring appropriate and timely treatment. Also, the soft tissue injury should be classified (see Table 8–1).

The role of the initial examiner is to evaluate and arrange treatment of these fractures in an expedient fashion. First, control hemorrhage with a sterile dressing. After a careful physical examination, the extremity is splinted, appropriate radiographs are obtained, intravenous antibiotics are begun (usually a cephalosporin), and tetanus prophylaxis, including tetanus immune globulin for large crush wounds, is administered. The patient is then referred for definitive treatment, which includes emergency surgical debridement in the operating room and often procedures for soft tissue coverage and internal or external fixation (Fig. 8–4).

CONSEQUENCES OF INJURY

Fractures of the tibial shaft initially prevent weight-bearing ambulation. If the fracture is open and is not treated adequately, serious infection may threaten life and limb. There is concern that malalignment of a tibial fracture may result in joint damage over time. However, this possibility has not been established. The location of the fracture is important. Distal fractures and deformities are more likely to have long-term symptoms than are more proximal fractures.[12]

FRACTURES OF THE TIBIA IN CHILDREN

Fractures of the tibia in children are the most common injuries of the lower limb. These fractures heal so readily that delayed union or nonunion is rarely seen.[3–14]

Physical examination and evaluation should be performed as in the adult. The

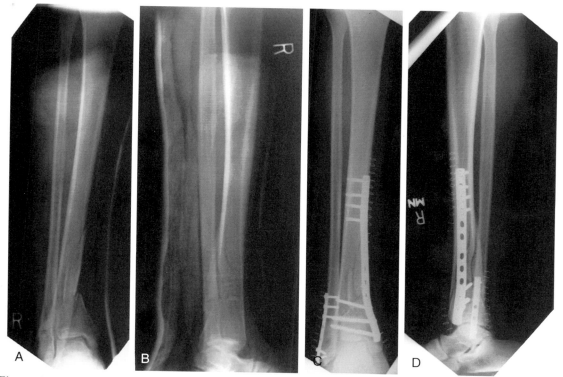

Figure 8–4. *A* and *B*, Anteroposterior and lateral radiographs of a butterfly fracture of the distal tibia. *C* and *D*, Anteroposterior and lateral radiographs after open reduction and internal fixation with plates and screws.

treatment of tibial shaft fractures in children is usually uncomplicated and can be treated by simple manipulation and long leg cast application.[6]

In children more than 8 years of age, one must attempt to achieve anatomic position. In younger children, the amount of shortening that may be tolerated after closed reduction is 5 to 10 mm between 1 and 5 years of age, and up to 5 mm between 5 and 8 years of age.

Postreduction radiographs must include both the ankle and knee joint so that the treating physician can see whether the ankle and knee joints are parallel. If rotational alignment is of concern, the treating physician should order a computed tomographic scan.[6]

Special Tibial Fractures

Toddlers' Fractures

In children up to the age of 6 years, torsion of the foot produces a spiral fracture of the tibia with no fibular fracture. Although these children have minimal pain, they fail to bear

weight on the affected limb. The treatment for this fracture is immobilization in a long leg cast for 4 to 5 weeks.

Proximal Metaphyseal Tibial Fractures

Fractures of the proximal tibial metaphysis may appear benign but may develop undesirable sequelae. The most common sequela is the development of a valgus deformity.

It must be emphasized to the family that with these fractures there may be overgrowth and angulation despite adequate appropriate treatment.

References

1. Bauer GCH, Edwards P, Windmark PH: Shaft fractures of the tibia; Etiology of poor results in a consecutive series of 173 fractures. Acta Chir Scand 124:386–395, 1962.
2. Bondurant FJ, Cotler HB, Backle R, et al: The medical and economic impact of severely injured lower extremities. J Trauma 28:1270–1273, 1988.
3. Chapman MW: Fractures of the tibia and fibula. *In* Chapman MW (ed): *Operative Orthopaedics.* Philadelphia, JB Lippincott, 1988.

4. Committee on Trauma, American College of Surgeons: *Advanced Trauma Life Support Program.* Chicago, American College of Surgeons, 1989.
5. Ellis H: The speed of healing after fractures of the tibial shaft. J Bone Joint Surg 40B:42–46, 1958.
6. Geiderman J: Fractures. *In* Harwood-Nuss A (ed): *The Clinical Practice of Emergency Medicine.* Philadelphia, JB Lippincott, 1991.
7. Grazier KL, Holbrock TL, Kelsey JL, Stauffer RN: *The Frequency of Occurrence, Impact, and Cost of Musculo-skeletal Injuries in the United States.* Chicago, American Academy of Orthopaedic Surgeons, 1984.
8. Gustillo RB, Merkow RL, Templemen D: Current concepts review. The management of open fractures. J Bone Joint Surg 72A:299–303, 1990.
9. Leach RE: Fractures of the tibia and fibula. *In* Rockwood CA Jr, Green DP (eds): *Fractures in Adults.* Vol 2. Philadelphia, JB Lippincott, 1984.
10. Marcus RE, Hansen ST Jr: Bilateral fractures of the tibia: A severe injury associated with multiple trauma. J Trauma 27:415–419, 1987.
11. Nicoll EA: Fractures of the tibial shaft; A survey of 705 cases. J Bone Joint Surg 46B:373–387, 1964.
12. Olerud C: The pronation capacity of the foot: Its consequences for axial deformity after tibial shaft fractures. Arch Orthop Trauma Surg 104:303–306, 1985.
13. Russell TA, Taylor JC, LaVelle DG: Fractures of the tibia and fibula. *In* Rockwood CA, Green DP, Bucholz RW (eds): *Rockwood and Green's Fractures in Adults,* 3rd ed. Philadelphia, JB Lippincott, 1991.
14. Trafton PG: Tibial shaft fractures. *In* Vol. 1. Browner BD, Jupiter JB, Levine AM, Trafton PG (eds): *Skeletal Trauma.* Philadelphia, WB Saunders, 1992.
15. Tscherne H, Gotzen L: *Fractures with Soft Tissue Injuries.* New York, Springer-Verlag, 1984.

Fractures and Ligamentous Injuries of the Ankle

- P A R T   I

Ankle Sprains

Daniel DiChristina
William P. Garth, Jr.

The most common ligament injuries of the body occur in the ankle.[12] Successful management depends upon an accurate diagnosis to rule out other injuries, followed by aggressive functional rehabilitation.

Knowledge of the ligamentous anatomy of the ankle is a prerequisite for diagnosing and managing ankle sprains (Figs. 9–1 and 9–2).[16] The lateral ankle ligaments are much weaker than the medial ligaments and are injured during the frequently seen mechanism of ankle inversion (Fig. 9–3). The medial ligament consists of the deep and superficial deltoid ligament, and it is injured during pronation and external rotation or eversion of the ankle (Fig. 9–4). Medial and lateral ligament injuries of the ankle are also seen in association with ankle fractures, the specifics of which may be found in Part II of this chapter.

The diagnosis of an ankle sprain is based on the history and physical examination. The patient will describe an injury of excessive inversion or eversion and, less commonly, excessive plantar flexion or dorsiflexion. Palpation of the principal ligaments reveals points of maximal tenderness and establishes the diagnosis. Palpation of anatomic areas that when injured may simulate an ankle sprain, or may be injured in association

with an ankle sprain, is also necessary to prevent a misdiagnosis (Table 9–1).

In all cases of a presumed ankle sprain, an anterior drawer test should be performed.[21] This is accomplished by stabilizing the tibia with one hand while directing an anterior force on the calcaneus with the other hand (Fig. 9–5). Abnormal motion and pain elicited by this maneuver indicate an ankle sprain of significant severity, with a complete tear of the anterior talofibular ligament. This can be documented on a lateral radiograph.

Inversion testing of the ankle, referred to as the talar tilt test, evaluates the anterior talofibular and calcaneofibular ligaments.[37] These two ligaments are the most commonly injured ligaments about the ankle. Instability or tibiotalar opening with this maneuver implies a complete tear of the lateral ligaments and can be seen on an anteroposterior radiograph. Eversion testing may reveal the rarely seen problem of medial tibiotalar gaping caused by complete deltoid disruption. External rotation of the ankle stresses the syndesmosis between the tibia and fibula above the ankle joint. Pain with this maneuver is suggestive of a syndesmosis sprain of the ankle.[40,43]

Standard radiographs of the ankle are indicated in nearly all ankle injuries causing

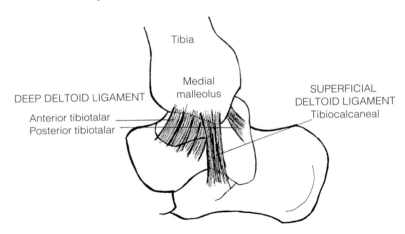

Figure 9–1. Medial ankle ligaments as viewed from the medial aspect of the right ankle.

a person to seek medical attention. When there is suspicion of a fracture, a radiographic examination should be performed prior to stress testing. Three views of the ankle (anteroposterior, lateral, and mortise) should be supplemented by additional radiographs of anatomic areas of tenderness. Most commonly this includes the proximal fibula and the lateral aspect of the foot.

Ankle sprains are graded on an increasing severity scale of mild, moderate, and severe,[32] or Grades I, II, and III.[25] In reference to an inversion ankle sprain, a Grade I injury is a partial tear of the lateral ligaments, with tenderness to palpation over the anterior talofibular or calcaneofibular ligament. The anterior drawer test is negative for tibiotalar subluxation, but it may elicit pain. Grade II injuries are characterized by a torn anterior talofibular ligament with an intact calcaneofibular ligament. The anterior drawer test results in anterior subluxation of the talus on the tibia. Grade III ankle sprains imply

a severe injury with torn anterior talofibular and calcaneofibular ligaments. The anterior drawer test and talar tilt are positive.[15]

Treatment of ankle sprains has evolved to the current standard of aggressive functional rehabilitation.[24,29,30,41] Studies comparing nonoperative versus operative treatment demonstrated no benefit from early surgical intervention.[5] The initial steps of functional rehabilitation are modalities to reduce pain and swelling, such as cold therapy, compressive dressings, and nonsteroidal anti-inflammatory medication. Range of motion exercises and weight-bearing as tolerated, with crutches if necessary, are the mainstays of early treatment. Strengthening exercises, particularly of the peroneal musculature for inversion sprains, and proprioceptive exercises should begin as soon as possible.

Return to activities largely depends on the severity of the initial injury, coupled with the patient's diligence in following treatment protocols. For athletes to return

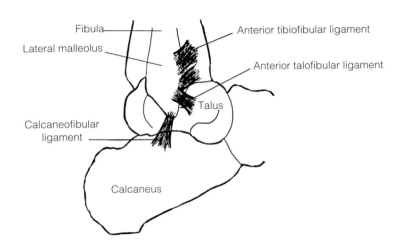

Figure 9–2. Lateral ankle ligaments as viewed from the lateral aspect of the right ankle.

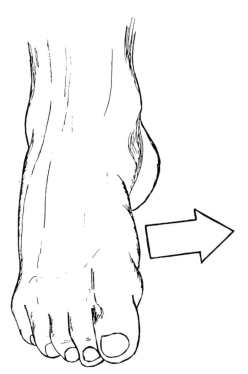

Figure 9–3. The arrow demonstrates the direction of force in an inversion ankle sprain.

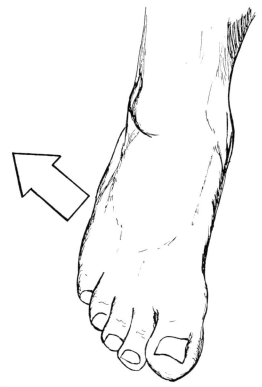

Figure 9–4. The arrow demonstrates the direction of force in an eversion ankle sprain.

to activities safely, they must pass a program of gradually increasing exercise. Walking without a limp is followed by jogging, then running. When running straight ahead without a limp is accomplished, cutting drills and sport-specific drills are implemented. The patients begin with figure of eight running over a 20-yard course, followed by figure of eight drills over an 8- to 10-yard course. When athletes complete these tasks at full speed, they may safely return to their sport. The time frame to return to competition varies. Most athletes with Grade I sprains should be capable of competing at full speed within 1 to 2 weeks. Athletes with Grade III sprains may require 4 to 6 weeks. During the rehabilitation period, the patients require additional support by ankle taping[44] or a brace for routine ambulation.[3,36] Upon returning to full activity, we advise ankle support by taping or a reusable lace-on brace for 6 months in stable ankles and permanently in ankles with residual laxity.

Failure of a patient to return to full activities within the predicted time period according to the severity of the injury should alert the physician to search for other injuries. Appropriate physical examination and radiographs should rule out other injuries (see

Table 9–1). Chronic problems secondary to ankle sprains should then be sought (Table 9–2). Chronic instability due to failure of ligamentous healing may be demonstrated on stress radiographs. A lateral radiograph of the ankle taken while an anterior drawer test is performed will determine anterior tibiotalar subluxation.[14] This is considered posi-

TABLE 9–1.
Injuries Simulating an Ankle Sprain

Avulsion of base of 5th metatarsal[7]
Jones' fracture[23,26]
Fracture of anterior process of calcaneus[18]
Osteochondral lesion of the talus[4,33]
Subluxation of the peroneal tendons[11,35]
Tibiofibular syndesmosis injury[40,43]
Subtalar joint sprain[19,28]
Salter I fractures of the lateral epiphysis
Subluxation of the cuboid[31]
Achilles tendon injuries[20]
Fracture of posterior lip of the distal tibia[17]
Fracture of trigonal process of the talus[17]
Sprain of the lateral tarsometatarsal joints (Lisfranc's)[17]
Fracture of the sustentaculum tali[17]
Sural nerve neuritis[25]
Peroneus brevis tendon lesion[38]

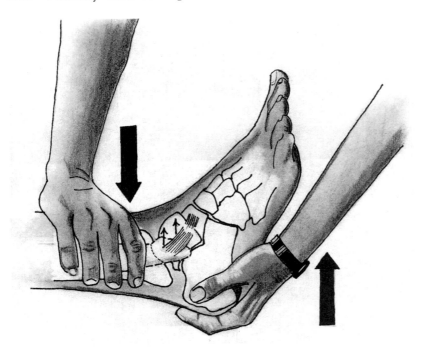

Figure 9–5. Anterior drawer testing of the right ankle, demonstrating anterior talar subluxation on the tibia.

tive if subluxation of more than 6 mm is seen between the posterior lip of the tibia and the articular surface of the talus (Fig. 9–6), or if a difference of more than 3 mm is seen compared with the uninjured ankle.[14] An anteroposterior radiograph taken with maximal inversion of the ankle is referred to as the talar tilt test. This is considered positive if a 10-degree difference of the tibiotalar angle is seen in comparison to the normal contralateral ankle (Fig. 9–7),[37] or if there is a 3-mm or greater separation of the lateral tibiotalar surface compared with the noninjured side.[22] If stress radiographs are positive, the patient may benefit from a ligamentous reconstruction of the lateral ankle.[6,13,42]

Osteochrondral lesions of the talus are another cause for failure of a patient to return to activities after an ankle sprain.[3] Plain radiographs taken at the time of the initial injury may not reveal an abnormality. Repeat radiographs performed when the

TABLE 9–2.
Pathology Associated with Recalcitrant Ankle Sprains

Chronic ligamentous instability[6,13]
Osteochondral lesions of the talus[4,33]
Anteroinferior impingement[2,27]
Reflex sympathetic dystrophy[34]

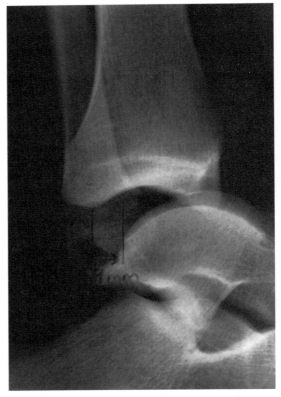

Figure 9–6. Positive anterior drawer test with 9 mm of tibiotalar subluxation.

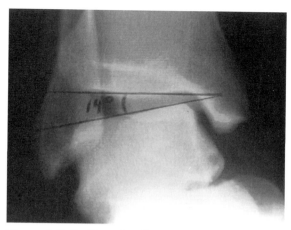

Figure 9–7. Positive talar tilt test with 14° of tibiotalar angulation.

patient has failed to return to activities may show changes in the dome of the talus (Fig. 9–8). For patients with negative results on radiographs and no other source of chronic ankle problems, bone scintigraphy is indicated to rule out osteochondral lesions of the talus.[1] Those who have a positive result on a bone scan should undergo further examination by magnetic resonance imaging (MRI). The reported advantage of MRI is the ability to stage the osteochondral lesion and assist in management decisions.[8] Lesions attached to the talus are capable of healing and may be managed nonoperatively. Partially attached and unattached lesions should be considered for surgical intervention. Arthroscopic management consisting of partial synovectomy, debridement of osteochondral lesions, and removal of loose fragments can yield a high percentage of excellent or good results.[33]

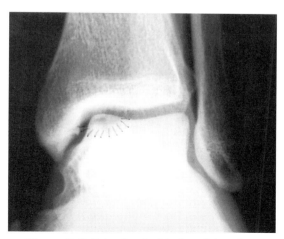

Figure 9–8. Osteochondral lesion of the talus.

Anterolateral ankle pain that prevents return to activity following an inversion ankle sprain may be due to anterior impingement of the talus secondary to a thickened distal fascicle of the anteroinferior tibiofibular ligament.[2] The symptoms may also be due to anterolateral ankle joint fibrosis and synovitis.[9,10,27] Resection of these abnormalities along with débridement of the abraded articular cartilage on the anterolateral aspect of the talus is usually successful in relieving the pain.

Reflex sympathetic dystrophy is a rare complication of ankle sprains. The diagnosis and treatment for this entity require a diligent and patient approach by clinicians specifically trained in this area (see Chapter 24). Factors such as personality traits and workmens' compensation claims have a negative effect on treatment results, whereas children and adolescents respond favorably to treatment directed toward alleviating symptoms.[34,39]

Ankle sprains are a common entity requiring a correct diagnosis and treatment plan. Familiarity with the ankle anatomy and injuries that may simulate an ankle sprain are key to successful management. Aggressive functional rehabilitation is the current standard of care for ankle sprains.

References

1. Anderson IF, Crichton KJ, Grattan-Smith T, et al: Osteochondral fractures of the dome of the talus. J Bone Joint Surg 71A:1143–1152, 1989.
2. Bassett F, Gates H, Billys J: Talar impingement by the anteroinferior tibiofibular ligament. J Bone Joint Surg 72A:55–59, 1990.
3. Bunch RP, Bednarshi K, Holland D, Macinati R: Ankle joint support: A comparison of reusable lace on braces with taping and wrapping. Physicians Sports Med 13:59–62, 1985.
4. Canale ST, Belding RN: Osteochondral lesions of the talus. J Bone Joint Surg 62A:97, 1980.
5. Cass J, Morrey BF, Katoh Y, Chao EYS: Ankle instability: Comparison of primary repair and delayed reconstruction after long-term follow-up study. Clin Orthop September 1985, No. 198 pp 110–117.
6. Chrisman OD, Snook GA: Reconstruction of lateral ligament tears of the ankle. J Bone Joint Surg 51A:904, 1969.
7. Dameron TB: Fractures and anatomical variations of the proximal portion of the fifth metatarsal. J Bone Joint Surg 57A:788–792, 1975.
8. Desmet AA, Fisher DR, Burnstein MI: Value of MR imaging in staging osteochondral lesions of the talus (osteochondritis dissecans): Results in 14 patients. AJR 154:555–558, 1990.
9. Ewing JW: Arthroscopic management of transchondral talar-dome fractures (osteochondritis dissecans) and anterior impingement lesions of the ankle joint. Clin Sports Med 10:677–687, 1991.

10. Ferkel RD, Karzel RP, Del Pizzo W, Friedman MJ, Fischer SP: Arthroscopic treatment of anterolateral impingement of the ankle. Am J Sports Med 19:440–446, 1991.
11. Frey C, Shereff M: Tendon injuries about the ankle in athletes. Clin Sports Med 7:103–118, 1988.
12. Garrick J: The frequency of injury, mechanism of injury and epidemiology of ankle sprains. Am J Sports Med 5:241–242, 1977.
13. Gillespie HS, Borcher P, Watson-Jones J: Repair of lateral instability of the ankle. J Bone Joint Surg 53A:920, 1971.
14. Glasgow M, Jackson A, Jamieson AM: Instability of the ankle after injury of the lateral ligament. J Bone Joint Surg 62B:196, 1980.
15. Grace DL: Lateral ankle ligament injuries: Inversion and anterior stress radiography. Clin Orthop 183:153–159, 1984.
16. Hamilton WG: Surgical anatomy of the foot and ankle. Clin Symposia 37:2–32, 1985.
17. Hamilton WG: Foot and ankle injuries in dancers. Clin Sports Med 7:143–173, 1988.
18. Harburn TE, Ross HE: Avulsion fracture of the anterior calcaneal process. Physicians Sports Med 15:73–80, 1987.
19. Harper MC: The lateral ligamentous support of the subtalar joint. Foot Ankle 11(6):354–358, 1991.
20. Hattrup SJ, Johnson KA: A review of ruptures of the Achilles tendon. Foot Ankle 6(1):34–38, 1985.
21. Hoppenfeld S: Physical Examination of the Spine and Extremities. Norwalk, Connecticut, Appleton-Century-Crofts, 1976, pp 221–222.
22. Johanssen A: Radiological diagnosis of a lateral ligament lesion of the ankle. Acta Orthop Scand 49:295, 1978.
23. Jones R: Fractures of the fifth metatarsal bone. Liverpool Med Surg J 42:103, 1902.
24. Kannus P, Renstrom P: Current Concepts Review. Treatment for acute tears of the lateral ligaments of the ankle. J Bone Joint Surg 73A: 305–312, 1991.
25. Laurin CA, Fleming LL, Hamilton WG, Hansen ST, Johnson KA: Symposium: Ligamentous injuries about the ankle. Contemp Orthop 25(1):81–100, 1992.
26. Lehman R, Torq J, Pavlov H, DeLee J: Fractures of the base of the fifth metatarsal distal to the tuberosity: A review. Foot Ankle 7(4):245–252, 1987.
27. Martin DF, Carl WW, Baker CL: Arthroscopic treatment of chronic synovitis of the ankle. Arthroscopy 5:110–114, 1989.
28. Meyer JM, Garcia J, Hoffmeyer P, et al: The subtalar sprain. A roentgenographic study. Clin Orthop 226:169–173, 1988.
29. Moller-Larsen F, Wetherlund JO, Jurik AG, DeCarvalho A, Lucht U: Comparison of three different treatments for ruptured lateral ankle ligaments. Acta Orthop Scand 59:564–566, 1988.
30. Molnar ME: Rehabilitation of the injured ankle. Clin Sports Med 7:193–204, 1988.
31. Newell S, Woodie A: Cuboid syndrome. Physicians Sports Med 9(4):71–76, 1981.
32. O'Donoghue DH: Treatment of ankle injuries. Northwest Med 57:1277–1286, 1958.
33. Parisien JS: Arthroscopic treatment of osteochondral lesions of the talus. Am J Sports Med 14:211, 1986.
34. Poplawski FJ, Wiley AM, Murray JF: Post-traumatic dystrophy of the extremities. J Bone Joint Surg 65:642, 1983.
35. Rosenburg ZS, Feldman F, Singson RD, et al: Peroneal tendon injury associated with calcaneal fractures: CT findings. AJR 149:125–129, 1987.
36. Rovere GD, Clarke TJ, Yates CS, Burley KP: Retrospective comparison of taping and ankle stabilizers in preventing ankle injuries. Am J Sports Med 16:228–233, 1988.
37. Gustav R, Witten M: The unstable ankle. Bull Hosp Joint Dis 25:179–190, 1964.
38. Sammarco GJ, DiRaimondo CV: Chronic peroneus brevis tendon lesions. Foot Ankle 9:163–170, 1989.
39. Schiller JE: Reflex sympathetic dystrophy of the foot and ankle in children and adolescents. J Am Podiatr Med Assoc 79:545–551, 1989.
40. Sclafani SJA: Ligamentous injury of the lower tibiofibular syndesmosis: Radiographic evidence. Radiology 156:21–27, 1985.
41. Sommer HM, Arza D: Functional treatment of recent ruptures of the fibular ligament of the ankle. Int Orthop 13:157–160, 1989.
42. St. Pierre R, Allman F, Bassett F, Goldner JL, Fleming LL: A review of lateral ankle ligamentous reconstructions. Foot Ankle 3:114–123, 1982.
43. Taylor DC, Englehardt DL, Bassett FH: Syndesmosis sprains of the ankle: The influence of heterotopic ossification. Am J Sports Med 20:146–150, 1992.
44. Wright KE, Whitehall WR: Comprehensive Manual of Taping and Wrapping Techniques. Skillman, New Jersey, Cramer Products, 1991, pp 21–25.

• P A R T II

Ankle Fractures

Jorge E. Alonso

The description of ankle fractures and their subsequent problems dates back to the fifth century B.C. Hippocrates recommended: "Closed fractures should be reduced by traction of the foot, but that open fractures should not be reduced or the patient would die from inflammation and gangrene within 7 days."[9]

An ankle fracture may be isolated or be a part of the multi-injured patient. In trauma cases, the evaluation and assessment of the patient have priority over the ankle injury, but the ankle must not be neglected as these injuries are often a source of permanent impairment.[2-9]

The ankle is a complex joint consisting of functional articulations between the tibia and fibula, tibia and talus, and fibula and talus, each supported by a group of ligaments. The tibia and fibula form a "mortise" providing a constrained articulation for the talus. This ankle joint provides some intrinsic stability, especially in weight-bearing.

The mortise is bordered laterally by the lateral malleolus. The fibula provides this lateral support, and the medial border of the fibula is covered by articular cartilage from the level of the tibial plafond to almost halfway down the remaining length. The medial malleolus is an extension of the distal tibia, and the inner surface is covered with articular cartilage and articulates with the medial facet of the talus. The entire tibial plafond is covered with articular cartilage.

The stability of the ankle joint is due to a combination of the bone architecture, joint capsule, and ligaments. Three distinct groups of ligaments are found in the ankle joint: the syndesmotic, medial collateral, and lateral collateral. These ligaments have been described previously in this chapter.

EVALUATION

Patients often can remember how they injured their ankle, but they may not remember or cannot describe the mechanism by which their injury occurred. The ankle joint can be injured by a fall, by axial loading, or by high-speed deceleration resulting in axial compression of the foot, ankle, and spine. Twisting also usually occurs, causing an external rotation injury.[3,5]

A careful physical examination and history can guide the examiner as to the type of ankle fracture. Injuries to the ankle result in many different combinations of bone and ligamentous injuries. In evaluation of the mechanism of injury, it is seen that the position of the foot influences the location of the initial stage of injury:[5] *supination* of the foot tightens the lateral structures, which are injured first; *pronation* of the foot tightens the medial structures, which then will be injured first. The injury pattern then moves around the ankle in the same direction as the deforming force. Injury to the lateral side (the fibula), can also be graded according to the force applied: *adduction* will result in injury to the

lateral collateral ligament or avulsion of the distal fibula. *Abduction* causes a bending fracture with comminution. *External rotation* produces a spiral fracture. Injury to the syndesmotic ligaments should be suspected when the fibula is fractured at or above the level of the ligaments.

A fractured fibula in the proximal one third can give rise to some ankle instability, even if the medial malleolus is intact (Maisonneuve's fracture).[7,9]

The injury to the medial side results from a direct injury from the talus or from tension as the talus rotates or moves laterally following the fibula. There are several possibilities: tear of the deltoid ligament, avulsion of the distal medial malleolus, fracture above the level of the ligamentous attachment, or fracture at the level of, or above, the tibial plafond.

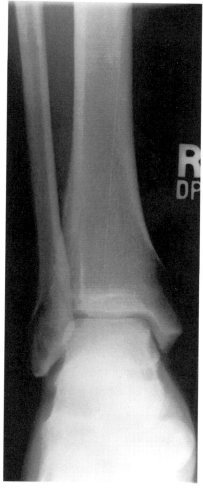

Figure 9–9. Anteroposterior radiograph of the ankle, used to evaluate medial and lateral malleolar fractures.

The tibia also has a posterior malleolus, and fractures of this area are caused by abduction/external rotation, posterior displacement of the talus, vertical loading, or a combination of these forces.[6,9,10]

These mechanisms account for most ankle injuries. It is very difficult to recreate, even in an experimental setting, as many variables are involved: outside forces, rates of loading, different degrees of weight-bearing, and the differences in the quality of bone and soft tissues.

A careful physical examination is important. Attention should be given to the soft tissues and to the neurovascular status of the foot. Without adequate perfusion, the foot will not survive. Therefore, it is crucial to recognize ischemia. Also, evaluation of the nerves is essential. The most disabling nerve injury of the ankle region is loss of the tibial nerve, which provides sensation for the sole. Because of the high risk of neurotrophic ulcers, some investigators have advocated primary amputation when adults sustain this injury along with an otherwise treatable arterial injury.[9]

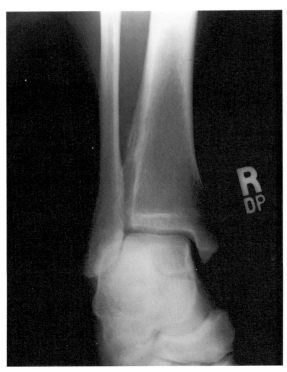

Figure 9–11. "Mortise view" of the ankle. This view is essential in evaluating stability of syndesmosis.

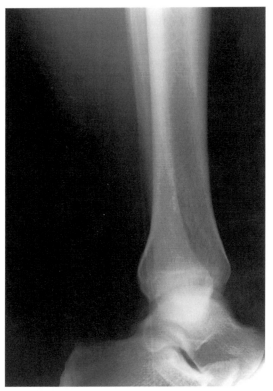

Figure 9–10. Lateral radiograph of the ankle, used to evaluate the posterior malleolus and anterior or posterior subluxation of the talus.

Marked deformity, usually resulting from a fracture dislocation, poses a threat to the local perfusion of the foot and should be aligned before radiographs are obtained. The ankle is then splinted to prevent additional soft tissue damage.

RADIOGRAPHIC IMAGING

Routine studies for the ankle include three views: the anteroposterior (AP) (Fig. 9–9), lateral (Fig. 9–10), and a mortise view (Fig. 9–11). The mortise view is an AP but with the foot internally rotated. Full-length views of the tibia and fibula (including the knee joint) are essential. If there is any suspicion of an additional injury to the foot, it should be x-rayed as well.

With these three views, virtually any type of ankle fracture can be diagnosed. Additional views can be helpful. Standard tomography in AP and lateral projections can aid in evaluating articular surface injuries, fracture comminution, and osteochondral lesions of the talus. Computed tomography (CT) is used to evaluate the fracture pattern when there is plafond involvement. These special tests should be obtained by the orthopaedic surgeon prior to surgery to preplan the surgical approach.[9]

DESCRIBING AN ANKLE FRACTURE

A myriad of classifications describe the fracture pattern by the forces of injury.[2,3,5,6,9] A simple way of looking at an ankle fracture is medial malleolus fracture, lateral malleolus fracture, posterior malleolus fracture, or a combination of these.

Malleolar Fractures
(Fig. 9–12)

This fracture involves the medial or lateral malleolus. On the medial side there may be a deltoid ligament injury, an avulsion fracture, or a fracture of the medial malleolus. On the lateral side there may be a lateral collateral ligament injury, avulsion of the distal fibula, comminution of the fibula, or a spiral fracture of the fibula. Injury to the syndesmotic ligament should be considered when the fibular fracture is at or above the level of the syndesmosis.

Bimalleolar Fractures
(Fig. 9–13)

Bimalleolar fractures are combinations of medial and lateral malleolus fractures.

These fractures can be displaced or undisplaced. They are usually displaced because the ankle joint loses the mortise effect.

Trimalleolar Fractures
(Fig. 9–14)

There is a fracture of the posterior tibial malleolus in addition to the bimalleolar fracture.

SPECIAL FRACTURES

The Maisonneuve fracture results from an external rotation injury. It produces a high fibular fracture with complete disruption of the interosseous membrane and syndesmotic ligaments and a deltoid ligament injury or a fracture of the medial malleolus. This injury should be suspected in a patient with an isolated medial malleolus fracture and pain in the lateral aspect of the leg. Full tibia and fibula radiographs should be obtained.[7]

Pilon fractures are complex intra-articular ankle fractures usually secondary to high-energy trauma (Fig. 9–15). These fractures have a high incidence of resultant disability secondary to post-traumatic arthritis.

Open fractures are also secondary to high-energy injuries and are usually associated with other injuries. Follow the management

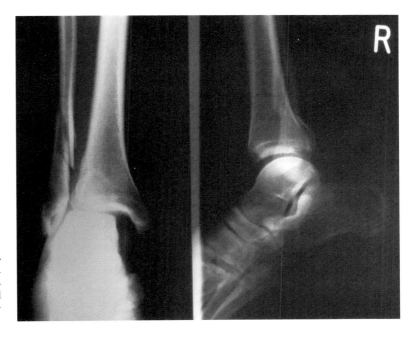

Figure 9–12. Anteroposterior and lateral radiograph of a malleolar fracture. The lateral malleolus is fractured with a deltoid ligament injury (the talus is shifting laterally).

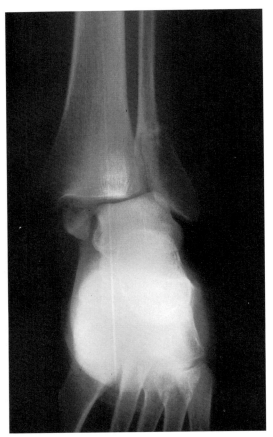

Figure 9–13. Anteroposterior radiograph of a displaced bimalleolar fracture. Fracture of the medial and lateral malleolus displaced the talus laterally.

of open fractures, and keep in mind that these are surgical emergencies.

TREATMENT

The goals of treatment are to obtain an anatomic reduction, maintain the reduction until the fracture heals, and return the patient to his or her preinjury level of function with a painless, mobile ankle.[1–3,8]

The indications for operative treatment have changed over the past 25 years. Closed reduction is indicated for undisplaced or stable fractures. The initial method of immobilization depends upon the amount of swelling and the condition of the soft tissues. A soft, bulky, Jones'-type of dressing with a posterior plaster splint usually provides adequate protection during the first few days after injury. If anatomic restoration has been achieved and operative treatment is not

expected, the extremity is placed in a long cast for 6 weeks, followed by a brace. During this treatment, the patient should be followed weekly to obtain radiographs so that any loss of reduction can be identified. If reduction is lost, then surgical fixation will probably be needed. Fractures not requiring reduction are usually stable and are treated with a walking cast and protected weight-bearing. Weight-bearing is advanced as comfort allows.

Circumferential casts should be applied several days later by the treating physician. The initial examiner should apply a simple bulky wrap and splint until the swelling has minimized.

Operative treatment is recommended for failure of closed reduction, reduction which requires a forced abnormal position, displaced or unstable fractures, and open fractures (Fig. 9–16). The current trend is to recommend open reduction and internal fix-

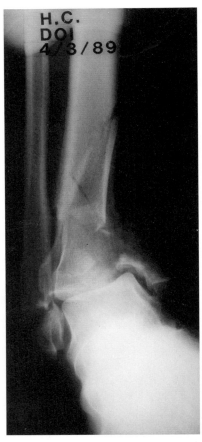

Figure 9–14. Anteroposterior radiograph of a displaced trimalleolar fracture of high energy with comminution of the metaphyseal area.

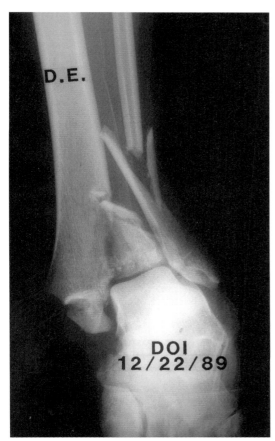

Figure 9–15. Anteroposterior radiograph of a "pilon" fracture. Not only has the medial and lateral malleolus fractured, but also the fracture line extends into the ankle joint.

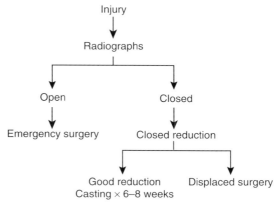

Figure 9–16. Management of ankle fractures.

ation for any displaced fractures that involve the articular surface within a week. The ideal time for operative intervention is immediately for open fractures and within days for closed fractures. The goals of operative treatment are to obtain a stable, anatomic reduction resulting in a healed fracture and return to normal function.

ANKLE FRACTURES IN CHILDREN

Ankle fractures in children are frequently caused by an indirect mechanism. Following careful examination of the injured ankle and detailed x-ray study, comparison radiographs should be obtained from the opposite ankle if there are any questions.

Closed reduction and casting is the treatment of choice; however, all Salter-Harris

Type III and IV fractures should be treated by open reduction and internal fixation in order to achieve a perfect reduction and decrease the incidence of physeal arrest.[9]

If the fracture is treated by closed methods, a long leg cast is applied and then changed at 3 weeks to a short leg cast until the fracture is healed. This usually requires another 3 weeks.[3]

References

1. Baur M, Bergstrom B, Hemborg J, Sandergard J: Malleolar fractures: Nonoperative versus operative treatment: A controlled study. Clin Orthop 199: 17–27, 1985.
2. Chapman MW: Fractures and Fracture-dislocations of the ankle. *In* Mann RA: Surgery of the Foot, 5th ed. St. Louis, CV Mosby, 1986.
3. Heim JL, Pfeiffer KM: Small Fragment Set Manual; Technique Recommended by the ASIF Group, 2nd ed. New York, Springer-Verlag, 1981.
4. Hughes JL, Weber H, Willenegger H, Kunner EH: Evaluation of ankle fractures. Non-operative and operative treatment. Clin Orthop 138:111–119, 1979.
5. Lauge-Hansen N: Fractures of the ankle. Analytic historic survey as basis of new experimental roentgenologic and clinical investigation. Arch Surg 60:957–985, 1950.
6. Mast JW, Spiegel PG: Complex ankle fractures. *In* Meyers MH (ed): The Multiple Injured Patient with Complex Fractures. Philadelphia, Lea and Febiger, 1984.
7. Pankovich AM: Maisonneuve fractures of the fibula. J Bone Joint Surg 58A:337–342, 1976.
8. Roberts RS: Surgical treatment of displaced ankle fractures. Clin Orthop 172:164–170, 1983.
9. Trafton PG, Bray TJ, Simpson LA: Fractures and soft tissue injuries of the ankle. *In* Browner BD, Jupiter J, Trafton PG, Levine J (eds): Skeletal Trauma. Philadelphia, JB Lippincott, 1991.
10. Yablon IG, Segal D, Leach RE: Ankle Injuries. New York, Churchill-Livingstone, 1983.

Fractures and Dislocations of the Foot

Victoria R. Masear

The foot is very susceptible to injury by virtue of being our contact point with the ground and of protruding forward from the body. Most commonly, it is injured from falls or jumps from heights, running or twisting injuries, automobile accidents, lawn mower injuries, and objects being dropped onto it. Since people do not have an efficient means of locomotion without the use of a foot, injuries to this area can be quite disruptive to one's lifestyle and livelihood.

The foot is composed of three units, all of which serve a separate function: the hindfoot, midfoot, and forefoot. The hindfoot consists of the calcaneus in the heel and the talus, which is the major articulation with the tibia. The midfoot consists of the navicular bone and just distal to that the three cuneiforms, and to the lateral side of the navicular and cuneiforms, the cuboid bone. The forefoot consists of five metatarsals and the phalanges of the toes. The great toe has two phalanges and the lesser toes normally have three phalanges. Frequently, the little toe has only two phalanges (Fig. 10–1). The hindfoot and forefoot provide the major weight-bearing areas, with about 50 percent of the weight distributed to each. Of that portion of the weight borne on the forefoot, the great meta-tarsal is responsible for twice as much support as each of the other four metatarsals. The midfoot area forms the arch. There are strong interligamentous and tendinous supports to this area to help maintain the arch. The midfoot is also responsible for the mobility between the forefoot and hindfoot. The multiple joints in the foot serve as shock absorption, as the forces that are placed upon the foot are several times that of body weight.

CALCANEUS FRACTURES

The primary mechanism of injury in fracture of the calcaneus is a fall or jump from a height, or an automobile accident. Ten to fifteen percent of calcaneus fractures have an associated vertebral body compression fracture. Therefore, an examination for tenderness in the spine is of utmost importance.

The patient will present with a large amount of swelling and tenderness over the heel. There will be pain with any motion of the subtalar joint into varus or valgus. Ecchymosis and blistering of the skin may develop early. The essential x-ray views include an AP and lateral and a Harris axial heel view (Fig. 10–2). The normal Böh-

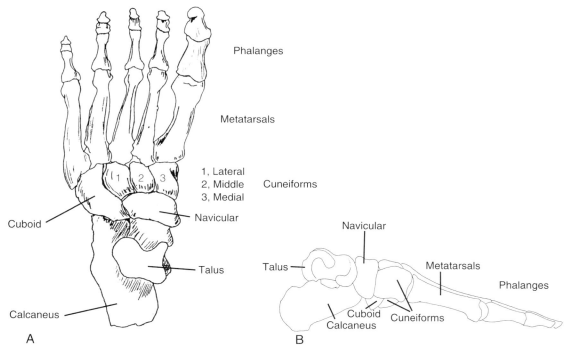

Figure 10–1. *A,* Anteroposterior view of the foot. *B,* Lateral view of the foot.

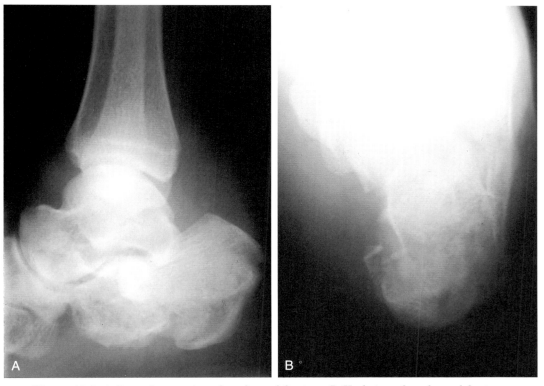

Figure 10–2. *A,* Lateral x-ray view of a calcaneal fracture. *B,* Heel view of a calcaneal fracture.

ler's angle is 20 to 40 degrees. With an intra-articular fracture, the posterior facet of the calcaneus is collapsed, and the angle will be decreased toward 0 degrees (Fig. 10–3). A CT scan in the coronal and transverse planes may be necessary to delineate the fracture further and to see the extent of intra-articular involvement.

The main determining factor in outcome is the extent of initial fracture displacement, which is intra-articular into the subtalar joint. Simple, nondisplaced fractures usually will have a good outcome, whereas very comminuted fractures often will have a poor result no matter what type of treatment is rendered.[51,54] If the fracture is extra-articular, the treatment of choice is a bulky dressing and posterior short leg splint. Early motion is begun within a few days to a couple of weeks, depending upon pain tolerance. The patient must remain nonweight-bearing for 10 to 12 weeks until there is radiologic evidence of bone union. If there is a significant displacement of the fracture, then an open reduction and internal fixation are indicated.

Most calcaneus fractures are intra-articular into the subtalar joint. Most of the best results have been obtained with anatomic reduction and fixation.[7,49,56,60] Non-operative treatment can be used, as in extra-articular fractures, for intra-articular fractures with minimal displacement, medi-

cal conditions that preclude surgery, soft tissue compromise such as severe blistering, and peripheral vascular disease. The complications of closed reduction include lateral impingement of either the fibula or peroneal tendons, flatfoot, difficulty in shoe wear, and chronic pain secondary to post-traumatic arthritis of the subtalar joint.[31,44,53,56] As with any other area of injury, open fractures should be taken to the operating room for surgical débridement. Primary arthrodesis of the subtalar joint is reserved for those fractures with severe intra-articular comminution.[24]

FRACTURES OF THE TALUS

Talar fractures usually result from a severe dorsiflexion injury, as with the floorboard in an automobile accident. Fractures of the talar neck are the most common (Fig. 10–4). There will be tenderness and swelling about the region of the talus just distal to the ankle joint. Radiographs should be obtained in the AP, lateral, and oblique projections.

The body of the talus is that portion articulating with the tibia. Just distal to this is the neck of the talus. Distally the talar head articulates with the navicular. An undisplaced talar neck fracture can be treated with a short leg cast for 6 to 8 weeks. When there is

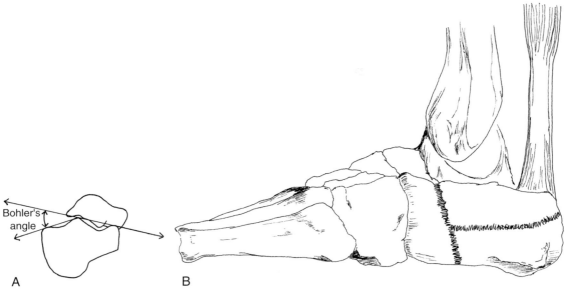

Figure 10–3. *A,* Böhler's angle measured on a lateral radiograph. The normal angle is 20 to 40 degrees. *B,* Artist's depiction of a calcaneal fracture with a depressed Böhler's angle.

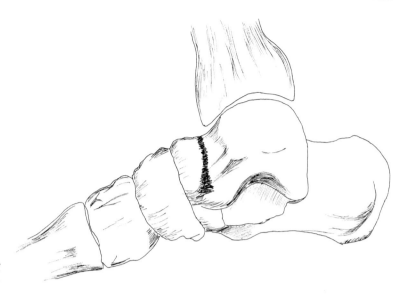

Figure 10–4. Artist's depiction of a nondisplaced talar neck fracture.

radiologic evidence of union, weight-bearing can be instituted.

Any intra-articular fracture, whether into the subtalar joint or ankle joint, requires an anatomic reduction to decrease the incidence of post-traumatic arthritis. This usually will necessitate an open reduction and internal fixation. The incidence of post-traumatic arthritis with intra-articular fractures of the talus is 30 percent.[40] Subsequently, this may necessitate an arthrodesis of the involved joint.[2]

The blood supply to the body of the talus enters from the distal aspect of the talus. Therefore, a displaced fracture of the talar neck associated with dislocation of the body (Fig. 10–5) has an increased risk for the development of avascular necrosis (AVN) of the talar body. This may be as high as 75 to 100 percent.[33] Early reduction of the displaced or dislocated fragment is imperative to prevent skin necrosis. Open reduction and internal fixation are usually required to give stability and to maintain the reduction.[36,55]

With the development of avascular necrosis, there will be an increased radiodensity in the talar dome just below the ankle joint. Hawkins' sign[27] is a subchondral radiolucency of the talar dome that occurs by 6 weeks following fracture. This is secondary to osteopenia from being immobilized in a cast, and it indicates that the blood supply to the talus is intact. If Hawkins' sign does not appear, then AVN of the talus is suspected. With AVN, protection for 12 to 18 months is recommended in a short leg cast

or patella-bearing brace. It may take up to 36 months for revascularization of the talus to occur.[36]

Some displaced fractures of the talus can be reduced with plantar flexion and pushing the foot backward. The foot is then casted in plantar flexion to maintain the reduction for 4 weeks. The ankle is then brought to neutral in the cast until the fracture is healed. Similarly, a dislocation of the talus usually can be reduced with traction on the forefoot and pressure applied directly to the talus with the examiner's thumbs.[36] Talar dislocations are treated in a long leg nonweight-bearing cast for 4 weeks, followed by a short leg cast with progressive weight-bearing for the next month.

SUBTALAR DISLOCATIONS

In subtalar dislocations, the tibiotalar relationship is maintained, but the talonavicular joint is dislocated. Most commonly this is a medial dislocation of the navicular on the talus.[3,10,14,23,61] Often there are associated fractures, and there is a marked deformity secondary to the severe inversion force to the foot. These should be reduced as soon as possible under spinal or general anesthesia. Countertraction is placed on the thigh by an assistant while the physician places traction on the foot with a slight accentuation of the deformity. Then after traction is applied, the foot is pronated, abducted, and dorsiflexed. If the dislocation is not reduced with this

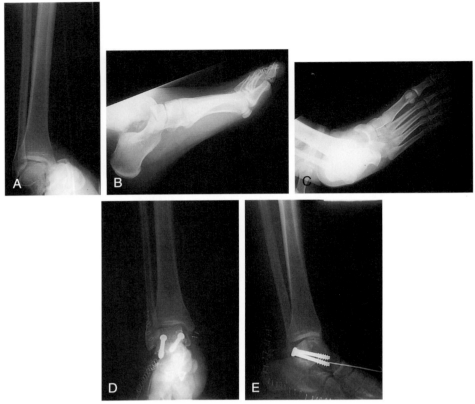

Figure 10–5. *A, B,* and *C,* X-ray views of talus fracture-dislocation. *D* and *E,* Status post-ORIF (open reduction, internal fixation).

maneuver, the patient needs to be transferred immediately to the operating room for an open reduction.[10,39]

Thirty percent of subtalar dislocations are everted at the time of injury, and a lateral dislocation of the navicular bone on the talus occurs. The reduction maneuver is opposite to that for a medial dislocation. The eversion deformity is accentuated and traction placed. The foot is then supinated, adducted, and plantar flexed. Posterior and anterior dislocations are rarer. They also should be reduced closed if possible, but if this is not possible, open.[23,45]

After reduction, the patient is placed in a nonweight-bearing bulky wrap and posterior splint for 3 weeks. Motion is begun at 3 weeks with progressive weight-bearing as tolerated.

Any delay in reduction can lead to severe swelling and skin blisters and possibly can compromise the circulation to the skin or neurovascular structures of the foot.[28] The risk of stiffness in the subtalar joint following subtalar dislocations is increased with an associated open injury, a delay in reduction, associated fractures, and soft tissue destruction.[17,37,58] Post-traumatic arthritis and limited subtalar motion may also occur. Any persistence of subtalar pain or swelling after several months of anti-inflammatory agents and physical therapy for strengthening is an indication for either subtalar or triple arthrodesis.[3]

MIDTARSAL INJURIES

These rare injuries occur at the talonavicular and calcaneocuboid joints. Fractures, fracture subluxations, or fracture-dislocations may be associated with injury in this area. The dislocation may be in any direction.[41] The navicular bone itself may dislocate, with the remainder of the joint articulations being in normal position.[20] Anteroposterior, lateral, and oblique radiographs are needed for a diagnosis. The reduction must be perfect since this is a potentially disabling injury. If the joint is not congruously reduced by closed reduction, then an open reduction and possibly internal fixation are needed. If the joint can be reduced closed, then the preferred treatment is a short leg cast with 6 weeks of nonweight-bearing followed by 2 weeks in a weight-bearing cast.

TARSOMETATARSAL FRACTURE-DISLOCATIONS

Fracture-dislocations through the tarso-metatarsal joints have been named after the French surgeon Lisfranc, who in the Napoleonic era was known for how quickly he could amputate feet through these joints. These injuries usually result from high-energy trauma. Initially they were described in calvary troops with equestrian injuries, but today they occur most frequently in motor vehicle accidents. Early diagnosis and treatment are essential as there is considerable associated morbidity.[26,38,48]

The mechanism of injury is secondary either to direct trauma to the metatarsal or a longitudinal force along the metatarsal ray. The second metatarsal is the primary stabilizer of the tarsometatarsal joint as it is recessed into a rigid mortis between the first and third metatarsals and cuneiforms. The strongest ligament maintaining this relationship is the oblique ligament between the medial cuneiform and second metatarsal base. This bone/ligamentous unit is disrupted in a Lisfranc dislocation. There may be associated cuneiform or cuboid fractures as well as metatarsal fractures. The subluxation may be in any direction.

Radiographs include AP, lateral, and oblique views. The most reliable sign is widening between the first and second metatarsal bases or at times between the second and third metatarsal bases, best seen on the oblique radiograph (Fig. 10–6). There may also be a small fracture on the base of the second metatarsal.

These dislocations are notorious for inadequate treatment as the diagnosis is often missed.[32,38,48] Treatment requires a stable anatomic reduction. Most of these will require open reduction and internal fixation, but a few may be treated with closed reduction and internal fixation with percutaneous pins.

METATARSAL FRACTURES

Most metatarsal fractures are secondary to crush injuries from a blow to the dorsum of the foot. One must keep in mind with this mechanism of injury that the degree of soft tissue damage is equal to that damage sustained by the bone. Direct blows will usually fracture the second through fourth metatarsal shafts or necks. Usually they will be comminuted secondary to the force of injury. Twisting injuries are more likely to cause a fracture of the fifth metatarsal shaft or base.[21]

With crush injuries, both skin necrosis and compartment syndromes of the intrinsic muscles of the foot are common complications. Initially the patient is placed in a bulky dressing and posterior plaster splint above the ankle for pain relief. The foot is elevated for several days and closely watched for any skin necrosis or compartment syndrome.

With minimally displaced fractures of the second through fourth metatarsals, a walking cast or rigid postoperative shoe is normally all the treatment that is needed. With a minimally displaced fracture of the first metatarsal, a short leg cast is indicated. Weight-bearing is begun after 2 weeks.[16,21]

Fractures that are shortened or seem to be displaced on the lateral radiograph will need fixation to maintain the proper weight-bearing distribution across the metatarsal heads (Fig. 10–7). Displacement on the AP x-ray film is not as critical, since the weight-bearing distribution across the metatarsal heads may still be maintained.[47] Healing in an abnormal position of shortening or angulation may cause either too much or too little weight-bearing on that metatarsal head. Too much weight will cause a callus to form over the metatarsal head and pain in that area. A metatarsal fracture either shortened significantly or angulated so that weight-bearing is not as prominent on that head will usually cause a transfer lesion. The weight from that metatarsal is then shifted to the adjacent metatarsal (transfer), where again a painful callus will develop.

The fifth metatarsal is unique in that healing of a fracture at the base of this metatarsal is difficult, and stress fractures often develop. Fractures of the neck or the mid-diaphyseal region of the fifth metatarsal are treated like other metatarsal fractures. Fractures of the metatarsal base often need additional consideration. A fracture that is

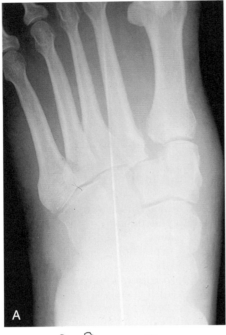

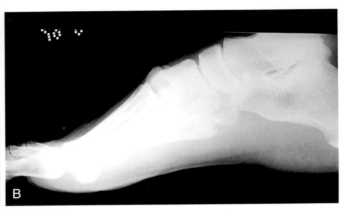

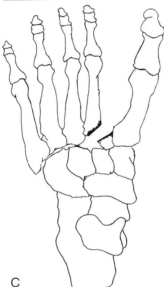

C

Figure 10–6. *A,* AP radiograph showing a widened space between the first and second metatarsal base. *B,* Lateral radiograph showing dorsal displacement of the second metatarsal base. *C,* Base of the second metatarsal fracture with lateral subluxation of the second through fourth metatarsals.

transverse through the proximal diaphysis (Jones' fracture) is notorious for reinjury, delayed union, and nonunion.[18,34,35,62] The Jones' fracture usually occurs when the fourth and fifth metatarsal heads are on the ground and the heel is elevated, frequently seen in basketball injuries.[34,35] These transverse, proximal diaphyseal fractures (Fig. 10–8) should be treated acutely with 6 weeks in a nonweight-bearing short leg cast. If they are not clinically and radiographically

healed by 6 weeks, a more aggressive surgical treatment with bone grafting or internal fixation or both is often recommended. The rate of delayed union increases when weight-bearing is allowed early.[62] The overall rate of delayed union and nonunion is 38 and 14 percent, respectively.[1,21]

Even in acute fractures, internal fixation is often indicated for competitive athletes.[18,35] The goal is to return them to competition at an earlier date. Following internal fixation,

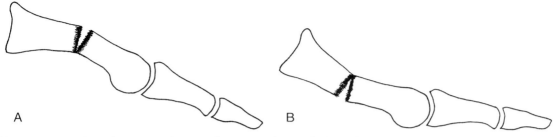

A   B

Figure 10–7. *A,* Dorsal apex angulation will increase the weight borne by this metatarsal, resulting in a painful plantar callus. *B,* Plantar apex angulation will decrease the amount of weight on this metatarsal head. The result will be a shift of the weight to the neighboring metatarsal head (transfer lesion).

they will remain nonweight-bearing for 2 weeks. They then begin progressive weight-bearing and light jogging by 6 weeks.[47,50] There is a 95 percent healing rate by 12 weeks if bone grafting is included.[62]

If there is any hint of prodromal symptoms or x-ray evidence of chronicity, then an open reduction and internal fixation with bone graft are probably indicated.[15,47] As many as 40 percent of Jones' fractures are probably actually a stress fracture.[35] The patients will have a history of several weeks of an aching pain in that area. An acute onset of increased pain occurs with an injury. Radiographs will show a wide fracture line with a periosteal reaction, including thickening of the lateral cortex and intramedullary sclerosis (Fig. 10–9).[18,47] When x-ray evidence shows chronicity, there is almost a 100 percent rate of nonunion in athletes not undergoing surgery.[35]

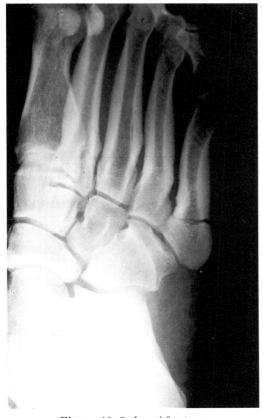

Figure 10–8. Jones' fracture.

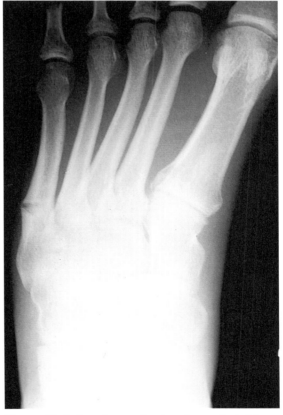

Figure 10–9. Jones' stress fracture demonstrated by a thickened lateral cortex.

Jones' fractures should not be confused with an avulsion fracture of the tuberosity. The tuberosity fractures are more proximal and may be intra-articular into the tarso-metatarsal joint (Fig. 10–10). They require symptomatic treatment only, as they do not carry the same risk of morbidity as the Jones' fracture. The tuberosity fracture is usually the result of an indirect force leading to avulsion by the peroneus brevis tendon as the peroneus brevis contracts on a plantar-flexed and inverted foot.[12,15,35] The tuberosity fractures usually require only a short leg walking cast, rigid-soled postoperative shoe, or Elastoplast dressing. Activities are increased as symptoms allow.[12,50] Most will heal without any residual dysfunction. If the tuberosity fracture is intra-articular and displaced, then internal fixation may be indicated.

METATARSAL STRESS FRACTURES

Stress fractures result from cumulative repetitive forces, usually secondary to either an increase in the amount of or change in the type of activity. Approximately 20 percent of stress fractures occur in the metatarsals, with most of these being the second or third metatarsals.[4,18,43]

Pain usually begins diffusely and is present only after training, exercise, or activity. Eventually the pain becomes more consistent and localized to one metatarsal where local tenderness is felt. Radiographs should be taken in the AP and lateral plane but often the x-ray pictures will remain negative for up to 2 months before the fracture line becomes radiographically visible. Eventually the radiograph will show a fracture line with surrounding fusiform proliferative callus (Fig. 10–11). A ^{99m}Tc bone scan is more sensitive than an x-ray film, and the findings will be positive for increased uptake as soon as symptoms occur. If it is imperative to make the diagnosis early, then a bone scan is indicated; treatment is directed toward a stress fracture if there is increased uptake in one of the metatarsals. A negative bone scan rules out a stress fracture.

When a stress fracture is either diagnosed or suspected, activities are first restricted. For early, nondisplaced stress fractures or those not showing by x-ray, exercise or training is restricted for 4 weeks. Running in a pool is begun for aerobic conditioning. If the stress fracture is displaced, then internal fixation should be considered. If the stress fracture does not heal with restriction of activities, then either a wooden shoe or a weight-bearing short leg cast is applied.

As discussed previously, fifth metatarsal fractures are notorious for nonunion or delayed union. They should be immobilized in a short leg nonweight-bearing cast or undergo internal fixation to decrease healing time.[18] Either weight-bearing casts or other nonsurgical methods of treatment for fifth metatarsal stress fractures give an increased incidence of nonunion or refracture.

SESAMOID INJURY

The sesamoids of the great toe bear the weight of the metatarsal head and therefore

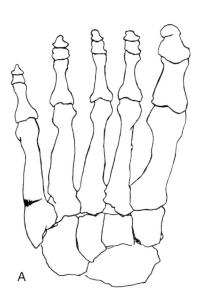
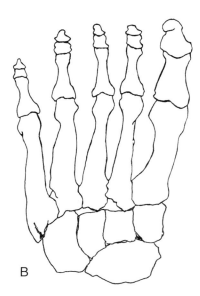

A   B

Figure 10–10. *A,* Typical location of Jones' fracture. *B,* Fracture of the fifth metatarsal tuberosity.

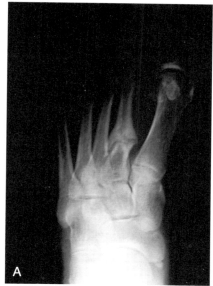
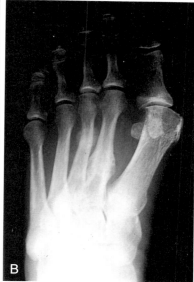

Figure 10–11. *A,* Stress fracture of the second metatarsal. *B,* Healed fracture of the second metatarsal, now with a third metatarsal stress fracture.

are subject to injury or overuse. Sesamoiditis and stress fractures are common in runners, other athletes, and aerobic dancers. Fractures may also occur from a fall.[25,57] The tibial (medial) sesamoid is the weight-bearing sesamoid and is more likely to be injured (Fig. 10–12).[9,11,29]

Patients with injury of the sesamoid will present with tenderness directly over the sesamoid, pain with push-off or rising on the tiptoes, and pain with dorsiflexion of the toes. Ten percent of sesamoids are bipartite and should not be confused with fractures.[11,29,52] The fractured sesamoid usually has irregular edges and is a normal size. The bipartite sesamoid has smooth edges, and two parts are larger than the other sesamoid and would not fit nicely into an oval or circle.

As with stress fractures elsewhere, stress fractures of the sesamoid may not show up initially on the routine radiographs, which may need to be repeated in several weeks.[63] Bone scanning is not specific for stress fracture of the sesamoid, as the bone scan will show an increased uptake with sesamoiditis as well (Fig. 10–13).

The treatment for sesamoiditis or sesamoid stress fracture is rest with protected weight-bearing by either an offloading shoe insert or, if the patient is severely symptomatic, a short leg walking cast. When comfortable, the patient progresses to a running shoe with a sesamoid pad to offload the weight from the involved sesamoid. This is worn for at least 3 months.[9,52] Stress fractures of the

sesamoid usually do not heal and may require either bone graft for the nonunion or excision of the sesamoid for pain relief. Excision of the sesamoid should be done only if the pain has been present for greater than 6 months.[63] With sesamoid excision, the weight-bearing is shifted to the condyles of the great metatarsal head and often symptoms persist.

METATARSOPHALANGEAL JOINT INJURIES

The metatarsophalangeal (MP) joints may be either sprained or dislocated. Turf toe is secondary to a forced hyperextension of the great toe as seen in football players on artificial turf.[5,6,13] These are usually the result of a flexible shoe on a relatively hard playing surface. Hyperflexion injuries of the great toe occur in ballet dancers with either an associated valgus or varus sprain.[57]

Treatment for sprains or strains of the great toe includes ice, elevation, and compression dressings. If symptoms are severe, immobilization in a cast or postoperative rigid-soled shoe or crutches for nonweight-bearing will assist in pain relief and rehabilitation. The pain may persist for several months. When the athlete is ready to resume competition, a stiff-soled shoe or orthosis to limit dorsiflexion and taping of the toe are beneficial.[13] Some complete tears of the joint capsule or volar plate may require surgical

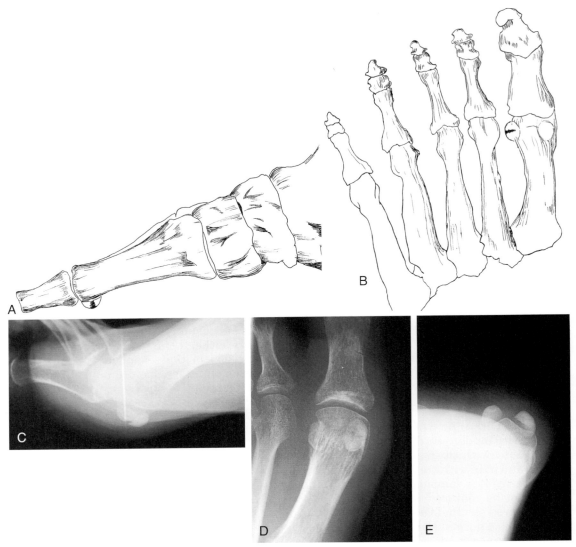

Figure 10–12. *A,* Lateral view of a sesamoid fracture. *B,* AP view of a sesamoid fracture. *C,* Lateral radiograph of a medial sesamoid fracture. *D,* AP x-ray of medial sesamoid fracture. *E,* Sesamoid view of a medial sesamoid fracture.

repair because of persistent discomfort and occasional instability of the joint.

Metatarsophalangeal dislocations are rare. Usually the proximal phalanx dislocates dorsal to the metatarsal head (Fig. 10–14). The most commonly dislocated MP joint is the great toe, but a dislocation may occur in other toes as well.[8,19,30]

The great toe may dislocate with the sesamoids. These are usually irreducible by closed means because the plantar plate becomes interposed between the metatarsal head and the proximal phalanx. This will require open reduction.[19,22,46] The sesamoids may fracture transversely or may separate.

When this occurs, the reduction is usually possible by closed means. Normally the difference can be seen on the x-ray film by localizing not only the dislocated joint but the position of the sesamoid in relation to the great metatarsal head.

The dislocation should be reduced early with distal traction while accentuating the deformity and then pushing the proximal phalanx over the metatarsal head. After reduction, an x-ray view is made to confirm a normal joint space and alignment. After reduction of the dislocation, the range of motion is also always checked to be sure that the joint is actually reduced. If the joint is

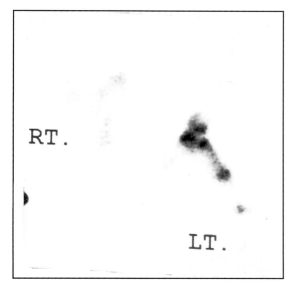

Figure 10–13. Although the bone scan will show increased uptake over the area of a sesamoid fracture, it is not specific for fracture.

not congruously reduced, then motion will be limited. Following the reduction, a short leg cast or rigid postoperative shoe is applied with weight-bearing as tolerated. Dislocations of the lesser toes are rarer and usually

are irreducible by closed means.[19,46] However, once reduced, they are usually stable and the only follow-up treatment is with buddy taping. One may also see a chronic dislocation with claw toes in some of the lesser toes. These will not be reducible by closed means and should be treated symptomatically with a deeper toe box in the shoe or surgically reduced if indicated by symptoms.

INJURIES TO THE TOES

Toes are frequently fractured but rarely require surgical treatment. The fracture is usually from a stubbed toe or an object dropped on the foot. Often the nail matrix will be damaged, and a subungual hematoma will develop. Pain can be relieved in these by piercing the nail with a cautery or a sharp, heated wire. This allows evacuation of the subungual hematoma and reduction in pressure and pain. If the nail matrix is lacerated, as occurs when the nail plate is torn loose or is cut, then a nail bed repair should be performed as is described in the hand in Chapter 15.

Toes with undisplaced or minimally displaced fractures are taped to the adjacent

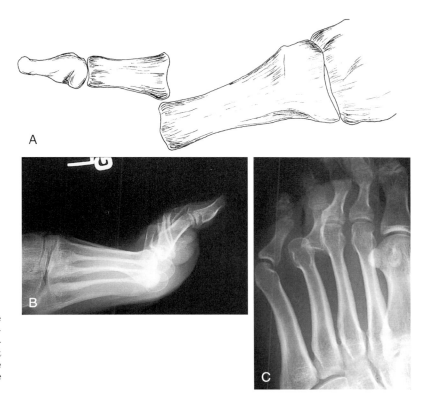

Figure 10–14. *A,* A great toe metatarsophalangeal (MP) dorsal dislocation. *B,* Dorsal dislocation of the fourth MP joint secondary to clawing. *C,* Oblique radiograph showing a fourth toe MP dislocation.

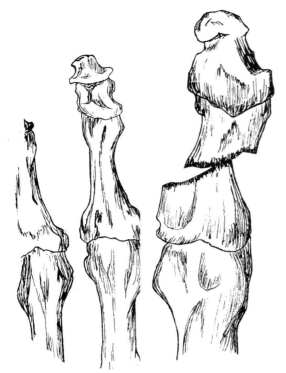

Figure 10–15. Displaced fracture of great toe proximal phalanx that would require reduction or fixation.

toe, and a firm shoe is worn for comfort. Displaced fractures are treated with either closed reduction and taping or percutaneous pinning (Fig. 10–15).

A displaced intra-articular fracture usually will require an open reduction and internal fixation for the great toe but probably can be treated by closed means and taping for the lesser toes. If the toe is angulated away from or overlaps its adjacent toes, this will usually require closed reduction and pinning or open reduction.

Interphalangeal dislocations also can occur in the toes. They are usually reduced with longitudinal traction and are then symptomatically treated with taping to adjacent toes and a rigid shoe.

References

1. Arangio GA: Proximal diaphyseal fractures of the fifth metatarsal (Jones's fracture): Two cases treated by cross-pinning with review of 106 cases. Foot Ankle 3:293, 1983.
2. Baker LD, Miller OL: Fracture and fracture dislocation of the astragalus. South Med J 32:125, 1939.
3. Barber JR, Brucker JD, Haliburton RA: Peritalar dislocation of the foot. Can J Surg 4:205, 1961.
4. Bernstein A, Childers MA, Fox KW: March fractures of the foot: Care and management of 692 patients. Am J Surg 71:355, 1946.
5. Bowers KD, Martin RB: Impact absorption: New and old Astroturf at West Virginia University. Med Sci Sports 6:217, 1974.
6. Bowers KD, Martin RB: Turf-toe: A shoe surface related to football injury. Med Sci Sports 8:81, 1976.
7. Braly WG, Bishop JO, Tullos HS: Lateral decompression for malunited os calcis fractures. Foot Ankle 6:90–96, 1985.
8. Brown TI: Avulsion fracture of the fibular sesamoid in association with dorsal dislocation of the metatarsophalangeal joint of the hallux: Report of a case and review of the literature. Clin Orthop 149:229, 1980.
9. Brugman JC: Fractured sesamoids as a source of pain around the bunion joint. Milit Surg 49:310, 1921.
10. Buckingham WW Jr: Subtalar dislocation of the foot. J Trauma 13:753, 1973.
11. Burman MS, Lapidus PW: The functional disturbance caused by the inconstant bones and sesamoids of the foot. Arch Surg 22:936, 1931.
12. Christopher F: Fractures of the fifth metatarsal. Surg Gynecol Obstet 37:190, 1923.
13. Coker TP, Arnold JA, Weber DL: Traumatic lesions of the metatarsophalangeal joint of the great toe in athletes. Am J Sports Med 6:326, 1978.
14. Coltart WC: Aviator's astragalus. J Bone Joint Surg 34B:535, 1952.
15. Dameron TB Jr: Fractures and anatomical variations of the proximal portion of the fifth metatarsal. J Bone Joint Surg 57A:788, 1975.
16. DeLee JC: Fractures and dislocations of the foot. *In* Mann RA, Couglin MJ (eds): *Surgery of the Foot and Ankle,* 6th ed. St. Louis, CV Mosby, 1993, pp 1465–1703.
17. DeLee JC, Curtis R: Subtalar dislocation of the foot. J Bone Joint Surg 64A:433–437, 1982.
18. DeLee JC, Evans JP, Julian J: Stress fractures of the fifth metatarsal. Am J Sports Med 11:349, 1983.
19. DeLuca FN, Kenmore PI: Bilateral dorsal dislocations of the metatarsophalangeal joints of the great toes with a loose body in one of the metatarsophalangeal joints. J Trauma 15:737, 1975.
20. Eichenholtz SN, Levine DB: Fractures of the tarsal navicular bone. Clin Orthop 34:142–157, 1964.
21. Giannestras NJ, Sammarco GJ: Fractures and dislocations in the foot. *In* Rockwood CA, Green DP (eds): *Fractures.* Philadelphia, JB Lippincott, 1975.
22. Giannikas AC, Papachristou G, Papavisilion N, et al: Dorsal dislocation of the first metatarsophalangeal joint. Report of four cases. J Bone Joint Surg 57B:384, 1975.
23. Granthan SA: Medial subtalar dislocations: Five cases with a common etiology. J Trauma 4:845, 1964.
24. Hall MC, Pennal GF: Primary subtalar arthrodesis in the treatment of severe fractures of the calcaneum. J Bone Joint Surg 42B:336–343, 1960.
25. Hamilton WG: Injuries in ballet dancers. Sports Med Dig 8:1, 1986.
26. Hardcastle PH, Reschauer R, Kutscha-Lissberg E, et al: Injuries to the tarsometatarsal joint. Incidence, classification and treatment. J Bone Joint Surg 64B:349, 1982.
27. Hawkins LG: Fractures of the lateral process of the talus. J Bone Joint Surg 47A:1170, 1965.

28. Horer DI, Fishman J: The early treatment of peritalar dislocation. Int Orthop 7:263–266, 1984.
29. Inge GL, Ferguson AB: Surgery of the sesamoid bones of the great toe. Arch Surg 21:456, 1933.
30. Jahss MH: Traumatic dislocations of the first metatarsophalangeal joint. Foot Ankle 1:15, 1980.
31. James ETR, Hunter GA: The dilemma of painful old os calcis fractures. Clin Orthop 177:112–115, 1983.
32. Jeffries TE: Lisfranc's fracture-dislocation. J Bone Joint Surg 45B:546, 1963.
33. Jergeson F: Open reduction of fractures and dislocations of the ankle. Am J Surg 98:136–150, 1959.
34. Jones R: Fracture of the base of the fifth metatarsal by indirect violence. Ann Surg 35:697, 1902.
35. Kavanaugh JH, Brower TD, Mann RV: The Jones' fracture revisited. J Bone Joint Surg 60A;776, 1978.
36. King RE, Powell DR: Injury to the talus. *In* Jahss MH (ed): *Disorders of the Foot and Ankle; Medical and Surgical Management,* 2nd ed. Philadelphia, WB Saunders, 1991, pp 2293–2325.
37. Lancaster S, Horowitz M, Alonso J: Subtalar dislocations: A prognostic classification. Orthopaedics 8/10:1234–1240, 1985.
38. LaTourlette G, Perry J, Patzakis M, et al: Fractures and dislocations of the tarsometatarsal joint. *In* Bateman JE, Trott AW (eds): *The Foot and Ankle.* New York, Grune & Stratton, 1980, pp 40–51.
39. Leitner B: Obstacles to reduction in subtalar dislocations. J Bone Joint Surg 36A:299, 1954.
40. Lorentzen JE, Christensen SB, Krogsoe O, Sheppes O: Fractures of the neck of the talus. Acta Orthop Scand 48:115–120, 1977.
41. Main BJ, Jowett RL: Injuries of the midtarsal joint. J Bone Joint Surg 57B:89, 1975.
42. Martinez S, Herzenber JE, Apple JS: Computed tomography of the hindfoot. Orthop Clin North Am 16:481–496, 1985.
43. Meurman KO: Less common stress fractures in the foot. Br J Radiol 54:1, 1981.
44. Miller WE: Pain and impairment considerations following treatment of disruptive os calcis fractures. Clin Orthop 177:82–86, 1983.
45. Monson ST, Ryan JR: Subtalar dislocation. J Bone Joint Surg 63A:1156–1158, 1981.
46. Murphy JL: Isolated dorsal dislocation of the second metatarsophalangeal joint. Foot Ankle 1:30, 1980.
47. Myerson MS: Injuries to the forefoot and toes. *In* Jahss MH (ed): *Disorders of the Foot and Ankle; Medical and Surgical Management,* 2nd ed. Philadelphia, WB Saunders, 1991, pp 2233–2273.
48. Myerson MS, Fisher RT, Burgess AR, Kenzora JE: Fracture dislocations of the tarsometatarsal joints: End results correlated with pathology and treatment. Foot Ankle 6:225, 1986.
49. Palmer I: The mechanism and treatment of fractures of the calcaneus. J Bone Joint Surg 30A:2–8, 1948.
50. Pearson JB: Fractures of the base of the fifth metatarsal. Br Med J 1:1052, 1962.
51. Pennal GF, Yadov MP: Operative treatment of comminuted fractures of the os calcis. Clin Orthop 4:197–211, 1973.
52. Powers JH, Traumatic and developmental abnormalities of the sesamoid bone of the great toes. Am J Surg 23:315, 1934.
53. Pozo JL, Kirwan OE, Jackson AM: The long-term results of conservative management of severely displaced fractures of the calcaneus. J Bone Joint Surg 66B:386–390, 1984.
54. Ross SDK, Sowerby MRR: The operative treatment of fractures of the os calcis. Clin Orthop 199:132–143, 1985.
55. Russotti GM, Johnson KA, Cass JR: Tibiotalocalcaneal arthrodesis for arthritis and deformity of the hind part of the foot. J Bone Joint Surg 70A:1304–1307, 1988.
56. Saint-Isister JF: Calcaneofibular abutment following crush fracture of the calcaneus. J Bone Joint Surg 56B:274–278, 1974.
57. Sammarco GI: Forefoot conditions in dancers: Part II. Foot Ankle 3:93, 1982.
58. Shelton ML, Pedowitz WJ: Injuries to the talar dome, subtalar joint, and midfoot. *In* Jahss MH (ed): *Disorders of the Foot and Ankle; Medical and Surgical Management,* 2nd ed. Philadelphia, WB Saunders, 1991, pp 2274–2292.
59. Smith RW, Staple TW: Computerized tomography (CT) scanning technique for the hindfoot. Clin Orthop 177:34–38, 1983.
60. Soeur R, Remy R: Fractures of the calcaneus with displacement of the thalamic portion. J Bone Joint Surg 57B:413–421, 1975.
61. St. Pierre RW, Velazco A, Fleming LL, Whitesides T: Medial subtalar dislocation in an athlete. J Sports Med 10:240–244, 1982.
62. Torg JS, Balduini FC, Zelko RR, et al: Fractures of the base of the fifth metatarsal distal to the tuberosity. Classification and guidelines for non-surgical and surgical management. J Bone Joint Surg 66A:209, 1984.
63. Van Hal ME, Keene JS, Lange TA, Clancy WG: Stress fractures of the great toe sesamoids. Am J Sports Med 10:122, 1982.

CHAPTER 11

Fractures and Dislocations of the Shoulder

Donald H. Lee

GENERAL PRINCIPLES

The purpose of these sections on shoulder, elbow, and forearm injuries is to provide guidelines for the examiner in assessing, recognizing, and treating injuries to the shoulder and upper extremity. A complete history and full physical examination of the patient, especially of the upper extremity, should be performed at the time of initial evaluation (see Chapter 1). Care must be taken to evaluate the patient fully and not focus on an obvious extremity injury. For the unresponsive patient, inspection, palpation, and passive mobilization of the injured extremity should be performed.

HISTORY

As with all injuries, a detailed history concerning the mechanism, the location, and the time lapsed from injury should be obtained. Facts concerning the injury will help determine the extent of injury and the course of treatment. What was the mechanism and nature (a fall vs. motor vehicle accident) of the injury? What was the neck, arm, or hand position at the time of injury? Was there any

loss of sensation in the extremity with the injury? Where did the injury occur (farmyard vs. inside the house)? What treatment has been performed since the injury (antibiotics, tetanus)?

INSPECTION

All clothing should be removed from the upper trunk and arms. Both sides of the upper trunk, extremity, and head and neck areas should be inspected. Areas of ecchymosis, abrasions, swelling, and asymmetry point to potential areas of injuries. The location and size of open wounds should be noted. Abrasions of the forehead may be suggestive of an extension injury to the neck. Abrasions of the shoulder may suggest a brachial plexus injury or acromioclavicular joint dislocation. Well-healed scars, abrasions, or muscle wasting may be suggestive of a chronic problem.

Active range of motion in the awake patient is noted and recorded. Loss of active motion may be secondary to pain associated with soft tissue, skeletal, or neurologic injuries. If the patient is unresponsive, gentle palpation of all areas should be performed to evaluate for crepitus and the patient's response to pain. Passive motion of all joints should be gently peformed and noted. Any alterations of joint motion may represent a fracture or joint dislocation; for example, loss of shoulder external rotation is seen with a posterior shoulder dislocation. When a patient has a history of an injury, a radiograph should be taken prior to passive mobilization of the injured extremity to rule out an obvious fracture or dislocation.

NEUROVASCULAR EXAMINATION

A vascular assessment should include observation for pallor or cyanosis, palpation of peripheral pulses, and assessment of digital capillary refill. Absence of brachial, radial, or ulnar pulses may be suggestive of an arterial injury or peripheral vasoconstriction. A Doppler ultrasound may be used to detect nonpalpable pulses. Normal capillary refill following blanching of the nail bed matrix should occur within 2 seconds. An Allen test (see Chapter 20) can be used to determine the relative contribution of the radial and ulnar arteries to hand perfusion. Arteriography is indicated with absent pulses associated with penetrating wounds (knife or gunshot wounds). Arteriography may also be indicated when the patient has absent pulses that do not return with reduction of a displaced fracture and dislocation (e.g., clavicular fractures, supracondylar humerus fractures, elbow dislocations).

A tense, swollen extremity or portion of the extremity must be assessed for a possible compartment syndrome (see Chapter 2). Pain should occur with passive stretch of the muscles in an involved compartment; passive extension of the thumb and fingers may elicit pain in the deep volar forearm compartment. If a compartment syndrome is suspected, all circumferential dressings should be removed. Compartmental pressures should be measured, especially in patients with an altered state of consciousness. An elevated compartment pressure or clinical symptoms consistent with a compartment syndrome warrant surgical release of the compartment.

The neurologic examination should include a careful assessment of brachial plexus status and peripheral nerve function in the upper extremity (see Chapter 18). Motor and sensory examination should be performed. Full excursion of the muscle is not needed to determine innervation of a given muscle in the injured patient. Simple palpation of a contracting muscle will indicate that the muscle is partially, if not completely, innervated. Sensory examination should include the assessment of sharp and dull touch or two-point discrimination in each peripheral nerve distribution (see Chapter 1).

FRACTURES AND DISLOCATIONS OF THE SCAPULA

The function of the scapula is to provide a stable link between the thorax and upper extremity. The scapula forms from the coalescence of the primary ossification centers of the body and spine of the scapula and multiple ossification centers forming the coracoid process, glenoid, and acromion. The time for fusion of these centers varies, but it is usually complete by the age of 22 years.

The brachial plexus, axillary artery, and several peripheral nerves lie in close proximity to the scapula. The suprascapular nerve travels through the scapular notch superiorly and around the spinoglenoid notch to supply the supraspinatus and infraspinatus muscles. The dorsal scapular nerve to the rhomboids travels near the medial border of the scapula. Because of the close proximity of these structures and the high energy required for scapular fractures, neurovascular injuries can be associated with scapular fractures.

Scapular fractures are classified according to the location of the fracture: body, scapular spine, glenoid neck, glenoid, coracoid, or acromion. Most fractures involve the body and glenoid neck of the scapula.[2,8]

Two rare injuries are scapular dislocation and scapulothoracic dissociation. With a scapular dislocation, the medial border of the scapula is lodged between the intercostal spaces. A more violent injury is associated with rib fractures. Scapulothoracic dissociation is a complete lateral displacement of the scapula and is frequently associated with brachial plexus, vascular, and muscular injuries.

Fractures of the scapula are not common.[2] Scapular body fractures usually occur from high-energy direct trauma, such as motor vehicle accidents. Acromial and coracoid fractures are usually secondary to direct trauma, such as a fall on the shoulder, and glenoid fractures can result from a fall on an outstretched arm. Shoulder dislocations and traction injuries can cause avulsion fractures of the glenoid rim and coracoid process.

The patient with a shoulder injury usually presents with the arm held against the chest wall. Motion of the arm may be painful. Localized tenderness is usually present. Due to the deep, intramuscular location of the scapula and the frequent occurrence of other associated injuries, scapular fractures can be easily missed. The presence of skin abrasions, ecchymosis, and swelling should alert the examiner to a potential scapular fracture. A scapular fracture should also be ruled out with the occurrence of clavicle fractures and thoracic injuries.

Injuries associated with scapular fractures have been reported to range from 35 to 98 percent. These injuries can include thoracic cage and pulmonary injuries (pneumothorax, pulmonary contusion). Other reported local injuries include fractures of the clavicle, brachial plexus injuries, and arterial injuries. Injuries to the ipsilateral upper extremity can also occur. Skull fractures and spinal, abdominal, and pelvic injuries have also been associated with scapular fractures.[2,6,8,9]

Radiographs should include an anteroposterior view of the scapula and of the glenohumeral joint (Fig. 11–1). An axillary lateral (Fig. 11–2) view of the glenohumeral joint should also be obtained to rule out dislocations of the joint or glenoid rim fractures. A transscapular lateral view or a radiograph taken parallel to the body of the scapula (Fig. 11–3) can be used if the arm cannot be moved. A chest x-ray film is made to help

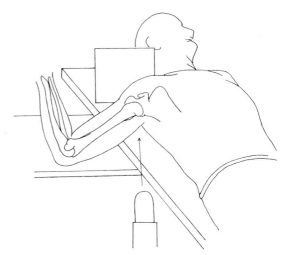

Figure 11–2. An axillary view of the glenohumeral joint is taken, with abduction of the arm.

rule out thoracic cage or pulmonary injuries. Oblique views may be needed to rule out rib, glenoid, coracoid, or acromial fractures. Tomography or computed tomography may be needed to evaluate glenoid fractures fully. These should be ordered by the treating physician who will determine the final treatment of these fractures.

In children, fractures of the scapula need to be differentiated from unfused growth centers. Helpful points to consider are that scapular fractures are relatively uncommon in children. Fracture lines tend to be sharp and well demarcated, and fractures on radiographs and clinical examination should correspond. A comparison view of the contralateral shoulder can be helpful in differentiating fractures and unfused growth centers.

Owing to the high incidence of associated injuries, care must be taken to evaluate carefully, recognize, and treat these injuries. Injuries requiring immediate treatment

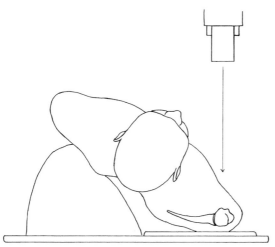

Figure 11–1. An anteroposterior view of the scapula and glenohumeral joint is taken perpendicular to the scapular plane.

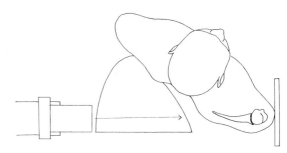

Figure 11–3. A transscapular (or Y lateral) view of the glenohumeral joint is taken parallel to the scapula.

include thoracic cage injuries (pneumothorax, flail chest, and so on). Arteriography may be indicated if a vascular injury is suspected. Vascular injuries compromising circulation to the extremity should be repaired as soon as possible.

Most scapular fractures can be treated nonoperatively with a shoulder immobilizer (Fig. 11–4). The rare scapular dislocation occasionally may require a closed reduction.

Large, displaced fractures of the glenoid, acromion, and coracoid process may require operative intervention, especially if there is instability or impingement of the glenohumeral joint. Open fractures require surgical debridement.

The indications for late surgical reconstruction may include an arthroplasty for post-traumatic arthritis of the glenohumeral joint; a shoulder fusion for brachial plexus injuries; or an above-elbow amputation for scapulothoracic dissociations associated with a vascular injury.

FRACTURES OF THE CLAVICLE

The function of the clavicle is to provide a link from the thorax to the scapula. It helps provide stability and power to the arm. The clavicle forms the fusion of the central with the medial and lateral ossification centers. The more radiographically detectable medial ossification center ossifies between 12 and 19 years and fuses between 22 and 25 years of age.

Because of its articulations with the sternum and acromion, the clavicle allows for a free range of motion of the shoulder. The clavicle acts as a scaffold to which several muscles are attached, including the deltoid, trapezius, sternocleidomastoid, pectoralis major, and subclavius. The clavicle also protects the brachial plexus, subclavian and axillary arteries, and upper lung.

Fractures of the clavicle are classified according to the location of the fracture: distal, middle, or proximal one-third shaft fractures (Fig. 11–5). Middle one-third fractures are the most common (Fig. 11–6), accounting for approximately 80 percent of clavicular fractures. Distal one-third fractures can be associated with injuries to the coracoclavicular ligaments and acromioclavicular joint. Proximal one-third fractures are associated with injuries to the costoclavicular and sternoclavicular ligaments. Fractures may extend into the sternoclavicular joint. In children and young adults whose medial physis has not fused, epiphyseal injuries can occur.

Clavicle fractures occurring at birth range from 2.8 to 7.2 per 1000 births. The incidence of birth fractures increases with larger babies, and with a midforceps delivery. Clavicle fractures do not occur with cesarean section.

Fractures of the clavicle may constitute up to 44 percent of shoulder girdle injuries. Fractures of the clavicle are usually secondary to either direct or indirect injuries. The fractures can occur from direct blows to the clavicle or lateral shoulder, resulting from a

Figure 11–4. *A* and *B,* A commercially available shoulder sling immobilizer. The hand should be included within the sling to prevent bending of the wrist over the edge of the sling. Compression of the wrist over the edge of the sling could cause ulnar neuropathy. (From: Lee DH, Neviaser RJ: Upper extremity fractures and dislocations. *In* Feliciano DV, Moore EE, Mattox KL (eds): *Trauma.* 3rd ed. East Norwalk, CT, Appleton & Lange, 1995.)

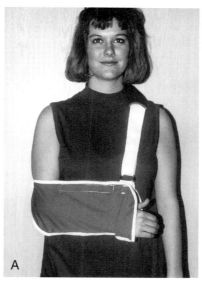
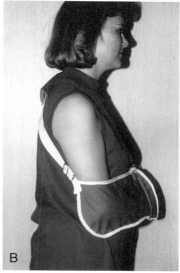

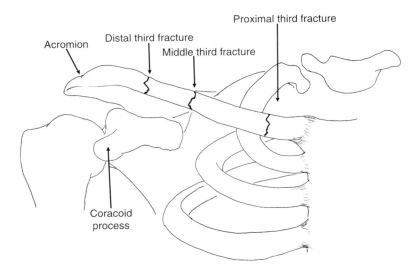

Figure 11–5. Fractures of the clavicle are classified by their location: proximal, middle, or distal third fractures.

fall or motor vehicle accident, or falls on an outstretched arm.

Birth fractures can be easily missed. The fracture may be noticed several days following injury as swelling in the clavicular region, representing a healing callus, occurs. There may be asymmetry of the neck line, localized swelling, and point tenderness. The child may present with pseudoparalysis of the affected arm, with limited voluntary movement of the arm due to pain. A brachial plexus injury, resulting in loss of motion, can occur with the clavicle fracture. The diagnosis of a clavicle fracture can be determined with a radiograph. In the young child, clavicle fractures may be incomplete and go undetected. Localized tenderness is usually present.

In the adult, due to the subcutaneous location of the clavicle, shaft fractures are usually easily detected. The affected arm will droop forward and downward. The proximal clavicular fragment is elevated superiorly by the pull of the sternocleidomastoid muscle. Undisplaced fractures or injuries to either the acromioclavicular or sternoclavicular joints may be less obvious.

Associated injuries include skeletal injuries, lung and pleural injuries, brachial plexus and vascular injuries, and head, neck, and mediastinal trauma. Skeletal injuries include injuries to the acromioclavicular and sternoclavicular joints and rib fractures.

Thoracic injuries include pneumothorax, pulmonary contusions, and tracheal or bronchial tears. Brachial plexus, subclavian or axillary artery, and subclavian vein injuries are also associated with clavicular fractures. With a suspected arterial injury, an arteriogram should be considered. Surgical exploration should be performed with major vessel injuries resulting in a life-threatening blood loss.[3,7,10,14,16,22]

Radiographs include an anteroposterior view of the clavicle. An AP view of the chest should be obtained to exclude any pulmonary or thoracic injuries. Anteroposterior and axillary (or transscapular) lateral views are obtained to evaluate the glenohumeral joint. With fractures that are obscured by underlying structures or in areas that are difficult to visualize, specific radiographs may be needed. To help determine the relationships of clavicle fracture fragments, 45-degree tilt views will be helpful. A cephalic tilt view will help determine injuries to the sternoclavicular joint. The x-ray is angled from below upward at a 45-degree angle. Anteroposter-

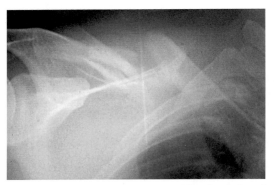

Figure 11–6. An example of a middle third clavicle fracture.

ior or PA views of both acromioclavicular joints with 10 pound weights strapped to each wrist will help determine any instability of the acromioclavicular joints or distal one-third clavicle fractures. However, care should be taken in using stress views that may displace previously nondisplaced fractures. Occasionally tomograms or CT scans are needed to evaluate injuries to the clavicle that are difficult to evaluate by plain radiographs, including injuries to the sternoclavicular joint.

Most clavicle fractures heal, especially in children, and can be treated nonoperatively. The injured extremity can be immobilized using a shoulder sling (see Figure 11–4), figure of eight sling (Fig. 11–7), or Velpeau immobilizer (Fig. 11–8). The simple immobilizer is probably the most comfortable for the patient.

Indications for immediate surgery include the debridement of open fractures, repair of vascular injuries, and reduction of a posteriorly displaced medial portion of the clavicle compromising the mediastinal structures. Severely displaced fractures that compromise the skin or neurovascular structures behind the clavicle and fail to respond to closed reduction may require operative treatment. Occasionally displaced, unstable distal one-third shaft fractures, and fractures of the clavicle associated with an unstable scapular fracture, may also require operative treat-

ment. Fractures of the clavicle in the multiply traumatized patient in whom closed treatment may not be possible may be a relative indication for surgery. Late surgical indications include the treatment of clavicular nonunions, malunions causing compression of the brachial plexus, and post-traumatic arthritis of the acromioclavicular and sternoclavicular joints.

DISLOCATIONS OF THE CLAVICLE

The clavicle articulates laterally with the acromion at the acromioclavicular (AC) joint and medially with the sternum at the sternoclavicular (SC) joint. Laterally, the clavicle is stabilized to the scapula by the acromioclavicular and coracoclavicular ligaments. Medially, the clavicle is stabilized to the sternum by the sternoclavicular and costoclavicular ligaments.

Immediately posterior to the SC joints are the innominate artery and vein, internal jugular vein, vagus and phrenic nerves, trachea, and esophagus.

Dislocations of the AC joint are classified according to the direction of the dislocation of the distal clavicle. The most common type occurs with superior dislocation of the distal clavicle (Fig. 11–9). The degree of superior dislocation of the clavicle increases with complete disruption of the acromioclavicular and

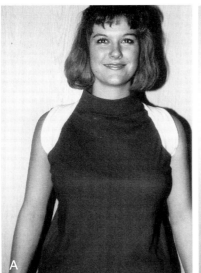
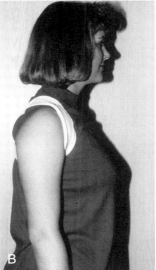
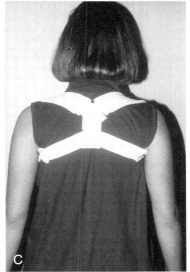

Figure 11–7. *A* to *C,* A commercially available figure-of-eight immobilizer used for immobilization of clavicle fractures. (From: Lee DH, Neviaser RJ: Upper extremity fractures and dislocations. *In* Feliciano DV, Moore EE, Mattox KL (eds): *Trauma.* 3rd ed. East Norwalk, CT, Appleton & Lange, 1995.)

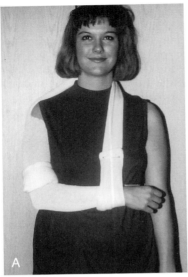
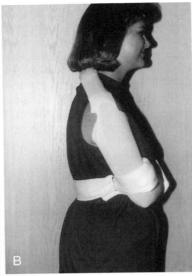
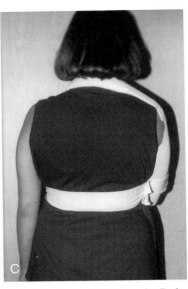

Figure 11–8. *A* to *C,* A Velpeau shoulder immobilizer made with a stockinette, safety pins, and ABD pads. Pads are used to provide soft padding around the neck, wrist, and arm areas. (From: Lee DH, Neviaser RJ: Upper extremity fractures and dislocations. *In* Feliciano DV, Moore EE, Mattox KL (eds): *Trauma.* 3rd ed. East Norwalk, CT, Appleton & Lange, 1995.)

coracoclavicular ligaments. Posterior dislocation of the distal clavicle through the trapezius muscle and inferior dislocation of the distal clavicle beneath the coracoid process are less common.

Dislocations of the SC joint are classified according to the direction of the displacement of the medial end of the clavicle, either anterior or posterior.

Injuries to the AC joint are more common in the second decade of life and usually in men. Superior and posterior dislocations of the AC joint are generally secondary to a direct blow on the lateral aspect of the shoulder. A less common mechanism of injury is

a fall on the outstretched arm. An inferior dislocation results from a fall on the outstretched arm. An inferior dislocation may be due to hyperabduction and external rotation of the arm combined with scapular retraction.

Dislocations of the SC joint are rare and can occur from direct trauma to the medial clavicle or indirectly by lateral compression on the shoulder combined with scapular protraction or retraction. Such injuries can occur in motor vehicle accidents or sporting injuries.

Panclavicular dislocations are rare and are the result of a high-energy injury with severe

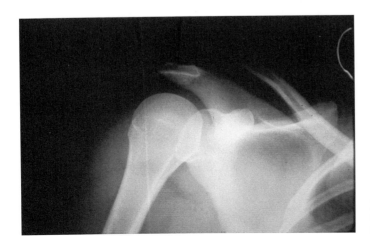

Figure 11–9. An example of a superior dislocation of the distal clavicle at the acromioclavicular joint.

protraction of the shoulder. With this injury, both the AC and SC joints are dislocated. Associated vascular and neurologic injuries should be identified.

Clinically, AC joint dislocations are associated with localized pain and tenderness. Mild subluxations or sprains of the acromioclavicular joint may have minimal deformity. Complete dislocations, associated with injuries to the acromioclavicular and coracoclavicular ligaments, usually produce a clinical deformity. With superior dislocations, the distal clavicle will appear superiorly displaced, and the shoulder will appear to droop.[15,16,20,23]

Sternoclavicular joint dislocations produce localized tenderness and pain with motion. Mild sprains or subluxations may not show any clinical deformity. Anterior dislocations may reveal a more prominent medial clavicle. The patient may support the injured arm, and the head may be tilted toward the affected side.

With posterior SC joint dislocations, the normally palpable medial clavicle may be less prominent. Localized tenderness is usually present. Symptoms associated with compression of mediastinal structures, such as difficulty in breathing and swallowing, venous congestion in the neck, and shortness of breath may be present.[18]

Associated injuries with AC dislocations include fractures of the clavicle, acromion, and coracoid process. Thoracic injuries, such as pneumothorax and pulmonary contusion, have also been described.

Few associated injuries are seen with anterior SC dislocations. However, with posterior SC dislocations, associated injuries include pneumothorax, injuries to the great vessels, esophageal and tracheal injuries, and brachial plexus compression. In the younger patient whose medial clavicular physis has not fully fused, physeal fractures may occur.

The recommended radiographs are similar to those for clavicular fractures, as noted earlier. To visualize the AC joint directly, a 10-degree cephalic tilt view, centered over the AC joint, is helpful. Stress views using weights are also helpful to determine the stability of the AC joint.

Radiographs of the SC joint are difficult to assess due to the underlying thoracic structures. The 45-degree tilt views are helpful, but tomograms or CT scans are frequently needed to evaluate this area fully.

Most acute injuries to the AC joint can be treated symptomatically in a shoulder sling (see Figure 11–4). Special slings or braces have been used, but most are usually poorly tolerated by the patient. Mild sprains of the SC joint, producing minimal clinical symptoms, also can be treated in a shoulder sling.

For the more severely displaced AC joint dislocations, reconstruction of the joint may be indicated as an elective procedure. Resection of the distal clavicle can be performed for post-traumatic arthritis. Any patient with a questionably severe injury of the AC joint should be referred.

For acute, complete SC joint dislocations, especially the posterior dislocation causing significant clinical symptoms, an attempt at closed reduction of the dislocation should be performed. Posterior SC joint dislocations causing vascular compromise that cannot be reduced in a closed manner should undergo an open reduction. Late surgical resection of the medial end of the clavicle can also be performed for post-traumatic arthritis.

FRACTURES OF THE PROXIMAL HUMERUS

The proximal humerus forms from the fusion of the primary ossification center of the proximal humerus and ossification centers for the greater and lesser tuberosities. Fusion of the proximal humeral physis occurs by 18 to 22 years of age.

The mobility of the glenohumeral joint is secondary to its minimal osseous constraints. Unlike the ball and socket hip joint, the stability of the glenohumeral joint is due to a complex relationship of the joint capsule, glenohumeral ligaments, muscles, and other soft tissues. The proximal humerus consists of the humeral head that articulates with the glenoid, the greater and lesser tuberosities, the bicipital groove, and the proximal humeral shaft. Between the two tuberosities is the bicipital groove, through which passes the long head of the biceps tendon as it proceeds to its insertion onto the superior glenoid. Overlying this entire complex is the deltoid muscle.

The blood supply to the humeral head is provided by a combination of anterior and posterior circumflex vessels from the axillary artery and by the muscle insertions into the tuberosities.

The brachial plexus and axillary artery lie medial, anterior, and inferior to the humeral head near the region of the inferior margin of the glenohumeral joint. The axillary nerve courses posteriorly along the humeral neck and is particularly vulnerable to injury with glenohumeral fractures and dislocations of the humerus.

Fractures of the proximal humerus are classified according to the location of the fracture (Fig. 11–10). Anatomic neck fractures are located between the humeral head articular surface and the greater and lesser tuberosities. Surgical neck fractures are located between the humeral tuberosities and humeral shaft. Fractures of either the greater or lesser tuberosities or both can occur. Depending on the number of displaced portions of the proximal humerus, fractures are termed two-, three-, or four-part fractures. A four-part fracture includes a displaced fracture of the humeral head, humeral neck, and both greater and lesser tuberosities. Displacement has been defined as greater than 1 cm of displacement or an angulation greater than 45 degrees between fracture fragments. Displacement of fracture fragments is usually secondary to injuries of the rotator cuff attachments to the tuberosi-

ties and pectoralis major attachment to the humeral shaft. Head-splitting fractures and fractures associated with dislocation of the glenohumeral joint can also occur. In children, fractures involving the physis can occur.

Approximately 45 percent of humeral fractures occur in the proximal humeral region, and the incidence increases to as much as 76 percent in patients over age 40 years. The most common mechanism of injury is a fall on the outstretched arm. A significant injury is not necessary to produce a humeral fracture in the osteoporotic elderly patient. Fractures or dislocations also can occur with direct blows to, or with excessive rotation of, the proximal humerus. Injuries, especially fracture-dislocations, can occur with electrical shock and seizures. In the newborn infant, fractures of the proximal humerus are usually due to hyperextension or excessive rotation during delivery.

Clinically, pain, swelling, and tenderness about the shoulder are noted. Crepitus may be present, and ecchymosis about the shoulder, arm, and chest wall develops within a day or two following the injury. The arm is usually held close to the chest, and active motion of the shoulder is painful. The neonate may present with a pseudoparalysis of

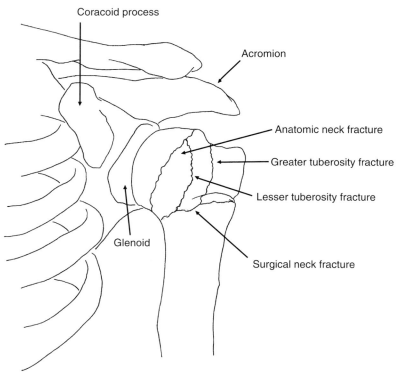

Coracoid process

Acromion

Anatomic neck fracture

Greater tuberosity fracture

Lesser tuberosity fracture

Glenoid

Surgical neck fracture

Figure 11–10. Fractures of the proximal humerus can be classified as anatomical neck, surgical neck, or greater or lesser tuberosity fractures.

the arm. The shoulder area is usually tender, and passive motion may elicit pain. Swelling and ecchymosis are usually limited.

Examination of distal pulses and motor and sensory testing should be performed. Deltoid muscle function and sensation along the lateral aspect of the shoulder should be tested to assess the status of the axillary nerve.

Associated injuries include brachial plexus and axillary artery injuries. The axillary nerve is the most commonly injured nerve, but injuries to the musculocutaneous and suprascapular nerve also have been described. Other associated injuries include thoracic cage and pulmonary injuries and other shoulder girdle injuries.[1,11-13]

Radiographs should include an anteroposterior view of the shoulder in the scapular plane. An axillary lateral view of the glenohumeral joint or, if for some reason this is unobtainable, a scapular lateral view of the glenohumeral joint should be obtained. Care must be taken to determine that the glenohumeral joint is not dislocated. Additional views may include special oblique views of the humeral head or glenoid to evaluate these areas better. In some instances, tomography or CT scans may be needed to evaluate glenoid fractures, which are difficult to evaluate by radiographs. Radiographs of the chest and entire humerus and elbow joint should be obtained. An arteriogram is indicated if an arterial injury is suspected.

In neonates, radiographs may not be helpful in detecting proximal humeral fractures due to incomplete ossification. Arthrograms and ultrasonography have been used to detect injuries in infants.

Most nondisplaced or minimally displaced proximal humerus fractures can be treated with shoulder sling immobilization (see Fig. 11–4). Follow-up radiographs should be obtained on a 1- to 2-week basis. Gentle range of motion exercises, including pendulum exercises, can be started when shoulder discomfort subsides, usually at 2 to 3 weeks. Exercises are then progressively increased. Sling immobilization is usually discontinued by 6 weeks. The use of a hanging arm cast is generally not advised because of the possibility of distracting fracture fragments. A nonunion may be produced by fracture fragment distraction.

Displaced fractures may require either a closed or open reduction and internal or pin fixation. Occasionally prosthetic replacement is used for severely comminuted or intra-articular fractures. Postoperatively, these fractures can be treated in a shoulder sling or swathe immobilizer. All fracture-dislocations require open reduction and internal fixation or prosthetic replacement. All open fractures require surgical debridement. Fractures associated with vascular and brachial plexus compromise may require surgical exploration. The indications for late surgical intervention include the treatment of post-traumatic arthritis, malunions, nonunions, and avascular necrosis of the humeral head.

In children, displaced fractures may require a closed reduction with or without pin fixation. An open reduction is usually not required. Immobilization is performed using a shoulder sling and occasionally a spica cast.

DISLOCATIONS OF THE SHOULDER (Glenohumeral Joint)

The glenohumeral joint is inherently mechanically unstable. The large, spherical humeral head articulates with the small, shallow glenoid. Stability of the joint is provided through a complex combination of capsular and ligamentous restraints, rotator cuff muscles, and bone restraints. In addition, motion of the shoulder is through a combination of glenohumeral and scapulothoracic motion. This requires motion not only of the glenohumeral joint but also the acromioclavicular and sternoclavicular joints and the scapulothoracic articulation.

Instability of the glenohumeral joint can be classified as a subluxation or dislocation. Subluxations of the glenohumeral joint occur when there is symptomatic translation of the humeral head beyond the normal physiologic translation that occurs with shoulder motion. With subluxations, the humeral head returns into the glenoid fossa without completely dislocating. Dislocations occur when there is a complete separation of the humeral head and glenoid.

Dislocations of the glenohumeral joint are classified according to the direction of displacement of the humeral head (e.g., anterior, posterior) and the final position of the humeral head (e.g., subcoracoid, subglenoid).

One of the most commonly dislocated joints in the body is the glenohumeral joint. Anterior dislocations (Fig. 11–11) are much more common than posterior dislocations. Up to

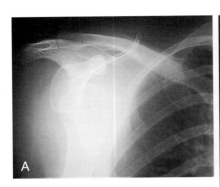
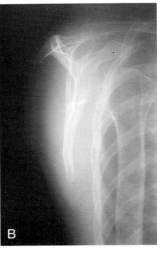

Figure 11–11. *A* and *B,* Anteroposterior and transscapular lateral views of an anterior dislocation of the glenohumeral joint. (Courtesy of Richard Cord, MD.)

60 to 80 percent of posterior dislocations are not diagnosed acutely. Inferior and superior dislocations are rare. Anterior dislocations usually occur with the arm in extension, abduction, and external rotation. Posterior dislocations occur with a fall on the flexed and adducted arm. Electrical shock injuries and seizures are also associated with posterior dislocations. Inferior dislocations are associated with a hyperabduction injury to the arm. A rare, severe inferior dislocation of the glenohumeral joint can occur as an open injury (luxatio erecta). Superior dislocations are secondary to a severe upward force on the adducted arm against the acromion.

Dislocations of the glenohumeral joint in children are very rare. The mechanism of injury is similar to that in adults. In neonates, a pseudodislocation or an epiphyseal separation can occur, usually from a birth injury.

Patients with shoulder dislocations are usually in severe pain. With an anterior shoulder dislocation, the arm is slightly abducted and externally rotated. The humeral head may be palpable anteriorly. There may be a hollowing of the shoulder contour posteriorly. There is an inability fully to rotate or abduct the arm internally. Care must be taken to assess the status of the axillary nerve owing to its high incidence of injury. This is performed by testing sharp/dull discrimination and light touch sensation over the lateral deltoid and by palpation of a contracting deltoid muscle. Its status should be known prior to any reduction maneuver.

Patients with a posterior shoulder dislocation may have no noticeable deformity. The humeral head may be palpable posteriorly with a hollowing of the anterior aspect of the shoulder. The patient will be unable to externally rotate or fully abduct the arm. With an inferior dislocation, the arm is slightly abducted, internally rotated, and shortened. With a severe inferior dislocation (luxatio erecta), the arm is held abducted about 110 or 160 degrees. Superior dislocations of the shoulder are associated with acromial fractures.

Associated injuries include vascular (axillary, thoracoacromial, subscapular, circumflex arteries), neural (axillary, radial, musculocutaneous, median, ulnar nerves, brachial plexus), soft tissue (glenohumeral joint capsule and/or ligaments, rotator cuff), and osseous (humeral head, greater or lesser tuberosity, glenoid rim, proximal humeral shaft) injuries.[5,13,17,19,21]

The radiographs taken are similar to those for proximal humerus fractures: an anteroposterior view of the glenohumeral joint in the scapular plane and an axillary (or transscapular) lateral view. Care should be taken to look specifically for tuberosity, humeral head, and glenoid fractures.

Computed tomography may be used to determine the extent of humeral head and glenoid rim fractures that are poorly seen by plain radiographs. Arthrography may be indicated in previously dislocated shoulders to detect rotator cuff tears. This method is reserved for patients with a painful shoulder that fails to respond to rest and rehabilitation.

After a careful clinical examination, determining especially the neurologic status, and after appropriate radiographs have been obtained, all glenohumeral dislocations should be quickly and gently reduced. In general, some form of anesthesia is needed. The degree and type of anesthesia may depend on several factors, such as the patient's overall status, duration of the dislocation, number of previous dislocations, other associated injuries, and so on. Several methods of reduction have been described. Most methods consist of the use of traction applied to the injured arm, with some form of countertraction applied across either the chest or axilla. A sheet can be placed around the chest and held by an assistant to provide countertraction. Longitudinal traction is then gently applied along the arm. The elbow is usually flexed at 90 degrees to provide additional leverage. For an anterior shoulder dislocation, with longitudinal traction the arm is then gently abducted and externally rotated until a reduction occurs. A palpable and audible clunk usually occurs when the joint reduces, and both passive and active joint motion are improved. For a posterior dislocation, in addition to longitudinal traction lateral traction is applied to the proximal humerus. Gentle internal rotation may unlock a locked posterior dislocation. Special care is taken not to rotate the arm forcibly with the reduction maneuver.

Another method of reduction for an anterior shoulder dislocation is performed with the patient lying in a prone position on a stretcher. The affected arm is placed over the edge of the stretcher, and approximately 5 to 10 pounds of weight are hung from the wrist. The process generally requires 10 to 20 minutes for the reduction to occur. The patient must be adequately anesthetized, relaxed, and supervised during this reduction technique. Multiple attempts at reduction or excessive force should not be used. General anesthesia and muscle relaxation should be used if reduction is not obtainable with intravenous sedation.

Anteroposterior and lateral postreduction radiographs should be taken to confirm adequate reduction of the dislocation and that fractures have not occurred or were not previously visible due to the dislocation. A neurologic examination should also be repeated. Following relocation of an anterior shoulder dislocation, the shoulder is immobilized in a shoulder sling and swathe shoulder immobilizer (Fig. 11–12). Abduction and external rotation of the shoulder are avoided. Following reduction of a posterior shoulder dislocation, the patient is placed with the shoulder in neutral rotation, not internal rotation. The long axis of the arm is placed slightly posterior to the long axis of the body. This can be accomplished with a long arm cast attached to a plaster band placed around the pelvis and abdomen, or with a commercially available splint (Fig. 11–13). For anterior dislocations, immobilization varies from 2 to 6 weeks. Shorter periods of immobilization are

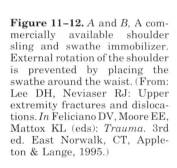

Figure 11–12. *A* and *B,* A commercially available shoulder sling and swathe immobilizer. External rotation of the shoulder is prevented by placing the swathe around the waist. (From: Lee DH, Neviaser RJ: Upper extremity fractures and dislocations. *In* Feliciano DV, Moore EE, Mattox KL (eds): *Trauma.* 3rd ed. East Norwalk, CT, Appleton & Lange, 1995.)

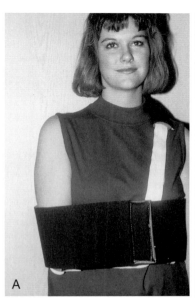

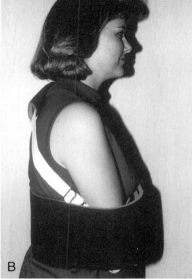

A   B

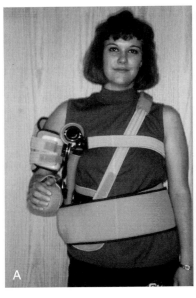
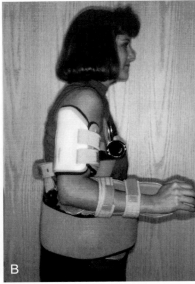

Figure 11–13. *A* and *B*, A commercially available shoulder brace can be used to immobilize the arm following reduction of a posterior shoulder glenohumeral dislocation. Notice that the arm is in neutral rotation and slightly posterior to the long axis of the thorax. Similar immobilization can be accomplished with a long arm cast attached to a pelvic band around the waist. (From: Lee DH, Neviaser RJ: Upper extremity fractures and dislocations. *In* Feliciano DV, Moore EE, Mattox KL (eds): *Trauma.* 3rd ed. East Norwalk, CT, Appleton & Lange, 1995.)

indicated for patients older than 30 years, who have a lesser tendency for recurrent dislocation and a greater tendency for shoulder stiffness. The elbow is placed through a range of motion several times a day. In the younger patient, external rotation beyond zero degrees and forward elevation greater than 90 degrees are avoided for 6 weeks. Heavy manual work or overhead activities are avoided for 3 months. Rehabilitation includes strengthening of shoulder girdle muscles, especially the internal rotators. For posterior shoulder dislocations, immobilization is maintained for 3 to 6 weeks. The post-immobilization rehabilitation is similar to that for anterior dislocations. Strengthening of the external rotators is emphasized.

Indications for surgery include debridement of open dislocations, open reduction of irreducible dislocations, repair of vascular injuries associated with dislocations, repair of large displaced fractures or soft tissue injuries (rotator cuff tears) associated with dislocations, or dislocations that are unstable following reduction. Late reconstruction is indicated for the treatment of chronic dislocations, recurrent dislocations or subluxations, and post-traumatic arthritis.

References

1. Bigliani LU, Craig EV, Butters KP: Fractures of the shoulder: *In* Rockwood CA, Green DP, Bucholz RW (eds): *Fractures in Adults,* 3rd ed. Philadelphia, JB Lippincott, 1991, pp 871–927.

2. Butters KP: Fractures and dislocations of the scapula. *In* Rockwood CA, Green DP, Bucholz RW (eds): *Fractures in Adults,* 3rd ed. Philadelphia, JB Lippincott, 1991, pp 990–1019.

3. Craig EV: Fractures of the clavicle. *In* Rockwood CA, Green DP, Bucholz RW (eds): *Fractures in Adults,* 3rd ed. Philadelphia, JB Lippincott, 1991, pp 928–990.

4. Curtis RJ, Dameron TB, Rockwood CA: Fractures and dislocations of the shoulder in children. *In* Rockwood CA, Wilkins KE, King RE (eds): *Fractures in Children,* 3rd ed. Philadelphia, JB Lippincott, 1991, pp 829–919.

5. DePalma AF: Dislocations of the shoulder girdle. *In* DePalma AF (ed): *Surgery of the Shoulder,* 3rd ed. Philadelphia, JB Lippincott, 1983, pp 428–511.

6. Hardegger FH, Simpson LA, Weber BG: The operative treatment of scapular fractures. J Bone and Joint Surg 66B:725–731, 1984.

7. Howard FM, Schafer SJ: Injuries to the clavicle with neurovascular complications: A study of fourteen cases. J Bone Joint Surg 47A:1335–1346, 1965.

8. Ideberg RJ: Fractures involving the glenoid fossa. *In* Bateman JE, Welsh RP (eds): *Surgery of the Shoulder.* Toronto, BC Decker, 1984, pp 63–66.

9. Imatani RJ: Fractures of the scapula. A review of 53 fractures, J Trauma 15:473–478, 1975.

10. Neer CS: Fractures of the distal third of the clavicle. Clin Orthop 58:43–50, 1968.

11. Neer, CS: Displaced proximal humerus fractures. Part I. Classification and evaluation. J Bone Joint Surg 52A:1077–1089, 1970.

12. Neer, CS: Displaced proximal humeral fractures. Part II. Treatment of three-part and four-part displacement. J Bone Joint Surg 52A:1090–1103, 1970.

13. Neviaser JS: Complicated fractures and dislocations about the shoulder joint. J Bone Joint Surg 44A:984–998, 1962.

14. Neviaser JS: Treatment of fractures of the clavicle. Surg Clin North Am 43:1555–1563, 1963.

15. Neviaser JS: Injuries of the clavicle and its articulations. Orthop Clin North Am 11:233–237, 1980.

16. Neviaser RJ: Injuries to the clavicle and acromioclavicular joint. Orthop Clin North Am 18: 433–438, 1987.

17. Neviaser RJ, Neviaser TJ, Neviaser JS: Concurrent rupture of the rotator cuff and anterior dislocation of the shoulder in the older patient. J Bone Joint Surg 70A:1308–1311, 1988.

18. Rockwood, CA: Injuries to the sternoclavicular joint. *In* Rockwood CA, Green DP, Bucholz RW (eds): *Fractures in Adults,* 3rd ed. Philadelphia, JB Lippincott, 1991, pp 1253–1307.

19. Rockwood CA, Thomas SC, Matsen FA III: Subluxation and dislocations about the glenohumeral joint. *In* Rockwood CA, Green DP, Bucholz RW (eds): *Fractures in Adults,* 3rd ed. Philadelphia, JB Lippincott, 1991, pp 1021–1179.

20. Rockwood CA, Williams GR, Young DC: Injuries to the acromioclavicular joint. *In* Rockwood CA, Green DP, Bucholz RW (eds): *Fractures in Adults,* 3rd ed. Philadelphia, JB Lippincott, 1991, pp 1181–1251.

21. Rowe CR: Acute and recurrent dislocations of the shoulder. J Bone Joint Surg 44A:998–1008, 1962.

22. Rowe CR: An atlas of anatomy and treatment of midclavicular fractures. Clin Orthop 58:29–42, 1968.

23. Tossy JD, Mead NC, Sigmond HM: Acromioclavicular separations: Useful and practical classification for treatment. Clin Orthop 28:111–119, 1963.

CHAPTER 12

Injuries to the Humerus and Elbow

Donald H. Lee

FRACTURES OF THE HUMERAL SHAFT

A general evaluation of upper extremity injuries is provided in Chapter 11. The shaft of the humerus is well enclosed by muscle. The humeral shaft extends from just below the neck of the humerus to the level of the supracondylar ridges of the distal humerus. At this level, the soft tissue envelope becomes thin, and open fractures in this area become more common.

The humeral shaft forms from a fusion of the primary ossification centers in the diaphyseal and metaphyseal regions and the secondary ossification centers on the proximal and distal ends of the humerus.

The radial nerve lies in the spiral groove adjacent to the bone along the posterior aspect of the humeral shaft and may be susceptible to injuries between the middle and distal thirds of the humeral shaft. Proximal to the elbow, the brachial artery curves laterally beneath the median nerve to lie lateral to the median nerve. At this level, the brachial artery, along with the median nerve, is susceptible to injury with a supracondylar fracture of the distal humerus. The profunda brachii artery courses with the radial nerve

in the posterior compartment and may be susceptible to injury with fractures of the humeral shaft.

Fractures of the humeral shaft are classified according to the location of the fracture (proximal, middle, or distal one third fractures), the configuration of the fracture (transverse, spiral, and so on), the status of the integument (closed or open), and the degree of the fracture (complete or incomplete). The fracture can also be classified as to whether it is associated with a dislocation of the shoulder or elbow joints.

Fractures of the humeral shaft are usually the result of direct blows to the arm, motor vehicle accidents, gunshot injuries, or crush injuries. Humeral fractures also can occur from indirect injuries, such as falls on an outstretched hand or on the elbow, and violent muscle contractions.[2]

In neonates, fractures of the humerus can occur from birth trauma. However, fractures of the proximal humerus are more common. In children, indirect twisting injuries can produce a long spiral fracture. Direct trauma produces a short spiral or transverse fracture of the humerus. Child abuse should be suspected with these types of injuries. Indirect trauma, such as a fall on an outstretched

156

arm, can produce an incomplete buckle fracture; more commonly, however, metaphyseal fractures occur near the elbow.

With complete fractures of the humerus, the arm appears shortened, and abnormal crepitus or motion or both at the site of the fracture are noted. Incomplete fractures may present with localized tenderness overlying the fracture site. Ecchymosis usually develops within 24 to 48 hours following injury.

In neonates, the arm may appear flail. Signs of swelling and ecchymosis are usually absent. Abnormal motion may be noted at the fracture site. Findings in the older child are similar to those in the adult. As with any injury, a careful neurovascular examination should be performed. Particular care should be taken to assess the status of the radial nerve. With a radial nerve injury, loss of wrist, finger, and thumb extension (dorsiflexion) and decreased sensation (sharp/dull and light touch) over the dorsal aspect of the thumb and index metacarpals will be noted. Approximately 5 to 10 percent of humeral shaft fractures may be associated with radial nerve injuries. Spiral fractures of the distal one-third of the humeral shaft appear to be particularly susceptible to radial nerve injuries.[3] Most radial nerve palsies are secondary to stretch injuries or bruising, and function usually returns within a few weeks to months. Brachial artery injuries have been associated with humeral shaft and supracondylar fractures. Arteriography may be indicated to determine the extent of arterial injury, if suspected.

Two radiographs of the humeral shaft, oriented perpendicular to one another, should be obtained. In addition, radiographs of the shoulder and elbow joint also should be made to rule out associated injuries to these joints.

Most fractures of the humeral shaft can be treated with immobilization.[8] Coaptation splints made of medial and lateral or U-shaped plaster arm splints (Fig. 12–1) are recommended for the initial fracture immobilization. Commercially available arm braces (Figs. 12–2 and 12–3) in conjunction with a shoulder sling can be used after swelling has subsided. Heavy hanging arm casts should be avoided because of the possibility of producing a nonunion. Splint removal is performed when fracture healing has occurred, usually 6 to 8 weeks. Radiographs are taken at 2- to 3-week intervals to assess fracture healing.

Surgery is indicated for debridement of open fractures. Surgical stabilization (internal or external fixation) of the humerus fracture is required for fractures associated with a vascular injury. Surgery may be needed for stabilization of humeral fractures in the multitraumatized patient who requires early use of the arm. Other conditions that may require surgical intervention include humeral nonunions, pathologic fractures, and fractures associated with radial nerve palsies.

FRACTURES ABOUT THE ELBOW

The distal humerus is composed of the supracondylar region and the medial and lateral columns. The medial column consists of the

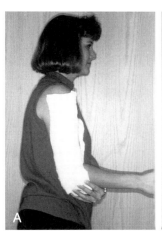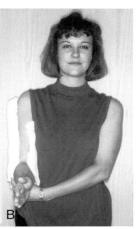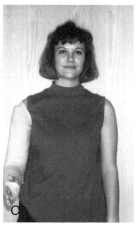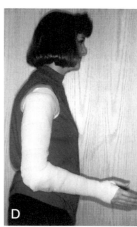

Figure 12–1. *A* through *D*, Most humeral fractures can be immobilized by using a U-shaped plaster splint or a coaptation splint (one medial and one lateral splint) placed around the humerus. Ace wrapping should include the hand and forearm to help prevent swelling in those areas. (From: Lee DH, Nevaiser RJ: Upper extremity fractures and dislocations. *In* Feliciano DV, Moore EE, Mattox KL (eds): *Trauma.* 3rd ed. East Norwalk, CT, Appleton & Lange, 1995.)

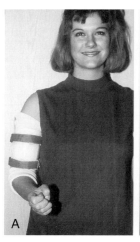 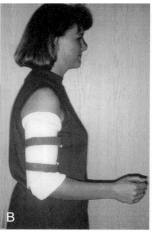 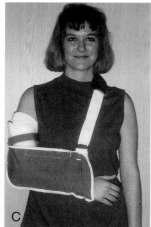 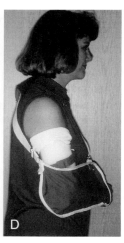

Figure 12–2. *A* and *B,* A commercially available plastic humeral fracture brace can be used to immobilize humeral fractures after the initial swelling has subsided. *C* and *D,* The brace can be used with a shoulder sling for comfort. (From: Lee DH, Nevaiser RJ: Upper extremity fractures and dislocations. *In* Feliciano DV, Moore EE, Mattox KL (eds): *Trauma.* 3rd ed. East Norwalk, CT, Appleton & Lange, 1995.)

medial condyle, trochlea, and medial epicondyle. The trochlea articulates with the greater sigmoid (semilunar) notch of the proximal ulna. The notch is composed of the olecranon process and the coronoid process. The articulation between the ulna and distal humerus allows for the hinge-like motion of the elbow. The lateral column consists of the capitellum and the lateral epicondyle. The capitellum articulates with the radial head and allows for forearm rotation. Additional stability to the elbow joint is provided by the medial and lateral collateral ligaments and the anterior and posterior joint capsule.

The distal humerus forms from the coalescence of multiple ossification centers. The ossification center for the capitellum (lateral condyle) is the first to ossify (6 to 12 months), followed by the medial epicondyle (5 to 6 years), the trochlea (9 to 10 years), and the lateral epicondyle (10 years) (Fig. 12–4). Fusion of the ossification centers occurs as the capitellum, lateral epicondyle, and trochlea fuse just before the completion of growth. The common epiphyseal center then fuses with the distal humeral metaphysis. The ossification centers of the proximal radius and ulna form as separate centers at 4 to 5

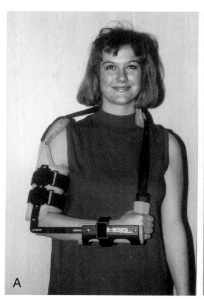 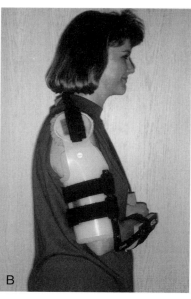

Figure 12–3. *A* and *B,* A commercially available humeral fracture brace with a hinged elbow and hand support. (From: Lee DH, Nevaiser RJ: Upper extremity fractures and dislocations. *In* Feliciano DV, Moore EE, Mattox KL (eds): *Trauma.* 3rd ed. East Norwalk, CT, Appleton & Lange, 1995.)

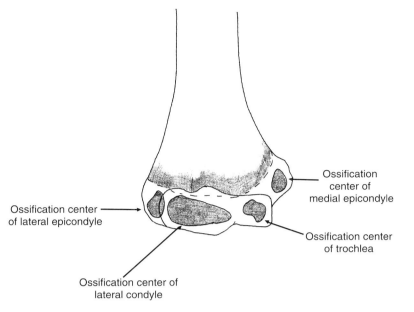

Figure 12–4. The distal humerus forms from the coalescence of multiple ossification centers. The ossification center for the capitellum (lateral condyle) is the first to ossify (6 to 12 months), followed by the medial epicondyle (5 to 6 years), the trochlea (9 to 10 years), and the lateral epicondyle (10 years).

years and 6 to 8 years, respectively, and fuse to their respective metaphyses around the same time that the common distal humeral epiphysis fuses with its metaphysis (at approximately 14 to 17 years of age).

Originating from the medial and lateral epicondyles and supracondylar ridges are the forearm flexor and extensor muscles, respectively. The flexor-pronator group is innervated by the median and ulnar nerves. The extensors and supinator are innervated by the radial nerve. The triceps attaches to the tip of the olecranon process, and the biceps attaches to the bicipital tuberosity of the proximal radius. The brachialis inserts into the coronoid process.

The median nerve crosses the elbow along the anteromedial aspect of the joint. The radial nerve courses along the anterolateral aspect of the joint. The ulnar nerve courses through the cubital tunnel posterior to the medial epicondyle.

Fractures about the elbow are classified according to the location of the fracture. The fractures are divided into extra-articular and intra-articular fractures. Extra-articular fractures include supracondylar (Fig. 12–5), supracondylar process, transcondylar, epicondylar, and radial neck fractures. The supracondylar process, a rare congenital variation, is a small bone process that arises from the anteromedial surface of the humerus about 5 cm proximal to the medial epicondyle. A fracture of this process can be associated with a median nerve injury. Intra-

articular fractures include condylar (Fig. 12–6), olecranon, and radial head or neck (Fig. 12–7) fractures. Coronoid fractures can be intra- or extra-articular, depending on whether the fracture extends into the joint. Radial head and neck fractures can be associated with disruption of the distal radioulnar joint (Essex-Lopresti fracture-dislocation). With this injury there is also a disruption of the forearm interosseous membrane connecting the radius and ulna. The distal radioulnar joint should be carefully assessed for pain, swelling, and tenderness when an elbow injury is evaluated.

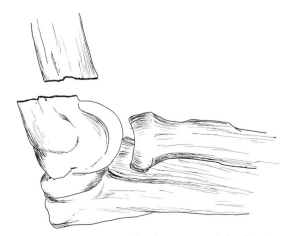

Figure 12–5. An example of a supracondylar fracture of the distal humerus.

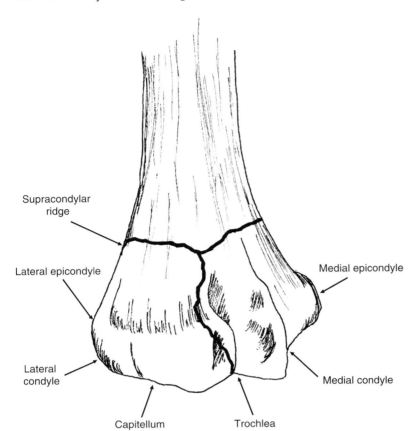

Supracondylar ridge

Lateral epicondyle

Medial epicondyle

Lateral condyle

Medial condyle

Capitellum

Trochlea

Figure 12–6. An example of an intra-articular distal humerus fracture involving both condyles.

Fractures about the elbow are frequently the result of falls on an outstretched arm (supracondylar, transcondylar, condylar fractures) or from direct blows to, or falls on, the elbow (intercondylar or condylar fractures). Factors that contribute to the type and location of the fracture include the age of the patient, the amount of varus or valgus stress, the degree of elbow flexion, and the association of an elbow dislocation that occurs at the time of the injury.[1,4,5,7]

Physeal injuries may occur in skeletally immature patients. The peak age for the location of the physeal injury varies according to the time of fusion of the various regions of the distal humerus and proximal radius and ulna. For instance, supracondylar fractures peak around the ages of 5 to 10 years, whereas medial epicondylar fractures peak around 11 to 15 years of age.

The normal elbow has several bone landmarks, including the tip of the olecranon and the medial and lateral epicondyles. With the elbow flexed to 90 degrees, these three structures should form a triangle in a plane parallel to the posterior surface of the humerus. The radial head, located laterally and just distal to the capitellum, is palpable as the forearm is pronated and supinated.

With a normal elbow fully extended, there is a valgus angulation varying from about 5 to 15 degrees. This carrying angle is usually slightly greater in females. The carrying angle, when compared with the other side, may be altered with various elbow fractures.

Patients with elbow injuries will present with varying degrees of pain, swelling, deformity, crepitus, and limited motion about the elbow, depending on the type of fracture and degree of displacement. As with all injuries, a careful neurologic and vascular examination is needed before and after any type of reduction maneuver is performed.

Associated injuries, especially with supracondylar fractures, include brachial artery and all three major peripheral nerves, the radial, median, and ulnar. The radial nerve is most commonly involved. Radial nerve function is assessed by having the patient actively extend (dorsiflex) the wrist, fingers, and thumb. The presence of sensation (sharp/dull and light touch) over the dorsal

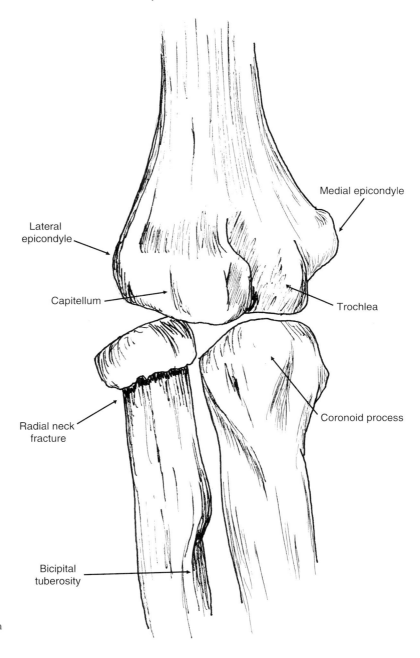

Lateral epicondyle

Capitellum

Radial neck fracture

Bicipital tuberosity

Medial epicondyle

Trochlea

Coronoid process

Figure 12–7. An example of an angulated radial neck fracture.

aspect of the thumb and index metacarpals is tested. Median nerve function is assessed by having the patient palmarly abduct the thumb, then palpation of a contracting abductor pollicis brevis muscle is performed. Sensation (two-point, light touch, sharp/dull) is tested on the pulp of the thumb and index and long and radial aspects of the ring fingers. Ulnar nerve function is tested by having the patient abduct and adduct the fingers. Sensation is tested along the pulp of the little and ulnar aspect of the ring fingers. Both radial and arterial pulses should be palpated, and capillary refill in the digits should be assessed (less than 2 to 3 seconds is normal).

Special care should be taken to examine patients with fractures about the elbow serially, especially in the pediatric population, because of the high potential for a compartment syndrome. Hospitalization of these patients for serial observation should be considered if neurovascular compromise is suspected. Ipsilateral extremity injuries, such as wrist injuries, should always be suspected. Because of the high possibility of neurovascular compromise with supracondylar fractures, especially in the pediatric population, referral to a specialist should be considered.

Good quality anteroposterior and lateral radiographs of the elbow joint are needed. Radiographs of the shoulder and wrist (the joint above and below the area of injury) should be taken. Radiographs of the humeral shaft and forearm may be needed if injury is suspected.

On the lateral radiograph, a subtle sign of an intra-articular injury is the fat pad sign. Distension of the joint capsule from fluid accumulation results in a lucent line over either the anterior or posterior surface of the distal humerus. This is due to the displacement of fat pads that overlie the capsule in the coronoid and olecranon fossas.

Occasionally, tomography or computed tomography (CT scan) may also be helpful in delineating complex fracture patterns about the elbow that are difficult to assess by plain radiographs. These tests should be ordered by the treating physician determining the need for surgery. Arteriography may be indicated if a vascular injury is suspected.

Most nondisplaced fractures can be treated with immobilization, followed by early range of motion exercises when discomfort diminishes (usually 1 week). A posterior long arm splint (Fig. 12–8) is used in addition to a shoulder sling. Displaced fractures, especially supracondylar fractures and fractures involving the articular surface, require closed or open reduction and internal fixation. Methods of immobilization can include posterior elbow splints, casts, or traction. Skin or skeletal traction is occasionally used in children for comminuted fractures or with fractures associated with significant swelling. Prior to definitive operative treatment, most fractures can be immobilized with a posterior long arm splint.

Surgical indications include the debridement of open fractures and repair of brachial arterial injuries. Stabilization of the fracture should be performed prior to arterial repair. This can be performed with internal or external fixation. The indications for open reduction and internal fixation include the treatment of displaced intra-articular fractures (e.g., olecranon, condylar, and comminuted fractures), unstable fractures (e.g., supracondylar and epicondylar fractures), and fracture-dislocations of the elbow. Indications for late surgical reconstruction include the treatment of post-traumatic arthritis, nonunions, malunions, avascular necrosis, instability, nerve injuries, and myositis ossificans.

DISLOCATIONS OF THE ELBOW

Dislocations of the elbow are classified according to the position of the proximal ulna

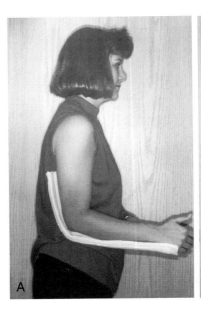
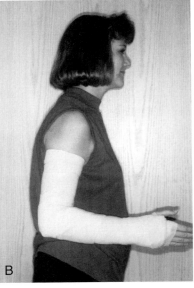

Figure 12–8. *A* and *B,* An example of a posterior elbow long arm splint. This splint can be used for distal humerus, elbow, and proximal forearm injuries. The splint can be combined with a humeral coaptation splint or a forearm sugartong splint. Ace wrapping of the hand is done to prevent swelling. (From: Lee DH, Nevaiser RJ: Upper extremity fractures and dislocations. *In* Feliciano DV, Moore EE, Mattox KL (eds): *Trauma.* 3rd ed. East Norwalk, CT, Appleton & Lange, 1995.)

and radius relative to the humerus. Most dislocations are posterior. With this dislocation, the radius and ulna dislocate together, posterior to the humerus. Pure medial or lateral dislocations are rare. In divergent dislocations, the ulna and radius dislocate in diverging directions—the ulna posteriorly and the radius anteriorly. Isolated ulnar dislocation, without the radius, is not common. Isolated dislocations of the radius are more common in the pediatric population and uncommon in the adult population. With longitudinal traction in the infant or young child, an isolated dislocation of the radial head (nursemaid's elbow or pulled elbow) can occur. The force to produce a pulled elbow may be minimal (such as lifting the child by the hand). The most common age of occurrence is in the 6-month to 3-year age group. Often the child does not complain until someone attempts to move the elbow.

The forearm is held in pronation and is reduced with gentle supination. Radiographs often are not diagnostic, but the dislocation is often reduced by the technologist attempting to position the elbow for the x-ray film. The child is then happy and able to move the elbow. Recurrences are common, and parents may be taught to perform the reduction and eliminate frequent visits to the emergency department. Immobilization following reduction is unnecessary, and long-term sequelae do not occur. Fractures of the proximal ulnar shaft are frequently associated with proximal radial head dislocations and are called Monteggia's fracture-dislocations (Fig. 12–9).

Most dislocations of the elbow are secondary to a fall on an outstretched hand. The more common posterior elbow dislocation is probably secondary to hyperextension of the elbow joint. The addition of varus or valgus stress at the elbow will determine whether the proximal radius and ulna displace medially or laterally. Anterior dislocations are probably secondary to a direct impact on the posterior forearm with the elbow in a position of some flexion. The rare divergent and isolated radial or ulnar dislocation probably requires some form of axial load associated with forearm rotation.

Associated injuries, as with fractures about the elbow, include brachial artery and nerve injuries. Damage to the median, ulnar, and radial nerves have all been reported. Entrapment of the median nerve following reduction of the dislocated elbow has been described. The ulnar nerve is usually injured by a valgus stretch injury. Associated fractures also can occur with elbow dislocations, including epicondylar fractures and coronoid process fractures. A compartment syndrome of the forearm should always be suspected with any elbow injury.[3,6]

Clinically, the appearance of the elbow is similar to that of fractures about the elbow. Palpation of bone landmarks may reveal a more prominent olecranon process with a posterior elbow dislocation, and a less prominent one with an anterior dislocation. Careful assessment of the neurovascular status of the extremity should be determined prior to any treatment.

As with fractures about the elbow, a minimum of two good-quality radiographs should be obtained prior to and after reduction of an elbow dislocation. The presence of fractures should be determined prior to closed reduction of the dislocation. Radiographs of the forearm, wrist, and humerus should be taken.

On the lateral view, the distal humeral trochlear groove should concentrically seat within the ulnar semilunar notch. A line drawn along the radial shaft and through the radial head should intersect the center of the capitellum. True anteroposterior and lateral radiographs centered over the elbow joint are needed to assess adequate reduction of the joint.

Most elbow dislocations can be treated with closed reduction and posterior long arm splint immobilization. Usually some form of anesthesia is needed to perform the reduction. The type of anesthesia may depend on other factors such as the age of the patient, the patient's overall status, duration of the dislocation, and other associated injuries. For posterior dislocations, a closed reduction is performed with longitudinal traction, placed along the forearm. The forearm segment is then translated anteriorly relative to the humerus. Pressure is gently applied to the olecranon process to translate the radius and ulna anteriorly. One method of reduction is performed by placing the patient in a prone position with the arm hanging over the side of the stretcher. Five to ten pounds of weights are hung from the wrist. After 10 to 20 minutes, gentle manipulation of the elbow is then performed. Return of the normal bone architecture of the elbow should occur following reduction. Anterior dislocations are also treated with longitudinal traction followed

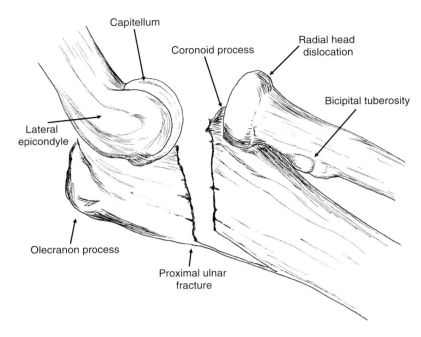

Figure 12–9. An example of a Monteggia fracture-dislocation consisting of a proximal ulnar fracture and a radial head dislocation.

by anterior translation of the humerus relative to the forearm. Medial and lateral dislocations are reduced with longitudinal traction on the forearm with direct medial or lateral pressure. Stability of the reduced elbow is checked with gentle flexion and extension of the elbow. An unstable posterior elbow dislocation will easily redislocate as the elbow is extended.

Radial head dislocations in the pediatric population require a closed reduction. An irreducible dislocation will need an open reduction. Appropriate anesthesia, frequently general anesthesia, is required. The patient should be referred to the appropriate treating physician.

Anteroposterior and lateral radiographs are needed to ensure an adequate reduction of the joint and absence of fractures following joint reduction.

Following reduction of a dislocated elbow, repeat assessment of the neurovascular status should be performed. A long arm posterior splint (see Figure 12–8) is used to immobilize the elbow. If the elbow joint stability is questionable following reduction, radiographs should be obtained in the splint to ensure that the joint is completely reduced.

The surgical indications include open elbow dislocations, dislocations associated with vascular injuries, irreducible dislocations, dislocations associated with fractures (e.g., Monteggia's fracture—see Chapter 13, Fractures of the Forearm), and entrapment of fracture fragments in the joint (e.g., epicondylar fracture). Late surgical indications include the treatment of post-traumatic arthritis, chronic dislocations, malunions, elbow contractures, and nerve injuries.

References

1. Cabanela ME, Morrey BF: Fractures of the proximal ulna and olecranon. *In* Morrey BF (ed): The Elbow. Philadelphia, WB Saunders, 1993, pp 405–440.
2. Epps CH, Grant RE: Fractures of the shaft of the humerus. *In* Rockwood CA, Green DP, Bucholz RW (eds): Fractures in Adults, 3rd ed. Philadelphia, JB Lippincott, 1991, pp 843–869.
3. Holstein A, Lewis GB: Fractures of the humerus with radial nerve paralysis. J Bone Joint Surg 45A:1382–1388, 1963.
4. Hotchkiss RN, Green DP: Fractures and dislocations of the elbow. *In* Rockwood CA, Green DP, Bucholz RW (eds): Fractures in Adults, 3rd ed. Philadelphia, JB Lippincott, 1991, pp 739–841.
5. Jupiter JB, Morrey BF: Fractures of the distal humerus in the adult. *In* Morrey BF (ed): The Elbow. Philadelphia, WB Saunders, 1993, pp 328–366.
6. Linscheid RL, O'Driscoll SW: Elbow dislocations. *In* Morrey BF (ed): The Elbow. Philadelphia, WB Saunders, 1993, pp 441–463.
7. Morrey BF: Radial head fracture. *In* Morrey BF (ed): The Elbow. Philadelphia, WB Saunders, 1993, pp 383–404.
8. Sarmiento A, Kinman PB, Calvin EG, Schmitt RH, Phillips JG: Functional bracing of fractures of the shaft of the humerus. J Bone Joint Surg 59A: 596–601, 1977.

CHAPTER 13

Fractures of the Forearm

Donald H. Lee

A general evaluation of upper extremity injuries is provided in Chapter 11. The forearm skeleton consists of the radius and ulna. Proximally, the radius and ulna articulate with the capitellum and trochlea of the distal humerus, respectively. Distally, the radius and ulna articulate with the carpal bones. The radius and ulna articulate with each other at only the proximal and distal radioulnar joints but are connected by a fibrous interosseous membrane. Forearm rotation occurs with the radius rotating about the ulna.

The radius and ulna form from a fusion of the primary ossification center with proximal and distal secondary growth centers. Both epiphyses are usually fused by the age of 17 to 18 years.

Forearm fractures are classified according to the location of the fracture—proximal, middle, or distal one third shaft fractures (Fig. 13–1). A fracture may involve one or both bones (Fig. 13–2). Fractures of a single forearm bone (radius or ulna) can be associated with a dislocation of the distal or proximal radioulnar joints. A Monteggia's fracture (Fig. 13–3) is a fracture of the proximal ulnar shaft that is associated with a radial head dislocation. A Galeazzi's fracture (Fig. 13–4) is a fracture of the distal third of the radius associated with dislocation of the distal radioulnar joint.[1–6]

In children, incomplete (greenstick) fractures and compression (buckle or torus) fractures frequently occur.

Fractures of the shafts of the radius and ulna are usually from a direct blow to the forearm, a motor vehicle accident, or a direct fall on an outstretched arm.

Findings on a physical examination will vary with the type and degree of fracture sustained by the patient. Most patients present with pain, swelling, and loss of function of the involved forearm and hand. Patients will feel tenderness in the region of the fracture. Abnormal motion, deformity, and crepitus at the fracture site may be noticed with complete fractures. Care should be taken to assess the neurovascular status of the extremity. Suspicion of a compartment syndrome should be high, especially with both bone forearm fractures.

Associated injuries may include nerves (median, ulnar, and radial) and arteries (radial and ulnar). Injuries, including dislocations or subluxations, of the proximal and distal radioulnar joints can occur with forearm fractures. Ipsilateral fractures of the arm, wrist, and hand can occur. A compartment syndrome (see Chapter 2) from soft tissue contusion, hematoma formation, or fracture may be present.

Radiographs should include two views of the entire forearm oriented at 90 degrees to

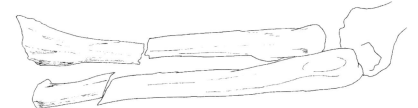

Figure 13–1. A distal one third shaft fracture involving both bones of the forearm.

one another. Radiographs of the elbow and wrist joints should be obtained to rule out injuries in these areas. Care should be taken to evaluate possible injury to the proximal or distal radioulnar joints.

Undisplaced fractures, common in children and uncommon in adults, can be treated with immobilization. Displaced fractures usually require more extensive treatment. In children, closed reduction of the fracture may be indicated. Some form of anesthesia is required for reduction. The method of anesthesia can vary from intravenous sedation, regional arm anesthesia, or general anesthe-

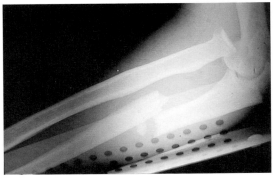

Figure 13–3. A Monteggia's fracture-dislocation.

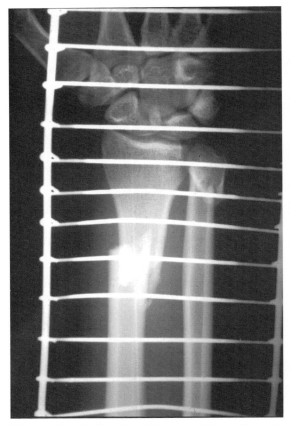

Figure 13–2. A distal third fracture of the radius and ulna.

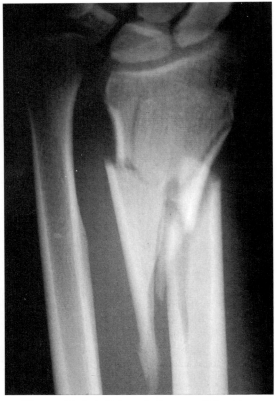

Figure 13–4. A Galeazzi's fracture-dislocation.

sia. Usually finger trap traction with use of 10 to 15 pounds of counterweight is used to provide distraction at the fracture. The fracture is then manipulated into proper alignment. In adults, displaced fractures generally require surgical intervention.

Immobilization of forearm fractures is provided with a sugartong splint (Fig. 13–5). Circumferential cast immobilization is generally not recommended as an initial form of treatment, especially if the patient is discharged from care. If the patient can be closely supervised, circumferential casting can be considered. Swelling from the fracture in association with constriction provided by

the cast may lead to a compartment syndrome. Immobilization of the forearm must include the wrist and the elbow joint to control rotation of the forearm. Repeat radiographs should be taken, especially following manipulation, to check adequacy of the reduction.

Immediate surgical indications include the treatment of open fractures and fractures associated with a compartment syndrome or vascular injury. Other indications for surgical treatment include displaced fractures in adults and fractures failing closed reduction in children. Unstable fractures and fractures associated with dislocation of either the prox-

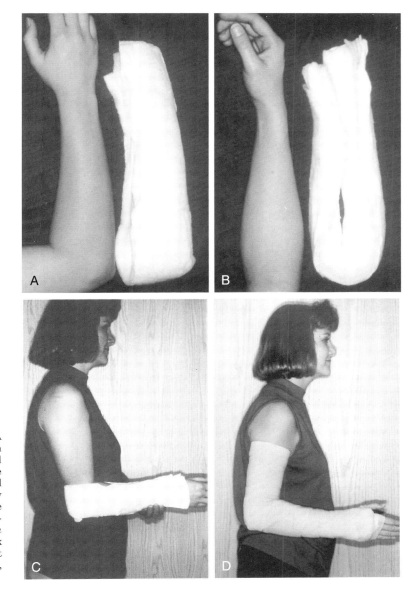

Figure 13–5. *A* through *D*, A sugartong splint. This splint can be used for forearm, distal radius, and wrist injuries. The splint should stop at the distal palmar flexion crease to allow full finger flexion. (From: Lee DH, Nevaiser RJ: Upper extremity fractures and dislocations. *In* Feliciano DV, Moore EE, Mattox KL (eds): *Trauma.* 3rd ed. East Norwalk, CT, Appleton & Lange, 1995.)

imal (Monteggia's fracture-dislocation) or distal radioulnar joints (Galeazzi's fracture-dislocation) also require surgical intervention. Indications for late surgical reconstruction include the treatment of malunions, nonunions, post-traumatic arthritis of the proximal or distal radioulnar joints, synostosis between the radius and ulna, and neurologic and other soft tissue injuries.

References

1. Anderson LD, Sisk TD, Park WI III, Tooms RE: Compression-plate fixation in acute diaphyseal fractures of the radius and ulna. J Bone Joint Surg 57A:287–297, 1975.
2. Anderson LD, Meyer LD: Fractures of the shafts of the radius and ulna. *In* Rockwood CA, Green DP, Bucholz RW (eds): Fractures in Adults, 3rd ed. Philadelphia, JB Lippincott, 1991, pp 679–737.
3. Bado JL: The Monteggia lesion. Clin Orthop 50:71–86, 1967.
4. Mikic ZD: Galeazzi fracture dislocations. J Bone Joint Surg 57A:1071–1080, 1975.
5. Mohan K, Gupta AK, Sharma J, Singh AK, Jain AK: Internal fixation in 50 cases of Galeazzi fracture. Acta Orthop Scand 59:318–320, 1988.
6. Reckling FW: Unstable fracture-dislocations of the forearm (Monteggia and Galeazzi lesions). J Bone Joint Surg 64A:857–863, 1982.

CHAPTER 14

Fractures and Ligament Injuries of the Wrist

Glenn Jonas

Victoria R. Masear

DISTAL RADIUS FRACTURES

Fractures of the distal radius are common injuries primarily affecting the elderly population. As a result of the effects of osteoporosis in this group, the energy required to cause a fracture is significantly less than that associated with fractures in the younger population. While many older patients will have a good outcome even with a residual deformity, a lesser deformity in a younger patient may lead to an unacceptable result. In addition, intra-articular involvement must be more aggressively treated in the younger population to avoid degenerative arthritis in the future.

There are many classification systems of distal radius injuries. They all attempt to define the injury, provide treatment options, and predict outcome. The treatment in these injuries is tailored to the patient more than to the specific injury. Rather than describing the injuries here by any one of the multitude of classifications, the fractures will be discussed by their well-known eponyms. When evaluating distal radius fractures, one should consider the direction and degree of *displacement* or angulation of the distal fragment, the degree of *comminution,* associated distal *radioulnar* or carpal injuries, and intra-articular radiocarpal involvement. Significant displacement, angulation, comminution, and intra-articular radiocarpal or radioulnar involvement may contribute to a poor result.

The majority of distal radius fractures can be evaluated for treatment with the use of standard posteroanterior (PA), lateral, and oblique radiographs. In addition, tomograms or computed tomography scans may be required to evaluate better the extent of intra-articular displacement. Three radiographic measurements are critical in the assessment of the distal radius: radial length, *radial inclination,* and *palmar slope.*[5] The radial length is normally 11 to 12 mm and is measured on the PA radiograph.[11] It is the length from the tip of the radial styloid to a perpendicular line drawn from the distal articular surface of the ulna. The radial inclination averages 23 degrees and is measured on the PA view.[9] It is the angle of projection of the articular surface of the radius toward the ulna. The palmar slope of the distal radius measures 11 to 12 degrees and is measured on the lateral.[9] This represents the amount of downward and forward bend to the distal radius (Fig. 14–1).

It has been shown that grip strength is impaired if a fracture heals with greater than 20 degrees of volar apex angulation, radial inclination less than 10 degrees, or radial shortening of more than 2 mm.[26] Failure to maintain length is associated with pain in the distal radioulnar joint and often will require future surgery to re-establish radial length or excise the incongruous distal radioulnar joint surface. Treatment of these fractures attempts to restore these measurements and restore intra-articular congruity. But, function should never be sacrificed in order to create a healthy-appearing radiograph! It may be better to accept a collapsed, angulated wrist in an elderly patient in order to begin early range of motion exercises to prevent stiffness.

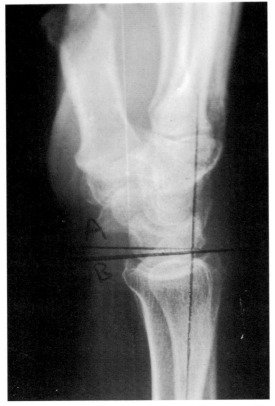

Figure 14–1. The volar tilt is the angle between a line connecting the dorsal and volar lips of the radius and a line perpendicular to the radial shaft.

Colles' Fracture

In the Colles' fracture, the distal radius fragment is displaced dorsally and proximally and the plane of the articular surface of the radial fragment tilts dorsally (Fig. 14–2). An associated ulnar styloid fracture may be present. Reduction of the fracture is greatly enhanced by the use of a Bier block or hematoma block. With the patient supine, finger traps are applied. With the elbow flexed at right angle, countertraction is applied through weight just proximal to the elbow crease. Traction is maintained for approximately 5 minutes. To reduce the fragment, the fingers of both hands are placed on the volar side of the forearm and both thumbs are used to push the distal fragment forward and toward the ulna.[4,5,21] Following reduction, a sugartong splint is applied with the forearm in neutral rotation. The wrist should not be placed in significant flexion, as this leads to median nerve compression and stiff fingers. The splint will allow slight wrist flexion and limited elbow motion without forearm rotation. Postreduction roentgenograms should show restored radial length, radial inclination, and palmar slope. An acceptable reduction is less than 2 mm of shortening, less than 2 mm of displacement of intra-articular fragments, and less than 5 degrees of dorsal tilt of the radius. In those fractures involving the ulnar styloid, the styloid often will remain displaced after reduction. The natural history of displaced ulnar styloid fractures is yet to be resolved.

These fractures may be treated with 2 weeks of splinting followed by 3 weeks in a short arm cast. Follow-up radiographs should be obtained weekly for the first 3 weeks to ensure that there is no loss of reduction. Some recommend a period of splinting after removal of the cast for additional support.[21] During the period of immobilization and subsequent splinting, motion of the fingers and shoulder is essential.

In comminuted Colles' fractures, dorsal redisplacement and shortening often occur following reduction. This is especially common in older adults with osteoporotic bone. In addition, often there is involvement of the distal ulna and distal radioulnar joint. The treatment for comminuted fractures may require external fixation, external fixation with K-wire fixation, or open reduction with

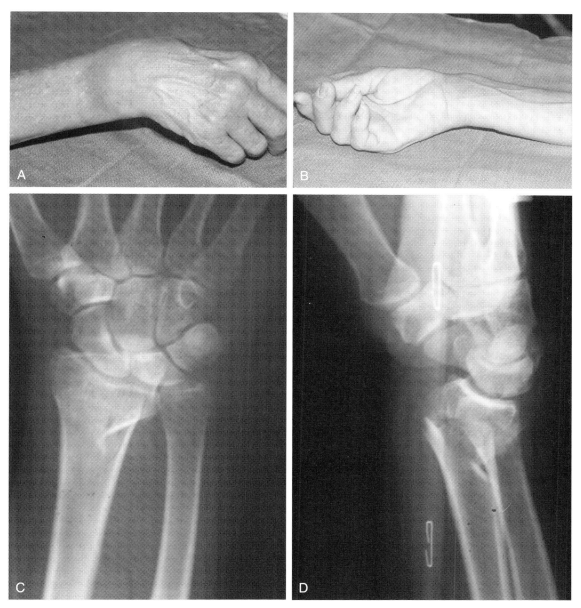

Figure 14–2. *A* and *B,* The classic "silver fork" deformity as described by Colles. *C,* PA radiograph of a distal radial metaphyseal fracture. *D,* Lateral radiograph confirms the volar apex angulation and loss of volar tilt typical of Colles' fractures.

internal fixation and bone grafting. Many of the patients will require surgical treatment in the future for a painful distal radioulnar joint. Definitive treatment must be individualized. Some collapse is acceptable in the physiologically older patient but these fractures should be treated more aggressively in the younger, more active patient.

Smith's Fracture

In contrast to the dorsally displaced Colles' fracture, the less common Smith's fracture displaces volarly and proximally (Fig. 14–3). The fracture line runs obliquely through the metaphyseal bone approximately 1 to 2 cm proximal to the articular surface. If mistak-

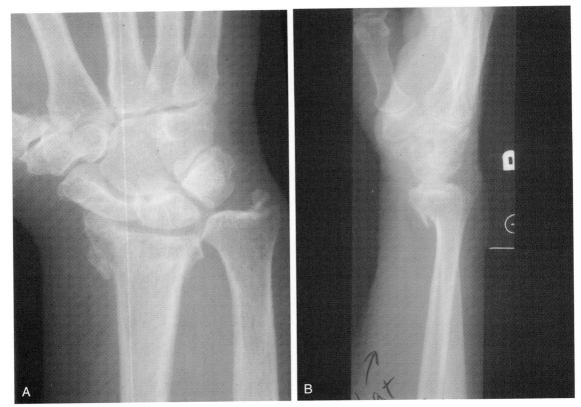

Figure 14–3. PA (*A*) and lateral (*B*) radiograph showing Smith's type of fracture.

enly treated as a Colles' fracture, significant disability may result. In these fractures, reduction is accomplished with the aid of traction as described for reduction of the Colles' fracture. While traction is maintained, the fingers of both hands support the proximal fragment. Both thumbs are used to press on the volar aspect of the distal forearm, pushing the distal fragment dorsally. A sugartong splint is applied with the wrist in slight dorsiflexion and ulnar deviation.[5,28]

Barton's Fracture

This is a fracture-dislocation in which a portion of the volar or dorsal articular surface of the distal radius is sheared off, displacing the carpus volarly or dorsally, and proximally (Fig. 14–4).[5] These fractures are extremely unstable and require a buttress fixation device to prevent recurrent disloca-

tion. A splint in neutral wrist position will suffice until surgery.

Chauffeur's Fracture

This is a fracture of the radial styloid process (Fig. 14–5). It often occurs in association with Colles'-type fractures and is important because it is intra-articular and displacement may lead to early arthritis. Large radial styloid fragments may displace even after satisfactory reduction, and therefore added fixation (K-wire or screw) to prevent displacement may be required.

Lunate Load or Die-Punch Fracture

This intra-articular fracture occurs with proximal migration of the lunate into the distal radius (Fig. 14–6). The fracture disrupts the distal radius articular surface and must

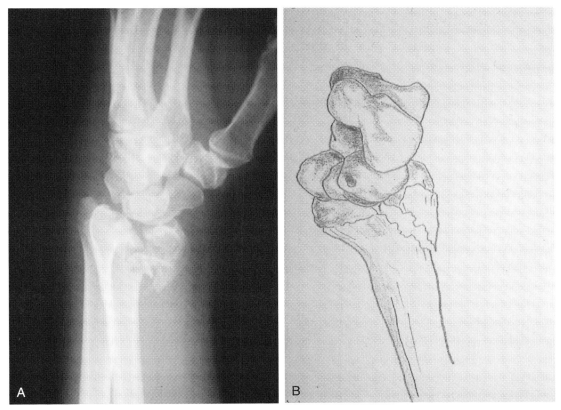

Figure 14–4. *A,* A volar Barton's fracture. *B,* Artist's depiction of a dorsal Barton's fracture.

be elevated to prevent arthritic changes in the joint. Unlike the displaced fracture fragments of the extra-articular Colles' fracture, which can be reduced with the use of traction and manipulation, depressed die-punch fragments must be surgically elevated and bone-grafted.[14,19] Depressions of the articular surface in younger people should be aggressively treated.

Complications of Distal Radius Fractures

The most common acute complication of distal radius fractures is median nerve compression. If a complete nerve lesion is present and no improvement is seen within 2 days following reduction, then surgical exploration and nerve release are justified. If the nerve lesion results or worsens from the reduction maneuver, then all bandages should be released and the wrist placed in neutral. With a partial nerve lesion, the fracture should be reduced, initially splinted

until the swelling begins to subside, and then casted. If no improvement is noted after 48 hours, surgical exploration and release may be required.[7,18] More commonly, patients will have loss of finger motion and loss of grip strength because of post-traumatic edema and weakness from disuse. Casting and splinting always should be applied in a way that does not restrict motion of the fingers. Elderly patients also should be instructed in shoulder exercises to prevent stiffness. Slings may be worn initially for comfort but should be discontinued after a few days. The extensor tendon function of the thumb should be checked initially and at follow-up visits. In a small number of cases the extensor pollicis longus tendon will rupture and require a tendon transfer for reconstruction.[13]

A significant number of distal radius fractures are associated with scaphoid fractures and scapholunate ligament injuries, especially in the younger population. These injuries are difficult to identify in the acute

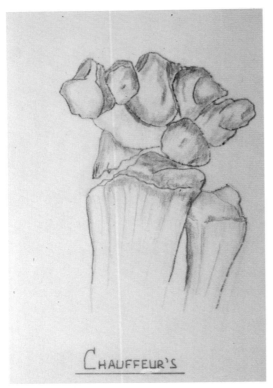

CHAUFFEUR'S

Figure 14–5. Radial styloid fracture (Chauffeur's).

setting and must be kept in mind in the evaluation of initial and follow-up radiographs. If an associated scaphoid fracture is identified, a long arm thumb spica cast is required for immobilization. Depending on the character of either fracture, surgical intervention may be required.

Post-traumatic arthritis and residual deformity must be treated on an individual basis. A high rate of distal radioulnar arthritis (19 percent) has been reported.[10] Corrective osteotomies, fusions, or arthroplasties may benefit the symptomatic patient. In summary, the treatment of distal radius fractures depends on the physiologic age of the patient, his or her functional requirements, the energy of injury, the fracture pattern, and the quality of bone.

Distal Radius Fractures in Children

The great majority of distal radius fractures in children may be treated with gentle reduction and 6 weeks of casting. These fractures are usually Salter Harris type II injuries (see Chapter 1) and will remodel significantly.[21] Therefore, reduction need not be anatomic

for the future result to be excellent. Avoid multiple rigorous reductions that may cause further injury. Be aware that these injuries may involve an element of crush to the growth plate and may result in a growth disturbance of the radial physis. Only time will tell, and patient and parent should be made aware of this possibility. If physeal plate damage has occurred, there are many operative procedures to aid in correcting or avoiding unequal growth of the distal radius and ulna.

CARPAL DISLOCATIONS AND INSTABILITIES

The wrist is made up of seven carpal bones (the pisiform is a sesamoid of the flexor carpi ulnaris and is not involved in carpal motion) arranged into two transverse rows connected by a complex arrangement of ligaments (Fig. 14–7). The bone and ligamentous architecture of the wrist allows for the considerable motion and stability of the carpus. Wrist ligamentous injuries upset this delicate balance and lead to predictable patterns of instability that can be identified on clinical and radiographic examinations. Four stages of progressive ligamentous injury have been described by Mayfield and associates.[16,17] These stages help explain the degree and direction of the injuring force. The range of wrist ligamentous injury begins with disruption of the scapholunate interosseous ligament and progresses to a dorsal perilunate and ultimately a volar lunate dislocation.

Routine x-ray views of the wrist include PA, lateral, and a 45-degree oblique with the wrist in 45 degrees of pronation. In the uninjured wrist, the scaphoid and lunate move in similar directions owing to competence of the interosseous ligament. Disruption of the interosseous ligament results in abnormal flexion of the scaphoid and extension (or dorsiflexion) of the lunate.

On the PA radiograph there should be no overlap of the carpal bones between the proximal and distal rows. Particular attention should be paid to the relationship between the lunate and capitate; overlap of these bones is highly suggestive of a carpal derangement. If the normally quadrilateral projection of the lunate appears triangular, this is suggestive of an abnormal position of the lunate relative to the rest of the carpus (Fig. 14–8). The scaphoid is normally elon-

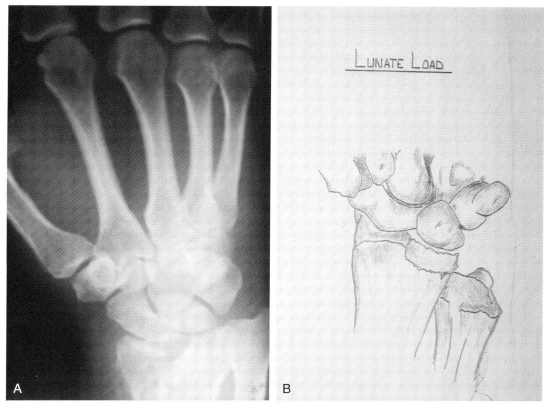

Figure 14–6. *A,* Die punch or lunate load fracture with severe intra-articular comminution. *B,* Compression of lunate fossa of radius as seen in a lunate load fracture.

gated. If the projection of the scaphoid appears foreshortened or there is a ring density in the body of the scaphoid, this may represent an abnormally flexed position of the scaphoid, commonly seen in scapholunate ligament tears (Fig. 14–9). Evaluate the space between the scaphoid and lunate. Widening of greater than 3 mm is significant for scapholunate ligament tears (Fig. 14–10).[23] Measure the carpal height.[29] The ratio of the length from the distal capitate to the radius divided by the length of the third metacarpal is known as the carpal height index and is normally 0.51 to 0.57.[29] Abnormal values are seen in carpal dislocations and advanced carpal collapse.

Make sure that the lateral x-ray view is a true lateral. That is, the metacarpals must be superimposed upon one another. In addition, the view must be taken with the wrist neither ulnarly nor radially deviated, because the position of the lunate and scaphoid are affected by the position of the wrist. As a result of wrist architecture, as the wrist

ulnarly deviates the lunate dorsiflexes and the scaphoid becomes more colinear with the long axis of the radius. As the wrist radially deviates, the lunate and the scaphoid palmar flex.[29] The long axes of the radius, lunate, and capitate are normally colinear or with a slight volar tilt of the lunate. If the lunate is tipped dorsally, this is suggestive of a scapholunate interosseous ligament tear. The lunate tipped volarly suggests a lunotriquetral tear (Fig. 14–11). Normally, there may be up to 15 degrees of lunate tilt in either direction. Check the relationship between the long axis of the scaphoid and the long axis of the lunate. The angle between them should range between 30 and 60 degrees (Fig. 14–12).[15] Abnormal values suggest carpal instability.

CARPAL INSTABILITY FROM SCAPHOLUNATE DISSOCIATION

Injury to the scapholunate interosseous ligament and possibly some of the secondary

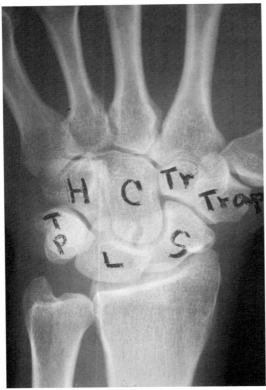

Figure 14–7. The normal wrist is composed of eight carpal bones: T = triquetrum, P = pisiform, H = hamate, C = capitate, Tr = trapezoid, Trap = trapezium, S = scaphoid, L = lunate.

lunate greater than 2 to 3 mm,[23] a foreshortened scaphoid (due to its abnormal flexion) demonstrating a cortical ring sign, and a triangular lunate. On the lateral radiograph, the lunate becomes dorsiflexed in relation to the radius and capitate, and the scapholunate angle increases to greater than 60 degrees (see Fig. 14–11A).

The treatment of scapholunate ligament tears is controversial. Most experts agree that reduction, whether closed with K-wires or open with primary ligamentous repair or reconstruction, is required. If ligament injury is suspected but not confirmed on standard radiographs, arthroscopic evaluation to visualize the scapholunate ligament is helpful. Closed cast treatment will not adequately reduce the scapholunate diastasis, and therefore the patient may be splinted in neutral in the acute setting but referred for surgical reduction and ligament repair. The patient first presenting as a SLAC wrist may require carpal arthrodesis (bone fusion) or arthroplasty (joint resurfacing) for pain relief.

restraining ligaments presents in numerous ways and with subtle radiographic and clinical findings. Acute injuries are rarely diagnosed in clinical practice. In general, most patients present with weeks or months of dorsal radial wrist pain localized to the scapholunate interval, which may limit wrist motion. There may also be pain in the anatomic snuffbox (area on radial side of the wrist between tendons that extend and abduct the thumb) and over the tubercle of the scaphoid. If left untreated, these patients may present with advanced arthritis of the wrist, known as scapholunate advanced collapse (or SLAC wrist). This is an arthritis secondary to scapholunate instability and associated abnormal motion of the carpal bones, with marked arthroses of the radioscaphoid and capitolunate joints and with marked migration of the capitate between the scaphoid and lunate bones (Fig. 14–13). On the PA radiograph of a wrist with a scapholunate instability, findings include an increased gap between the scaphoid and

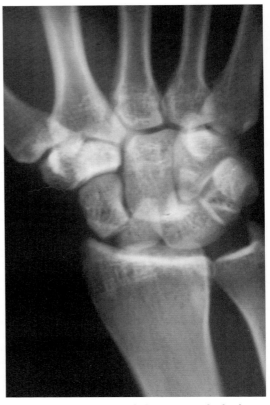

Figure 14–8. Perilunate dislocation, with the lunate taking on a triangular shape on the PA radiograph.

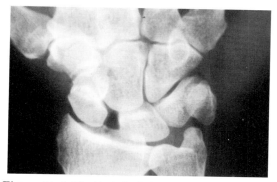

Figure 14–9. "Cortical ring" sign over the distal pole of the scaphoid in a patient with a scapholunate diastasis.

Triquetrolunate Dissociation

A less common carpal instability occurs with injury to the ligament between the lunate and triquetrum.[22] The history is most commonly that of hyperpronation or dorsiflexion with subsequent dorsal ulnar-sided wrist pain. On physical examination, pain may be elicited by stabilizing the lunate with one hand while the triquetrum is moved palmarly and dorsally with the other hand. Although there are many causes of ulnar-sided wrist pain, the lateral radiograph can be diagnostic of lunotriquetral ligament injury. This view will demonstrate a volar (palmar) tilting of the lunate (see Fig. 14–11*B*). These injuries often require surgical fixation.

Triangular Fibrocartilage Injuries

The triangular fibrocartilage complex (TFCC) is the major stabilizer of the distal radioulnar joint and ulnar carpus. It is made up of ligaments that extend from the ulnar portion of the distal radius into the ulnar styloid and distally into the lunate, triquetrum, and base of the fifth metacarpal, creating a sling that supports forces crossing the ulnar portion of the wrist joint. Injury to this complex occurs in association with fractures involving the distal radioulnar joint and ulnar styloid, with dorsal or volar dislocation of the distal ulna in respect to the radius, and as isolated tears with no evidence of dislocation or instability. The patient will describe wrist pain over the ulnar head, often associated with a "clicking" of the wrist, with radial-ulnar deviation or pronation-supination of the wrist.[3] Treatment of these injuries

may require arthroscopic evaluation of the TFCC and possible debridement or repair. In cases of displaced ulnar styloid fractures, an attempt at reduction and casting in a short arm cast in neutral with mild ulnar deviation may correct the deformity.[3] If this is unsuccessful and the patient is symptomatic, surgical correction may be performed later.

Distal Radioulnar Dislocations

Dislocations of the distal radioulnar joint may be treated with cast immobilization for 6 weeks. An ulnar volar dislocation is reduced by pronating the forearm and applying a long arm cast or sugartong splint. Dorsal dislocations are reduced by full supination and immobilization (Fig. 14–14). These injuries may be associated with radial head fractures, distal radioulnar joint fractures, or soft tissue disruption at the radioulnar interosseous membrane and distal radioulnar joint. Therefore, the evaluation must include the elbow, forearm, and wrist.

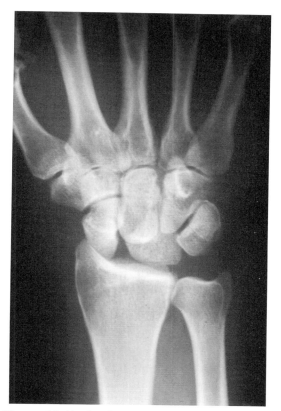

Figure 14–10. Scapholunate diastasis with greater than 3-mm width between the scaphoid and lunate.

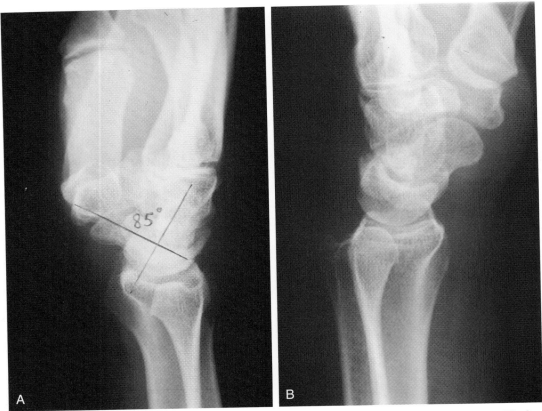

Figure 14–11. *A,* Dorsal intercalary segment instability (DISI) with an 85-degree scapholunate angle. The lunate is dorsiflexed relative to the long axis of the radius. *B,* Volar intercalary segment instability (VISI) with volar tilting of the lunate.

Reduction may require regional anesthesia. Associated injuries and irreducible dislocations may require operative intervention. Reduction should be documented by PA and true lateral x-ray views of the wrist.

CARPAL DISLOCATIONS AND FRACTURE DISLOCATIONS

The diagnosis of acute, severe ligamentous injury with concomitant carpal dislocation is relatively obvious. The radiographs display either a dorsal perilunate dislocation or a volar dislocation of the lunate into the carpal canal. The capitate and the rest of the carpal bones lie dorsal to the lunate on the lateral radiograph of the wrist (Fig. 14–15). These dislocations are commonly associated with fractures of the scaphoid. Clinically, the patient presents with acute wrist pain, weakness, and wrist swelling. In some cases of volar lunate dislocation, carpal tunnel symptoms are present.

These high-energy injuries require immediate reduction. The technique described by Green includes longitudinal traction in finger traps with 10 to 15 lbs of counterweight.[12] Ideally, this should be performed under adequate anesthesia. During this traction period a PA x-ray view of the wrist should be performed to delineate injuries that may have been missed on previous films. After 10 minutes the finger traps are removed, and the lunate is stabilized volarly by the physician's thumb while the other hand is used to push the capitate over the dorsal pole of the lunate.[5,12] Flexion of the wrist may aid in bringing the capitate distally. After reduction, the patient should be placed in a thumb spica splint. Postreduction roentgenograms should demonstrate reduction of the dislocation. It is generally accepted that these injuries, with or without scaphoid fractures, will require operative fixation. The best results

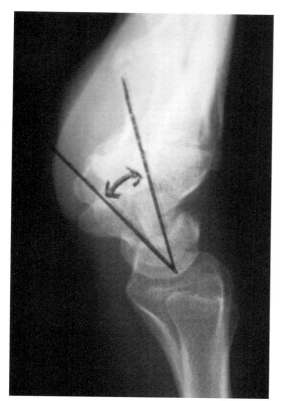

Figure 14–12. The normal scapholunate angle is between 30 and 60 degrees. The lines drawn are a perpendicular one to the tangential line of the lunate and a line along the long axis of the scaphoid.

radiographs at 2 to 4 weeks to allow for resorption at the fracture line. If the presence of fracture is not evident on these repeat films but the patient still has pain or tenderness in the anatomic snuffbox, the next step may include bone scanning (which is highly sensitive but not specific) or computed tomography. Another option is to continue casting for up to 6 weeks, by which time the fracture line should be evident on plain films.[23] These fractures are at times difficult to diagnose and may lead to poor outcomes if not immobilized initially.

The initial treatment of these injuries is cast immobilization. A generally accepted method is a well-fitting long arm thumb spica cast leaving the fingers free. At 6 weeks the cast is converted to a short arm thumb spica cast. In general, fractures of the carpal bones are casted until there is radiologic evidence of union (trabeculae bridging the fracture site). Then range of motion and graduated exercises for strengthening are begun.

are achieved with definitive operative treatment within 1 to 2 weeks.

CARPAL FRACTURES

Scaphoid

The most frequently seen clinical picture is that of a young adult with a history of a fall on the outstretched hand and subsequent radial-sided wrist pain. The pain may be localized more specifically to the anatomic snuffbox (area on radial side of the wrist between tendons that extend and abduct the thumb) (Fig. 14–16). The radiographic examinations that best delineate the presence of fracture are the standard PA, an ulnar deviation PA, a true lateral, and a 45-degree pronation PA view[1] (Fig. 14–17). If these radiographs do not display a fracture but there is a strong clinical suspicion of fracture, the patient still should be casted, with repeat

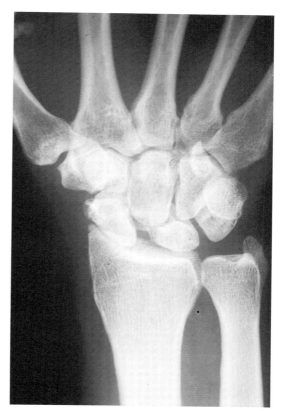

Figure 14–13. Scapholunate advanced collapse (SLAC) wrist with scapholunate diastasis and arthritic changes in the radioscaphoid, scaphocapitate, and capitolunate intervals (as demonstrated by the narrowed joint spaces).

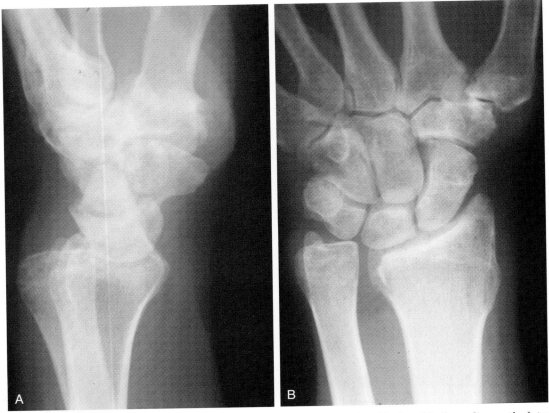

Figure 14–14. Dorsal dislocation of the distal radioulnar joint. The ulnar head is dorsal to the radius on the lateral radiograph (*A*), and the radioulnar joint is widened on the PA radiograph (*B*).

Cast treatment of undisplaced fractures for 8 to 12 weeks results in consistently successful results. If the fracture involves the proximal one third of the scaphoid, the length of immobilization may need to be increased to 16 to 24 weeks. The scaphoid is known to have a tenuous blood supply that enters the bone distally. Disruption of the blood supply to the proximal pole of the scaphoid leads to a high incidence of nonunion (Fig. 14–18). Factors that correlate with poor results are late diagnosis, proximal location of fracture line, fracture displacement, and fracture angulation. In these instances, immobilization may not be adequate, and open reduction with internal fixation may be required.

Lunate

Traumatic fracture of the lunate is extremely rare. However, lunate fracture and collapse are associated with a clinical entity known as *Kienböck's disease,* which is an avascular necrosis of the lunate thought to be the result of chronic microtrauma to the lunate. Classically, the patient is a young man with dorsal central wrist pain and swelling and loss of grip strength and wrist motion.[1] The diagnosis is made on standard wrist views that display an increased lunate density suggestive of lunate avascular necrosis and collapse. The disease progresses radiologically from a subtle linear density to a pattern of sclerosis, loss of lunate height, fragmentation, and finally wrist collapse and arthritis (Fig. 14–19). The disease is often associated with patients whose ulnas are shorter than the radius on the PA radiograph of the wrist. This has been termed an ulnar negative wrist. It has been suggested that, in the ulnar negative wrist, shear forces are increased on the lunate due to its less supported position. If there is clinical suspicion without evidence of fracture or sclerosis, technetium bone scanning and MRI may be helpful, or the wrist may be splinted or casted with repeat plain x-ray views after one month. It is gener-

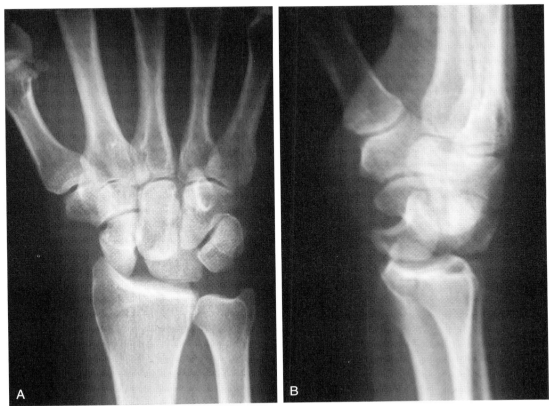

Figure 14–15. A dorsal perilunate dislocation. There is increased space between the scaphoid and lunate, and the lunate is triangular on the PA view (*A*). The lateral radiograph (*B*) shows the other carpal bones dorsal to the lunate. Continued force would push the lunate into the carpal tunnel (a volar lunate dislocation).

ally accepted that advanced cases will require surgical procedures to unload the lunate or fuse the carpal bones or wrist joint.

Triquetrum

Fractures of the triquetrum are the third most common carpal fracture, after those of the scaphoid and lunate.[23] The most common mechanism of injury is a forced hyperextension of the ulnarly deviated wrist, with impingement of the ulnar styloid into the dorsal proximal aspect of the triquetrum. The fracture is best seen on lateral or oblique radiographs of the wrist and responds well to 4 to 6 weeks of short arm splinting or casting with the wrist in neutral (Fig. 14–20). This fracture most commonly is seen as a flake of bone on the lateral radiograph, but it may also present as fracture through the body of the triquetrum. Similar cast treatment is employed for these body frac-

tures, but if markedly displaced, they may require operative reduction.

Trapezium

Fractures of the trapezium are uncommon injuries. They occur as a result of a direct blow, such as a fall onto an outstretched hand, or they may result from thumb axial compression or hyperabduction. These injuries are often associated with fractures of the thumb metacarpal or radius. There are two major types: one occurs through the body of the trapezium, and the other through the trapezial ridge. Standard wrist radiographs should demonstrate a body fracture, but trapezial ridge fractures require carpal tunnel views and Bett's view, obtained with the hypothenar eminence resting on the plate, the thumb extended and abducted, and the hand pronated slightly from neutral. Undisplaced body fractures may be treated in a

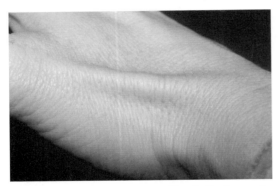

Figure 14–16. The anatomic snuffbox is the depression just volar to the extensor pollicis longus tendon.

short arm thumb spica cast for 3 to 6 weeks.[23] Displaced body fractures are usually intra-articular and may require surgical reduction. Fractures of the trapezial ridge can be initially treated with casting of the thumb in full abduction. It is not uncommon for these ridge fractures to result in a painful non-union requiring future surgical excision.

Trapezoid

Trapezoid fractures are rare. They occur as a result of force applied through the index metacarpal and may be associated with dorsal dislocation of the trapezoid or metacarpal.[1] These fractures are difficult to visualize and may require computed tomography for further delineation. While minimally displaced fractures can be treated with short arm cast immobilization, displaced fractures or dislocations may require operative treatment.

Capitate

Capitate fractures are uncommon and often lead to unsatisfactory outcomes. These fractures are often the result of a hyperdorsiflexion of the wrist, and it is hypothesized that the dorsal lip of the radius impinges upon the capitate, causing its fracture. Scaphoid wrist fractures are often associated with these injuries and should be sought when

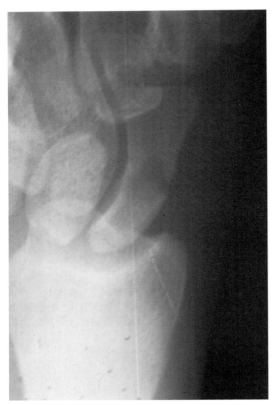

Figure 14–17. Scaphoid fractures are best seen on the "scaphoid view."

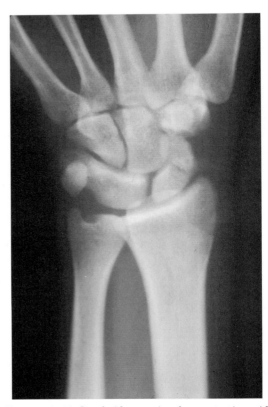

Figure 14–18. Scaphoid nonunion demonstrating widening and cystic changes around the fracture site. There is a coincidental lunatotriquetral coalition.

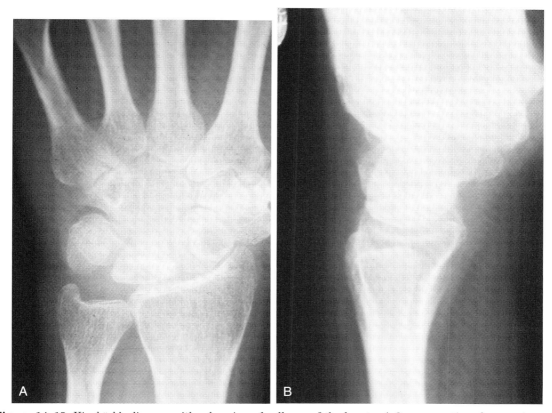

Figure 14–19. Kienböck's disease, with sclerosis and collapse of the lunate. A 3-mm negative ulnar variance is seen on the PA view *(A)*.

evaluating capitate injuries. Isolated fractures of the capitate that are nondisplaced may be treated with a short arm cast, but some have been reported to progress to avascular necrosis. Displaced fractures and those associated with scaphoid fractures (known as the scaphoid-capitate syndrome) require open treatment.

Hamate

Fractures of the body of the hamate are uncommon and usually are associated with injury to the ring and little metacarpal bases. Fractures of the hamulus process *(hook of hamate)* are not uncommon and occur with blunt trauma to the ulnar base of the wrist. This injury occurs in golf, racquet sports, baseball, and other activities in which the ulnar base of the hand is subjected to blunt trauma. Patients commonly describe a dull, aching pain that can be elicited by deep palpation at the base of the hypothenar emi-

nence and with abduction of the little finger against resistance. Ulnar nerve involvement as well as rupture of the flexor tendon to the little finger has been associated with this injury.[1] The diagnosis is made with a carpal tunnel profile view, or with a 45-degree supination oblique view in which the hand is held in 45 degrees of supination, mild radial deviation, and dorsiflexion. If these views do not display the fracture, computed tomography or a CT scan can be used. Hamate hook fractures may be treated acutely with cast immobilization but often do not heal and may require surgical excision or internal fixation.

Pisiform

Fractures of the pisiform occur from blunt trauma to the hypothenar eminence. They are difficult to visualize radiographically and may require computed tomography for diagnosis. Casting is recommended initially, but continued pain may necessitate surgical exci-

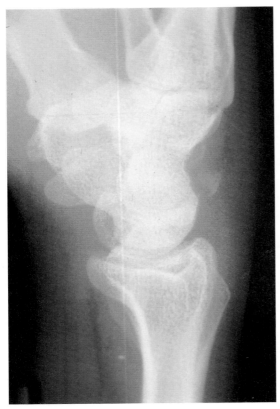

Figure 14–20. Triquetral fractures are best identified by the dorsal fragment on the lateral radiograph. PA radiographs are usually unremarkable.

sion. Excision does not seem to have any effect on grip strength or wrist motion.

References

1. Amadio PC, Taleisnik J: Fractures of the carpal bones. *In* Green DP (ed): Operative Hand Surgery, 3rd ed. New York, Churchill Livingstone, 1993, pp 799–852.
2. Bednar J, Osterman L: Carpal instability: Evaluation and treatment. J Am Acad Orthop Surg 1:10–18, 1993.
3. Bowers WH: The distal radioulnar joint. *In* Green DP (ed): Operative Hand Surgery. New York, Churchill Livingstone, 1993, pp 973–1019.
4. Charnley J: The Closed Treatment of Common Fractures, 3rd ed. Edinburgh, Churchill Livingstone, 1961, pp 128–143.
5. Connolly JF: The Management of Fractures and Dislocations. Philadelphia, WB Saunders, 1981, pp 1008–1134.
6. Cooney WP III, Agee JM, Hastings H II, Melone CP, Rayhack JM: Management of intraarticular fractures of the distal radius. Contemp Orthop 21:71–104, 1990.
7. Cooney WP III, Dobyns JH, Linscheid RL: Complications of Colles fractures. J Bone Joint Surg 62A:613–619, 1980.
8. Cooney WP III, Linscheid RL, Dobyns JH: Scapholunate dissociation. *In* Rockwood CA, Green DP (eds): Fractures in Adults, 3rd ed. Philadelphia, JB Lippincott, 1991, pp 609–620.
9. Friberg S, Lindstron B: Radiographic measurements of the radiocarpal joint in normal adults. Acta Radiol (Stockh) 17:249, 1976.
10. Frykman G: Fracture of the distal radius including sequelae—shoulder hand finger syndrome, disturbance in the distal radioulnar joint and impairment of nerve function. A clinical and experimental study. Acta Orthop Scand (Suppl) 108:1–155, 1967.
11. Gartland JJ, Jr, Werley CW: Evaluation of healed Colles' fractures. J Bone Joint Surg 33:895–907, 1951.
12. Green DP: Carpal dislocations and instabilities. *In* Green DP (ed): Operative Hand Surgery, 3rd ed. New York, Churchill Livingstone, 1993, pp 861–919.
13. Hirasawa Y, Katsumi Y, Akiyoshi T, Tamai K, Tokioka T: Clinical and microangiographic studies on repair of the EPL tendon after distal radius fractures. J Hand Surg 15B:51–57, 1990.
14. Knirk JL, Jupiter JB: Intraarticular fractures of the distal end of the radius in young adults. J Bone Joint Surg 68A:647–659, 1988.
15. Linscheid RL: Kinematic considerations of the wrist. Clin Orthop 202:27–39, 1986.
16. Mayfield JK: Patterns of injury to carpal ligaments; A spectrum. Clin Orthop 187:36–42, 1984.
17. Mayfield JK: Wrist ligamentous anatomy and pathogenesis of carpal instability. Orthop Clin North Am 15:209–216, 1984.
18. McMurtry RY, Jupiter JB: Fractures of the distal radius. *In* Browner BD, Jupiter JB, Levine AM, Trafton PG (eds): Skeletal Trauma. Philadelphia, WB Saunders, 1992, pp 1063–1094.
19. Melone CP: Open treatment for displaced articular fractures of the distal radius. Clin Orthop 202:103–111, 1986.
20. Moneim MS: Management of greater arc carpal fractures. Hand Clin 4:457–467, 1988.
21. Palmer AK: Fractures of the distal radius. *In* Green DP (ed): Operative Hand Surgery, 3rd ed. New York, Churchill Livingstone, 1993, pp 929–971.
22. Regan DS, Linsheid RL, Dobyns SH: Lunotriquetral sprains. J Hand Surg 9A:502–514, 1984. Orthopedics 21:71–104, 1990.
23. Ruby L: Fractures and dislocations of the carpus. *In* Browner BD, Jupiter JB, Levine AM, Trafton PG (eds): Skeletal Trauma. Philadelphia, WB Saunders, 1992, pp 1025–1062.
24. Sennwald G: Fractures of the distal radius. *In* The Wrist. St. Gallen, Springer-Verlag, 1987.
25. Taleisnick J: Carpal instability. J Bone Joint Surg 70A:1262–1267, 1988.
26. Van der Linden W, Ericson R: Colles' fracture: How should its displacement be measured and how should it be immobilized? J Bone Joint Surg 63A:1285–1288, 1981.
27. Wilson AJ, Mann FA, Gilula LA: Imaging the hand and wrist. J Hand Surg 15B:153–167, 1990.
28. Woodward JE: A review of Smith's fractures. J Bone Joint Surg 51B:324–329, 1969.
29. Youm Y. Flatt AE: Kinematics of the wrist. Clin Orthop 149:21–32, 1980.

CHAPTER 15

Bone and Soft Tissue Injuries of the Hand

Ekkehard Bonatz

GENERAL PRINCIPLES

The hand has complex mechanical and sensory functions. Thus, injuries to the hand compromise the function of the entire upper limb. Fractures of the metacarpals and phalanges constitute 10 percent of all fractures, and more than one-half are work related. Motor vehicle accidents, recreation, and household injuries are less frequent. Distal phalanx fractures are the most common, followed in frequency by metacarpal fractures, proximal phalanx fractures, and fractures of the middle phalanx.

A fracture is described in terms of the bones involved (carpal bones, metacarpals, phalanges), and its location is determined by the region of bone involved, e.g. the base, shaft, neck, or head of the metacarpal. The prognosis is worse if there is intra-articular displacement of 1 mm or more, whereas such displacement at the shaft level may be acceptable. Most open fractures constitute orthopaedic emergencies. For further management of such injuries, see Chapter 2.

A deformity following fracture is apparent in rotational malalignment of a digit, or in angulation. For a description of fracture terminology, see Chapter 1.

It is important to assess associated injuries. These may affect the circulation, skin condition, and nerves. Restoration of joint anatomy is critical to regain function, and injuries about joints should be examined particularly carefully. Tendon injuries can occur as isolated injuries or in conjunction with bone injury. They may not be obvious on initial examination because of the pain, swelling, deformity, and reluctance to move the finger due to fractures.

Children's fractures frequently involve the physeal plate. The epiphyses are located proximally in the phalanges and in the thumb metacarpal. They are located distally in the index, long, ring, and small finger metacarpals. Sometimes a proximal epiphysis appears on the metacarpals, most commonly on the index (or distally on the thumb metacarpal). This is known as a *pseudoepiphysis* and should not be confused with the true growth center or with a fracture (Fig. 15–1). The prognosis of an epiphyseal injury depends on its location. If the fracture line crosses the physeal plate or extends into the

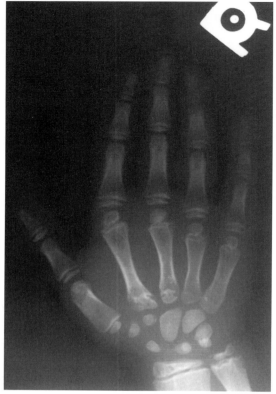

Figure 15–1. Pseudoepiphysis. A radiolucent line is seen across the proximal aspect of the index metacarpal and the distal thumb metacarpal, while the true epiphyseal lines are at the opposite end of each bone. (Courtesy of Gregory T. Odrezin, MD.)

articular surface, accurate reduction of the fracture must be obtained.

EVALUATION

A careful history of the force producing the injury and an assessment of the soft tissue involvement should be documented. Local tenderness, swelling, or rotational or angulatory deformity may indicate a fracture or dislocation. The active or gentle passive range of motion as well as the neurovascular status should be evaluated. Two-point discrimination can be tested with a paper clip, and is normally 4 to 5 mm. The two points are gradually brought closer together until they feel like one point. If a nerve is injured, the patient will not be able to tell one from two points, or the two-point discrimination will be widened. Only a gentle, brief touch of the finger pulp on either side, in a longitudinal direction, is applied, and care is taken that

the underlying skin not blanch. Sharp from dull discrimination is a less sensitive test but is valuable in areas other than the finger pulps and in patients unable to understand a two-point test. Compression of the nail or nail bed normally will lead to capillary refill within 2 seconds. This time is faster in venous injuries and delayed in arterial injuries. For further discussion on nerve injuries, see Chapter 16, and for vascular injuries, Chapter 20.

Once a fracture is suspected, radiographs are required. These should be an anterior/posterior and a true lateral view of the individual digit. When a fracture is close to a joint, oblique views will aid in the assessment of overall alignment. Oblique views are also valuable in the hand, where multiple bones overlie one another on the lateral radiograph.

MANAGEMENT

Associated soft tissue injury will aggravate the prognosis—for example, an open fracture of the proximal phalanx will take longer to heal than a closed fracture. A delay in diagnosis sometimes will make fracture reduction difficult, as fractures in the hand will form early callus within 7 to 10 days and are then difficult to manipulate. Associated diseases, such as diabetes mellitus, rheumatoid arthritis, or malnutrition, may alter the outcome. Patient motivation is a critical factor in rehabilitation after hand injuries and often can be enhanced by a brief physical therapy program. Socioeconomic factors, such as the patient's occupation, and future expectations must be carefully considered.

The principles of treatment involve accurate fracture reduction, movement of the uninvolved fingers to prevent stiffness, and elevation of the extremity to limit edema.[3] An injured hand should be placed in the intrinsic positive or safe position (Fig. 15–2). This position maintains 70 degrees of metacarpophalangeal (MP) joint flexion to avoid the stiffness that would otherwise occur with MP extension. For the proximal interphalangeal (PIP) joints, extension is maintained, as the PIP joints are more likely to get stiff if held in flexion. Early mobilization of the injured finger is important and can be enhanced by an exercise program directed toward the characteristic fracture problems.

Open fractures must be converted to clean wounds through thorough debridement. If

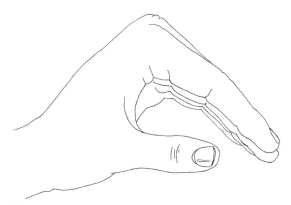

Figure 15–2. The intrinsic plus or "safe" position of the hand: The metacarpophalangeal joints are held in 70 degrees of flexion, and the interphalangeal joints are held in extension.

necessary, open packing of the wound and repeat debridement after 2 to 3 days must be performed. Gunshot wounds are usually of low velocity and usually cause minimal damage to tendons and nerves. It is important to clean the entrance and exit wounds, but no formal exploration of a bullet track is necessary. For extensive open injuries with multiple fractures, the primary goal is restoration of skeletal stability as soon as possible (such as with immobilization, K-wire fixation, or external or internal fixation). This will allow easier soft tissue management. Severe fractures involving joint surfaces may obviate any form of fixation and may require primary arthrodesis.

For closed, nondisplaced fractures of the phalanges and metacarpals, motion usually can be started after 21 days, depending on stability. Fracture consolidation usually will have taken place by then and will allow unprotected motion without fear of displacement. However, fractures of the tapered midshaft diaphyseal region of the phalanges or metacarpals may require a longer time to consolidate and will require intermittent splinting for a longer time (proximal phalanx, 5 to 7 weeks; middle phalanx, 10 to 14 weeks). Comminuted fractures and those requiring open reduction because of the more severe nature of the injury will take longer to consolidate. The fracture is usually consolidated and motion begun prior to radiologic evidence of healing. The diagnosis of a consolidated fracture usually can be made clinically. Typically, there is loss of fracture line tenderness, no motion felt by the examiner

while pushing on either side of the fracture, and a palpable mound of callus.

Early management in stable fractures may require simple measures such as buddy taping or splinting, with repeat radiographs obtained at 7 to 10 days to rule out further displacement. Initially, unstable fractures should be reduced and immobilized. This can be accomplished using a cast with or without metal outrigger splints or percutaneous pinning, in order to prevent displacement and to allow early motion. In fractures that cannot be reduced or remain unstable, open reduction and internal fixation are necessary. Surgical options include K-wire fixation, interosseous wiring, interfragmentary screws, or plates and screws (Fig. 15–3). Such fractures are difficult to treat and should be referred to a specialist early. In fractures with segmental bone loss, the primary treatment for the soft tissue wounds includes surgical debridement. Every effort must be made to maintain bone length, and this can be achieved with K-wire fixation or external fixation. Delayed bone reconstruction with bone grafts and future surgery requiring flap coverage in addition to tendon, nerve, or bone surgery may become necessary.

DISTAL PHALANX FRACTURES

The tip of the finger is often injured by crushing forces that cause a fracture of the distal phalanx and frequently a hematoma under the nail bed. Most commonly the middle finger and thumb are involved.

Reduction is usually not necessary unless the articular surface is involved and shows a step-off of more than 1 mm on radiography. Splinting is used only for protection and comfort. It is important to mobilize the PIP and MP joints as soon as possible. The splints are usually discontinued by 3 to 4 weeks. Epiphyseal plate injuries in children are treated by closed reduction with hyperextension of the phalanx, returning the nail to its place under the nail fold after the wound has been cleansed (Fig. 15–4). After reduction, these fractures usually will be stable, but prompt follow-up with a radiograph is necessary to confirm this.

Nail bed injuries are often associated with distal phalanx fractures (Fig. 15–4). Decompression of the subungual hematoma may be necessary to relieve pain. If the hematoma

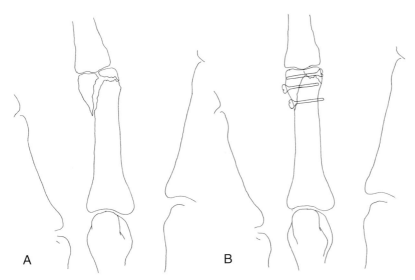

Figure 15-3. *A* and *B,* An unstable intra-articular fracture of the proximal interphalangeal joint may require surgical fixation with screws.

occupies greater than 50 percent of the area under the nail, repair of the nail bed should be undertaken to minimize nail bed complications. The nail plate must be removed in order to expose the laceration of the nail bed. Meticulous repair of the nail bed is performed with fine, absorbable suture (e.g., 7-0 chromic). The nail fold should be kept open by reinserting the cleansed nail, petrolated gauze, or a piece of rubber from a sterile glove or Penrose drain for a few days. If the hematoma is less than 50 percent of the nail

surface area, drilling a hole in the nail bed with a heated paper clip or an 18-gauge needle may be performed, which will allow the hematoma to drain. This method converts a closed fracture of the distal phalanx into an open fracture. A brief course of prophylactic antibiotics should be administered (e.g., first-generation cephalosporin orally for 2 to 5 days) after nail bed repair or evacuation of a nail bed hematoma.

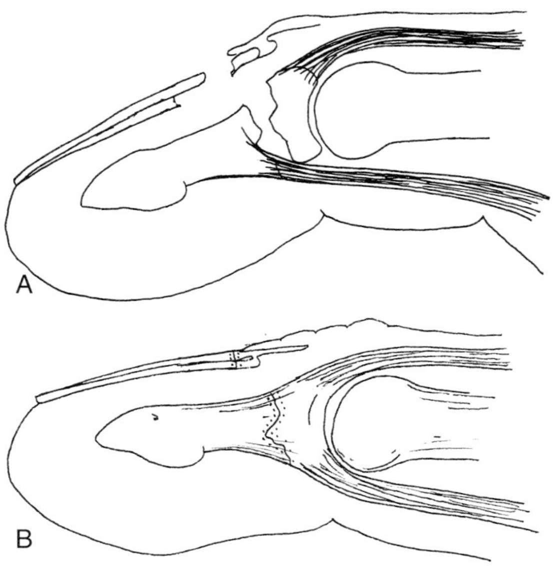

PROXIMAL AND MIDDLE PHALANX FRACTURES

Middle phalanx fractures are displaced by the forces of the central slip attachment dorsally and proximally and the flexor digitorum superficialis (FDS) insertion volarly and distally (Fig. 15–5). Fractures proximal to the FDS insertion will angulate with the apex dorsally, whereas fractures distal to the FDS insertion will angulate with the apex volarly. Proximal phalanx fractures generally will angulate volarly, because the interosseous muscles flex the proximal fragment at their proximal insertion, while the central slip insertion about the PIP joint extends the distal portion. The major problem in fractures of the middle and proximal phalanges is adherence of the flexor and extensor tendons during callus formation. This may impair joint motion.

For stable, nondisplaced, or impacted fractures, temporary protection with a splint and mobilization to tolerance can be started. The

Figure 15-4. *A* and *B,* Distal phalanx fractures are usually stable after reduction of the fracture. Repair of the nail bed is often necessary.

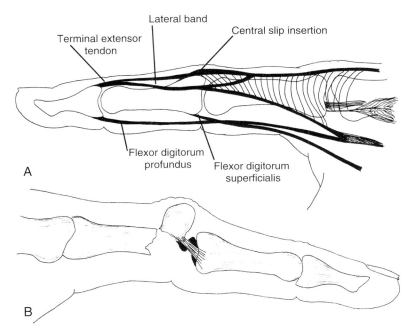

Figure 15–5. Phalangeal fractures. *A,* Soft tissue attachments to the phalanges. The central slip of the extensor tendon mechanism inserts into the middle phalanx dorsally, while the flexor digitorum superficialis tendon inserts volarly. *B,* Proximal phalanx fractures generally will angulate volarly, because the interosseous muscles flex the proximal fragment at their proximal insertion, while the central slip insertion about the PIP joint extends the distal portion.

splint should include the joints on either side of the fracture (in the intrinsic plus position). Displaced or angulated fractures are reduced under digital block by longitudinal traction and realignment of the fragments. Early x-ray follow-up (within 4 to 5 days) is mandatory to detect early redisplacement. If closed reduction is necessary, the forearm, wrist, and injured digit, as well as the adjacent digit, must be enclosed in a plaster cast or gutter splint. Sometimes a short arm cast with a metal outrigger is used, because it allows easier x-ray evaluation of the fracture through the splint. External fixation and other surgical modalities are used for markedly comminuted fractures, fractures with significant bone loss, as in gunshot wounds, or those that cannot be reduced and reduction maintained.

Complications of phalangeal fractures usually result from tendon adherence and contracture, particularly at the PIP joint level. Further surgery, such as tenolysis or tendon excision, may improve PIP joint motion. In severe contractures, a PIP fusion is used as a salvage procedure. Malunion, in the form of volar angulation, occurs mostly after fractures at the base of the proximal phalanx. This may require an osteotomy.

Reduction of fractures of the phalanges or metacarpals requires correct rotational as well as longitudinal alignment. In the normal hand, the tips of flexed fingers point toward the tuberosity of the scaphoid (Fig. 15–6). This alignment should be checked before and after reduction of the fractures. Malrotation or scissoring of the digits is often due to fractures of the metacarpal or phalangeal shaft with a spiral or oblique pattern. Even minimal displacement may lead to significant malrotation—that is, supination or pronation of more than 15 degrees. These fractures are unstable and may not maintain their reduction in a splint or cast. In acute

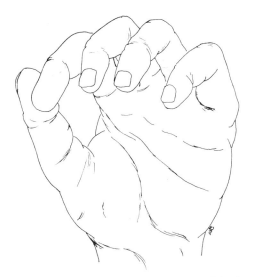

Figure 15–6. In the normal hand, the tips of the flexed fingers point toward the tuberosity of the scaphoid.

fractures, surgical fixation will then become necessary. When malrotated fractures are seen late, an osteotomy at the metacarpal or phalangeal levels may become necessary.

Infection rarely occurs and is usually seen after pin fixation or external fixation. Nonunion is infrequent and is most likely seen in severe open injuries, injuries with soft tissue interposition, or in those with insufficient immobilization or distraction at the fracture site.

METACARPAL FRACTURES

Metacarpal fractures are treated according to their location. Fractures with any degree of comminution or intra-articular displacement should be referred for possible operative treatment to obtain satisfactory reduction. Collateral ligament avulsions will require operative intervention if the bone fragment is displaced or involves more than 20 to 30 degrees of the joint surface. In rare cases, epiphyseal arrest may result in shortening of the metacarpal, but it is usually of no functional consequence.

Metacarpal neck fractures usually result from a direct blow with comminution of the volar cortex and subsequent dorsal apex angulation. This is the most common form of metacarpal fracture. It is often called the boxer's fracture or street fighter's fracture (Fig. 15–7).

Metacarpal neck fractures are usually treated with closed reduction and immobili-

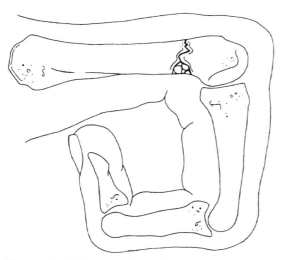

Figure 15–7. Metacarpal neck fractures usually result from a direct blow. They have volar comminution and are often dorsally angulated.

zation in an ulnar gutter splint holding the MP joint in 70 to 90 degrees of flexion (Fig. 15–8). Most of these fractures will heal satisfactorily. It is important to assess rotational alignment by asking the patient to flex the fingers slightly (see Fig. 15–6). Some residual dorsal apex angulation may be acceptable, especially on the ulnar side of the hand, since the ulnar side of the hand is more flexible and can adapt to a slight deformity. The most common sequela is a depressed knuckle, but this will usually be of no functional consequence. With excessive angulation, often there will be a residual inability to completely extend the MP joint. If angulation greater than 20 degrees is present after reduction, percutaneous pinning or open reduction is usually preferred. If rotational malalignment exists, operative treatment also may become necessary. Although the finger may appear reduced in the splint, this is deceiving. Rotational alignment is almost impossible to control without surgical fixation. In the index and long finger metacarpal, a residual dorsal angulation of greater than 15 to 20 degrees may become unacceptable because of the lack of compensatory carpometacarpal motion, and further operative treatment may be needed.

Most transverse fractures of the metacarpal shaft are angulated dorsally by the pull of the intrinsic muscles of the hand. The central metacarpals of the middle and ring finger are stabilized by the adjacent border metacarpals and the deep transverse metacarpal ligaments. They do not generally shorten significantly even if the fracture is comminuted. However, oblique or spiral fractures of the metacarpal of the border digits occasionally will shorten or displace, as they have no adjacent splinting structures. Shortening of 2 to 3 mm is acceptable.

The reduction maneuver for metacarpal fractures involves longitudinal traction on the proximal phalanx with the MP joint flexed for improved leverage through the collateral ligaments. Any rotation leading to scissoring of the digits when the fingers are flexed into the palm is not acceptable. Treatment of most metacarpal fractures is with plaster immobilization for about 4 weeks. The MP joint should be flexed at 70 degrees, with the PIP joint in full extension. This will relax the pull of the intrinsic muscles and allows the physician to check for length and rotational alignment of the metacarpals. Operative treatment may become necessary

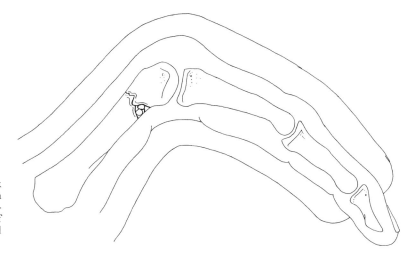

Figure 15–8. Metacarpal neck fractures are immobilized with a splint, holding the metacarpophalangeal joints in 70° to 90° of flexion with the interphalangeal joints extended.

in the case of any persistent rotational deformity, shortening of more than 3 mm, and dorsal angulation of 10 degrees in the index and long fingers or 20 degrees in the ring finger and little finger metacarpal. Multiple displaced metacarpal fractures are also an indication for surgical fixation. Open fractures are treated surgically as well, and on an emergency basis.

With any fracture of the metacarpal head or neck area, the physician must search carefully for a laceration over the adjacent metacarpophalangeal joint caused by the impact of a tooth. These lacerations can lead to severe infections with marked disability if not treated promptly. For a further discussion of bite injuries, see Chapter 23.

The complications of metacarpal fractures include malunion, usually resulting in dorsal angulation with prominence of the metacarpal head in the palm, and pain with gripping. Rotational malunion also can occur and may be corrected with a rotational osteotomy if necessary. Nonunion is rare but may follow a gunshot wound, severe open fractures, or distraction of the fracture. Most metacarpal fractures will heal in 4 weeks. Diaphyseal (shaft) fractures may take longer. Less frequent complications include metacarpophalangeal joint extension contractures, tendon adherence to the metacarpals, and refracture.

Because of its independent position and greater range of motion, most thumb metacarpal fractures do not need an anatomic reduction. Most extra-articular fractures can be treated with splinting in a thumb spica until the fracture is healed. Fractures involving the proximal one-fourth of the thumb

metacarpal may result in adduction and supination of the distal fragment (Fig. 15–9). This requires an attempt at closed reduction, with a thumb spica immobilization for about 4 weeks.

ARTICULAR FRACTURES AND JOINT INJURIES

Fracture of the Base of the Thumb Metacarpal (Bennett's Fracture, Rolando's Fracture)

Mobility of the carpometacarpal (CMC) joint of the thumb is paramount for adequate hand function. All fractures of the thumb CMC joint, therefore, should achieve and maintain good reduction and alignment. The thumb CMC joint is a saddle joint with a variable degree of flexion and extension, also allowing lateral motion and rotation. Its main ligamentous support is volarly, between the first metacarpal and the trapezium and index metacarpal. The dorsal and radial ligaments are weaker. In any injury, the abductor pollicis longus and adductor pollicis are the major displacing forces (Fig. 15–9). When obtaining an x-ray film, it is important to show a true AP view of the joint. This is usually done with the hand in maximal pronation (so-called Robert's view).

Type I intra-articular fracture (Bennett's fracture) is often associated with proximal subluxation of the metacarpal shaft. The abductor pollicis longus tendon, which inserts on the base of the metacarpal of the thumb, tends to abduct and pull the metacar-

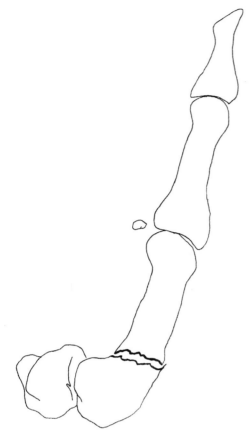

Figure 15–9. Fractures of the proximal one fourth of the thumb metacarpal may result in adduction and supination of the distal fragment, because of the deforming forces of the abductor pollicis longus and adductor pollicis tendons.

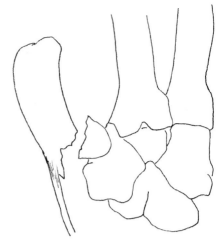

Figure 15–10. A Type I intra-articular fracture (Bennett's fracture) of the thumb metacarpal is often associated with proximal subluxation of the metacarpal shaft. The abductor pollicis longus tendon, which inserts on the base of the metacarpal of the thumb, tends to abduct and pull the metacarpal shaft proximally.

pal shaft proximally (Fig. 15–10). The volar ligament maintains the alignment of the proximal fragment with the trapezium. Because of the strong pull of the abductor pollicis longus tendon and its counterforce, the adductor pollicis, reduction is often difficult to maintain in a cast. If the ulnar fragment of the metacarpal base is small, the dislocated metacarpal can be easily reduced by traction and holding the thumb in abduction. However, this will often require supplemental fixation with a percutaneously inserted Kirschner wire or even open reduction and internal fixation if the intra-articular fragment is large. Closed reduction alone often will not be maintained. It is important to recognize that the Bennett's fracture is a fracture dislocation rather than just an intra-articular fracture, and that achieving and maintaining adequate reduction are paramount.

Type II intra-articular fracture (Rolando's fracture) involves a comminuted fracture of the articular surface of the thumb metacarpal. In contradistinction to Bennett's fracture, there is no significant proximal displacement of the remaining metacarpal. Comminution is often quite extensive, and restoration of the joint surface may not be possible (Fig. 15–11). Immobilization in a thumb spica splint or cast until fracture healing would be appropriate. Osteoarthritis of

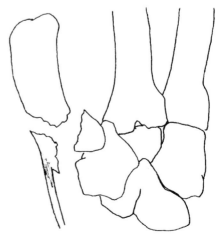

Figure 15–11. A Type II intra-articular fracture (Rolando's fracture) involves a comminuted fracture of the articular surface of the thumb metacarpal. In contradistinction to Bennett's fracture, there is no significant proximal displacement of the remaining metacarpal.

the carpometacarpal joint may later require arthrodesis or arthroplasty to relieve pain.

Extra-articular fractures of the thumb metacarpal can be treated with closed reduction and immobilization and rarely require surgery. Reduction is usually easily accomplished by longitudinal traction, downward pressure on the apex of the fracture, mild pronation of the distal fragment, and thumb extension. The reduction is usually stable and can be maintained in a thumb spica cast, excluding the distal phalanx. Angulation of less than 20 to 30 degrees is well compensated because of the abundant motion of the CMC joint. Angulation of more than 30 degrees may require surgical treatment.

In children, injuries involving the proximal metacarpal epiphyses are usually Salter-Harris Type II fractures, with the metaphyseal fragment on the ulnar side. These can also be treated closed and rarely require surgery.

Finger Carpometacarpal (CMC) Joint Injuries

The metacarpal bases articulate with the distal carpal row through a complex interlocking anatomic configuration. There is good soft tissue support through intermetacarpal dorsal and volar ligaments. There is very little motion at the index, long, and ring finger CMC joints but up to 30 degrees at the small finger CMC joint. Sprains of the CMC joints are usually evident by local tenderness and laxity on stress. These are usually a result of flexion and torsion forces applied to the individual finger. Treatment consists of 6 weeks of immobilization with a short arm splint or cast, if the injury is seen acutely. Sometimes chronic CMC joint injuries will respond to steroid injections or splinting. If this fails, referral for surgical joint fusion may be contemplated. The main complication of CMC sprains is persistent pain and carpal bossing (dorsal osteophyte formation of the proximal metacarpal).

CMC fractures and dislocations in the fingers are less frequent than in the thumb. They are usually the result of direct or longitudinal blows and are displaced dorsally more commonly than volarly. The ulnar side of the hand tends to be affected more frequently, and multiple dislocations are frequent. Many x-ray views, including oblique views of the hand, are often necessary to detect these subtle injuries. Because of the vicinity of the motor branch of the ulnar nerve immediately deep to the small finger carpometacarpal joint and the deep palmar arch in the vicinity of the long finger carpometacarpal joint, injuries to the ulnar nerve and vascular injuries must be ruled out. The treatment usually can be initiated with closed reduction, using longitudinal traction and pressure over the joint. CMC subluxations or dislocations are difficult to hold in a reduced position. Postreduction radiographs are crucial to assure that the reduction is indeed maintained. Often, specialist referral is necessary to maintain reduction with percutaneously inserted K-wires or open reduction and internal fixation.

The little finger metacarpal/hamate fracture dislocation is also known as the reverse Bennett's fracture. Displacement is produced by the pull of the extensor carpi ulnaris tendon with the hypothenar muscles as the counterforce. Longitudinal traction on the small finger metacarpal will restore joint alignment but often will require supplemental K-wire fixation. Open reduction is reserved only for large fragments and irreducible dislocations.

Soft Tissue Injuries to the Metacarpophalangeal Finger Joints

Dorsal dislocations of the MP joints are usually seen in the index or small finger and are caused by hyperextension. The volar plate may become interposed in the dislocated joint, thus preventing a closed reduction. The finger is held slightly in extension at the level of the MP joint and often deviates toward the middle finger. X-ray views will show a widened joint space (interposition of the volar plate). It is important to look for chip fractures on radiographs, as they will indicate a volar plate injury. With a simple dislocation or subluxation, closed reduction under local anesthesia, consisting of one attempt of longitudinal traction and accentuation of the deformity, will result in reduction. Multiple, repeated attempts at closed reduction should not be made as this will likely cause joint damage and residual stiffness. Once the MP joint is reduced, active motion is allowed in a dorsal extension block splint, permitting extension only to neutral.[1]

If the dislocation is irreducible with an interposed volar plate, then open reduction with volar plate release will become necessary. Complications of such dislocations include traumatic arthritis, decreased motion, or nerve damage, because the digital nerve is sometimes entrapped in the joint.

Volar dislocations are rare. Isolated metacarpophalangeal joint radial collateral ligament ruptures are usually seen in the index finger. These are evident by local tenderness and swelling. Reduction and immobilization in 30 degrees of flexion for 3 weeks, with protection by a splint or buddy taping for another 2 to 3 weeks often will resolve symptoms.

Metacarpophalangeal Thumb Joint

Acute injuries to the ulnar collateral ligament are common among skiers and ball-handling athletes and are much more common than radial collateral ligament injuries. The mechanism is forced radial abduction. Associated injuries may involve the surrounding soft tissues or a proximal phalanx fracture. Occasionally, the adductor aponeurosis may become interposed distally between the avulsed ligament and its insertion point, and this will prevent healing with closed treatment (Fig. 15–12).

Ulnar collateral ligament injuries present with pain, swelling, and tenderness over the ulnar side of the joint. Stress testing can be done under adequate anesthesia and should be compared with the opposite thumb. The joint should be stressed into radial deviation both in extension and flexion. A 30-degree difference indicates an ulnar collateral ligament injury. In partial tears, a thumb spica or splint for 6 weeks may suffice. Complete tears with laxity of over 30 degrees, articular fractures involving more than 20 percent of the articular surface, or avulsion fractures

displaced more than 2 mm will require surgical referral.

A chronic sprain of the ulnar collateral ligament, also known as gamekeeper's thumb, may require treatment for pain or functional instability. A protective brace holding the joint in a corrected position will consist of a thumb spica and may help symptomatically. Surgical treatment often will become necessary in the form of fusion or ligament reconstruction.

Radial collateral ligament injuries of the thumb metacarpophalangeal joint are caused by forced adduction and rotation of a flexed MP joint. As with the ulnar collateral ligament, stress testing and radiographs will yield the diagnosis. Immobilization for 4 to 6 weeks is needed. Patients are often left with some degree of residual pain.

A dorsal dislocation of the MP joint of the thumb is caused by hyperextension. The collateral ligaments usually remain intact, but the volar plate may become entrapped between the joint surfaces. Gentle closed reduction through dorsal pressure with flexion of the thumb MP joints and interphalangeal joints to relax the flexor pollicis longus tendon may effect a reduction. The collateral ligaments should be stress tested once the reduction is achieved. If the reduction fails, an open reduction is needed. After reduction, if there is significant lateral instability (over 30 degrees), then referral for surgery is warranted.

Proximal Interphalangeal Joint Injuries

The patient presents with pain, swelling, and a decrease in motion at the PIP joint. Evaluation of the PIP joint includes true AP and lateral radiographs of the joint and func-

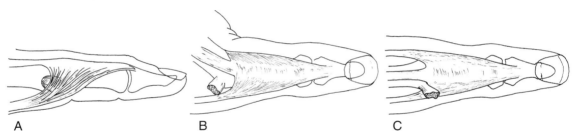

| A | B | C |

Figure 15–12. *A* to *C,* In the thumb metacarpophalangeal joint, the adductor aponeurosis may become interposed distally between the avulsed ulnar collateral ligament and its insertion point. This will prevent healing with closed treatment.

tional stability testing. For suspected collateral ligament injuries, stress testing may have to be performed.

Condylar fractures of the PIP joint are commonly seen in athletes and are best diagnosed on an oblique x-ray view. They are often misdiagnosed as a sprain. Angulation of the finger and any joint irregularity should be sought on the radiographs. Referral and surgical treatment become necessary if the fragments are displaced more than 1 mm. A permanent loss of motion is anticipated with many of these injuries. Extensively comminuted phalangeal head fractures are best treated closed in a position of extension. Mobilization with a removable protective splint may start at 10 to 14 days. Middle phalanx dorsal base avulsion fractures require open reduction if they are 2 mm or more displaced. A subtle subluxation may be associated with these fractures (Fig. 15–13). Large displaced avulsion fractures of the collateral ligaments should be referred for surgery. Similarly, a spiral shaft fracture of the proximal phalanx may remain displaced with a proximal spike of bone blocking PIP joint motion. Either early reduction or late excision of the bone prominence will improve motion.

Proximal Interphalangeal (PIP) Joint Dislocations

PIP dislocations may be acute or chronic and may involve a fracture. Acute dislocations usually occur due to hyperextension and longitudinal compression. In pure ligamentous injuries, the volar plate is avulsed from the middle phalanx, and the joint surface remains intact. Intra-articular impaction fractures render the fracture/dislocation sta-

ble if less than 40 percent of the middle phalanx base is involved and unstable if there is more than 40 percent bone involvement of the joint surface. In a pure dorsal dislocation, the finger can be immobilized in a dorsal splint with 20 to 30 degrees flexion for 3 to 5 days and then started on an active flexion/ extension program, using buddy taping for recreational activities. Unstable dislocations may require placing the joint in considerable flexion, about 75 degrees, to maintain reduction initially. If the radiographs show any fracture fragments well approximated and the remaining dorsal articular surface congruently reduced, a dorsal block splint can be applied (the splint is placed dorsally to block extension, but flexion is allowed). The amount of flexion is gradually decreased over 4 to 5 weeks by about 10 to 15 degrees each week. With PIP dislocations, only the PIP joint is splinted; the distal interphalangeal joint and MP joint are left free. Operative fixation is indicated for unsuccessful closed reductions or large middle phalanx base fractures.

Chronic PIP joint dislocations (those over 2 weeks old) may lead to a swan neck deformity secondary to chronic hyperextension of the PIP joint (Fig. 15–14). These should be referred for surgical reconstruction of the volar plate mechanism. Similarly, chronic PIP fracture/dislocations (those over 2 weeks old) should be referred for surgical treatment.

Lateral PIP joint dislocations are the result of lateral shear stress in extension with disruption of the collateral ligaments. The radial collateral ligaments are six times more commonly involved than the ulnar ones. There may be an associated injury of the volar plate or the extensor mechanism, or a fracture of the phalangeal base. The diagnosis is usually made on stress testing or from an appearance of joint asymmetry on radiographs. Immobilization for 3 weeks— usually buddy taping to the adjacent finger— with progressive mobilization is the treatment of choice.

Volar PIP dislocations are rare and are often unstable and irreducible. Often a condyle of the phalanx is buttonholed between the central slip and the lateral band. One attempted closed reduction with traction and flexion of the MP and PIP joints to reduce tension on the flexor tendons is warranted. The active range of motion after reduction should be tested to assure integrity of the

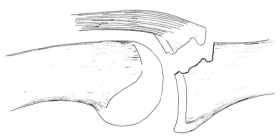

Figure 15–13. Dorsal avulsion fractures of the middle phalanges require open reduction if they are 2 mm or more displaced. Subtle subluxation of the joint may be associated with these fractures.

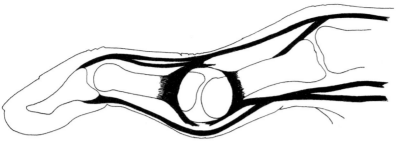

Figure 15–14. Chronic PIP joint dislocations with volar plate injury can lead to a swan neck deformity secondary to chronic hyperextension.

extensor slip. After that, continuous PIP extension splinting for 6 weeks with active DIP motion is recommended. A hand/occupational therapist will be helpful in enforcing such exercises. An open reduction is necessary if closed reduction fails.

Thumb Interphalangeal and Finger Distal Interphalangeal Joints

These dislocations are similar to the PIP joints, but the injuries are less frequent. The skin, however, may be torn open, rendering the dislocation open. Occasionally, interposed structures such as the volar plate, flexor tendon, or sesamoids will hinder reduction. Closed reduction by longitudinal traction is usually successful, and immobilization for 10 to 21 days in extension will suffice. Fractures consisting of less than 30 to 40 percent of the dorsal joint surface of the distal phalanx with displacement of less than 2 mm can be treated with a mallet splint. This holds the distal interphalangeal joint in extension. These splints are commercially available or can be custom fabricated. Care is taken not to hyperextend the joint for fear of skin necrosis over the distal interphalangeal joint. If there are larger fragments or greater displacement, open reduction may be

needed. Occasionally, such a mallet fracture will lead to volar subluxation of the distal fragment. This should be re-evaluated on the lateral x-ray view after application of a splint with the DIP joint in extension. Persistent volar subluxation will require surgical reduction and fixation.

Rarely, a volar fracture may be associated with avulsion of the profundus tendon. This will require operative fixation of the intra-articular distal phalanx fracture as well as tendon repair.

Rupture of the terminal extensor tendon at its insertion into the distal phalanx frequently occurs during recreational activities (baseball, basketball). The patient will be unable to extend the DIP actively (mallet finger). If untreated, the resulting deformity may lead to secondary hyperextension of the PIP joint (swan neck deformity) (Fig. 15–15). Active PIP flexion, while the DIP joint is immobilized in an extension splint, is therefore mandatory during rehabilitation.

FINGERTIP INJURIES

Fingertip injuries are the most common hand injuries. Since the fingertip is the most sophisticated organ of touch, its injury may lead to significant disability. Generally, the

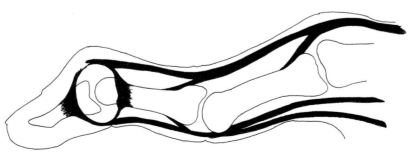

Figure 15–15. Mallet finger. Rupture of the extensor tendon insertion into the distal phalanx may lead to a secondary hyperextension deformity of the PIP joint if left untreated.

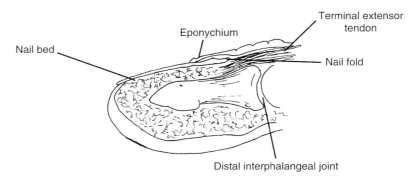

Figure 15–16. Anatomy of the fingertip.

fingertip is designated as that portion of the digit distal to the insertion of the extensor and flexor tendons. The volar pulp is covered by highly integrated skin. The skin is anchored to the phalanx by fibrous septa. The nail fold is made of a dorsal roof and ventral floor and contains the germinal matrix, and the remaining nail bed is distal to this. The lunula marks the transition zone between the two (Fig. 15–16).

The goals of treatment are restoration of adequate sensation, minimal tenderness, satisfactory appearance, good joint motion, and maximum length consistent with these goals. Factors in the choice of treatment must take into consideration the patient's age, occupation, and the involved digit.

Most commonly, the wounds are allowed to heal by contraction and epithelialization. This will most predictably lead to a satisfactory result and has few complications.[2] It works best in children, or in adults with defects of 1 cm or less. It is a simple procedure and involves thorough cleansing of the wound followed by debridement of any necrotic or compromised tissue. The bone may need to be shortened, always to the level of the distal extent of the nail bed (and not beyond). Care should be taken to remove enough bone to allow future granulation tissue to cover the bone sufficiently (Fig. 15–17). A dressing change should then be done at 3 to 5 days, followed by dressing changes every week until the wound is healed. The disadvantages of this treatment are prolonged healing, sometimes taking 4 to 6 weeks, and an unpredictable incidence of stump tenderness.

Replacement of amputated parts, as a composite graft, has been advocated in children. It is most useful using distal tissue, after a sharp amputation. It will give the best appearance when successful. However, it is unpredictable, and recovery is delayed when this method fails.

When the fingertip is severely crushed, referral for possible amputation may be necessary. Amputations are also considered in

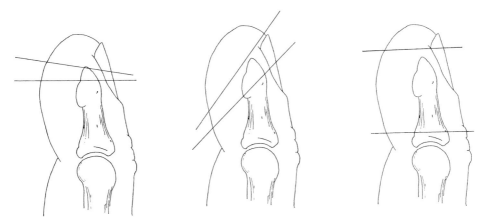

Figure 15–17. Various levels of fingertip injuries or amputations. Most can be treated with thorough cleansing, debridement, and secondary granulation, with frequent dressing changes. *Left lines:* Wound can be treated by dressing changes. *Proximal lines:* Bone is exposed and needs surgical coverage.

digits with multiple levels of injuries or in severe infections. If there is exposed bone and an intact dorsal, volar, or lateral skin flap, local tissue rearrangements can sometimes afford coverage. For instance, in situations with more volar than dorsal skin loss of the fingertip (Fig. 15–17), advancing the entire volar skin of a digit or thumb may allow tip coverage, if the advancement flap can be matched with dorsal skin.

REPLANTATION

Microvascular replantation may be indicated if the distal part is still available. The best results have been described at amputations distal to the insertion of the flexor digitorum sublimis (midmiddle phalanx). Because of its critical function in the hand, any level of amputation of the thumb should be considered for microvascular replantation.

The amputated part is wrapped in a cloth moistened with Ringer's lactate or normal saline. This is then sealed in a plastic bag or sterile specimen cup and placed on a bed of ice (see Chapter 2). It is important *not* to ligate or clamp vessels and *not* to use dry ice. The amputated part can be considered for replantation if its warm ischemia time is less than 6 hours. For cold ischemia, replantation may be considered after up to 12 hours, or even later in digits (up to 30 hours if cool).

X-ray views of both ends of the injured extremity should be obtained. Tetanus prophylaxis, if indicated, and a first-generation cephalosporin or synthetic penicillin are given parenterally. After gentle cleansing of the amputation stump, a sterile dressing followed by a pressure dressing is applied for patient transportation to a replant center. Near-complete amputations with preserved skin bridges, however small, should *not* be completed, because the skin bridge may contain critical veins.

Replantation should be considered for severed thumbs, multiple digits, amputation at the metacarpal level through the palm, almost any body part in a child, and an amputation through the wrist or distal forearm. At the level of the elbow or proximal arm, only sharp or moderately avulsed injuries may offer a chance for replantation. A short ischemia time is critical. Indications are set wider in children or younger patients. For individual digits, replantation distal to the flexor digitorum superficialis tendon insertion may be a consideration, and a more proximal replant in a single digit may be considered in children or women, but the patient must understand that there will be severe functional and aesthetic limitations.

Contraindications for replantation include severely crushed or mangled parts, amputations at multiple levels, amputations in patients with other serious diseases, arteriosclerotic vessels, mentally unstable patients, a prolonged warm ischemia time, and severely contaminated wounds.

References

1. Dray GJ, Eaton RG: Dislocations and ligament injuries in the digits. *In* Green DP (ed): Operative Hand Surgery. New York, Churchill Livingstone, 1993, pp 767–798.
2. Stevenson RT: Fingertip and nailbed injuries. Orthop Clin North Am 23(1):149–160, 1992.
3. Wilson RL, Carter MS: Management of hand fractures. *In* Hunter JM, et al. (eds): Rehabilitation of the Hand. St. Louis, CV Mosby, 1990, pp 284–303.

Suggested Reading

Bowers WH: The proximal interphalangeal volar plate. II. A clinical study of hyperextension injury. J Hand Surg 6:77–81, 1981.
Smith RJ: Post-traumatic instability of the metacarpophalangeal joint of the thumb. J Bone Joint Surg 59A:14–21, 1977.
Wilson RL, Liechty BL: Complications following small joint injuries. Hand Clin 2:239, 1986.

C H A P T E R 16

Injuries to the Peripheral Nerves

Richard Meyer

Nerves are the wiring harness of the body. They carry electrical signals to and from the central computer (brain) to the various peripheral organs (muscles, sensory nerve endings, and so on). They are subject to injury from a variety of mechanisms. There are often predictable responses to these injuries. By knowing the areas the nerves innervate and their response to trauma, the clinician can diagnose and begin treatment of the nerve injury. The most common mechanisms of injuries to nerves are traction, penetrating wounds (lacerations, blast), and blunt trauma. Knowledge of the mechanism of injury will influence initial treatment, and in many instances this can determine the outcome.

A peripheral nerve is actually a bundle of individual nerves (Fig. 16–1). The smallest unit in a nerve is a single axon. This would correspond to a single wire. Multiple axons group together to form fascicles (bundle of wires), and several groups of fascicles combine to form the nerve (cable). These "cables" originate in the spinal cord, and then exit from the cord and combine with each other ultimately to innervate a particular area (Fig. 16–2).

Most individual axons are surrounded by an important material known as myelin; this is created and maintained by Schwann cells. Integrity of the myelin is necessary for conduction of an impulse along the nerve. If there is very mild trauma to a nerve, it temporarily ceases to function or conduct; this is an injury to the myelin mechanism in a local area. When this area repairs itself, the nerve will conduct and thus function. The remainder of the nerve is uninvolved. This is called neuropraxia, or Grade I injury.[4] It is the mildest of injuries. Recovery time depends on the severity of the local conduction block (Fig. 16–3).

If the nerve is subjected to a greater degree of injury, the axons may be disrupted within the nerve while the nerve is structurally intact. This is called axonotmesis, or a Grade II injury (Fig. 16–3). Since the entire nerve is affected, the nerve must degenerate and then regenerate along its course. Since nerves regenerate at approximately 1 mm per day (or 1 inch per month), the time can be calculated from injury until the expected return of function begins. Complete normal return of function may or may not return. In the most severe injuries, the entire nerve is disrupted. This is neurotmesis, or a Grade III injury, and no spontaneous recovery is expected.[4] The patient should be referred

199

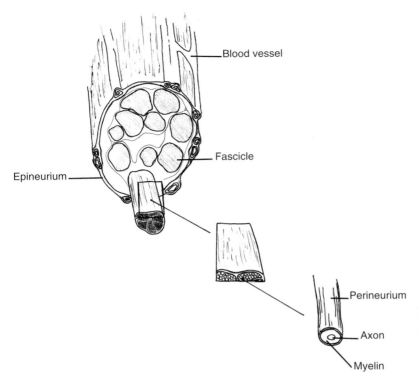

Figure 16–1. Anatomy of a nerve. A nerve consists of many bundles (fascicle groups). The smallest unit is the axon; the axons actually transmit impulses.

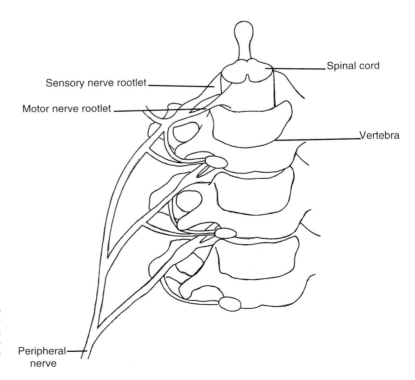

Figure 16–2. Nerve pathway. A peripheral nerve is a combination of axons that may arise from multiple levels and be a combination of both motor and sensory fibers.

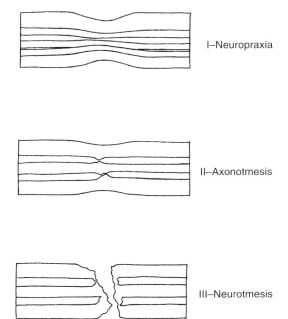

Figure 16–3. Injury grades. Seddon divided injury into three grades. However, an injury to a specific nerve may include components of all three grades.

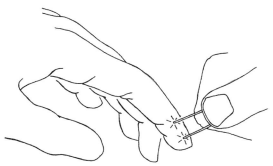

Figure 16–4. Two-point discrimination. The ability to discriminate two points of touch, 4 to 5 mm apart, assures a normal functioning nerve to both the finger and the nerve pathway involved.

within a few days to a surgeon who specializes in the treatment of nerve injuries.

The most important item in establishing the nature of the injury is a good history and physical examination. This should be done carefully before any analgesics or local anesthetics are given. The physical examination should be documented preferably before the patient is moved or splinted, if circumstances allow. The ability to move each finger, toe, hand, foot, arm, leg, and so on—even a little—should be documented. In the case of numbness, use a paperclip bent into a U to test for two-point discrimination (Fig. 16–4—see Chapter 15). If there is less than 15 mm of two-point discrimination, the nerve to the finger is intact. The feet, legs, arms, or trunk also should be examined for sharp-dull sensation (Fig. 16–5). It is important to establish an initial sensory level, which can then be followed for the return of function. Knowing the basic areas innervated by the nerves will help define the lesion (Fig. 16–6).

The median nerve supplies the muscles that flex the wrist, fingers, and tip of the thumb; the ulnar nerve also supplies some finger flexors but also the majority of the small muscles to the hand. Without ulnar nerve function, the patient is unable to spread the fingers against resistance and is unable to cross the fingers. The radial nerve supplies muscles that extend the elbow, wrist, and fingers (Figs. 16–7 and 16–8). Distally, the digital nerves in the palm and fingers supply sensation to the individual fingers.

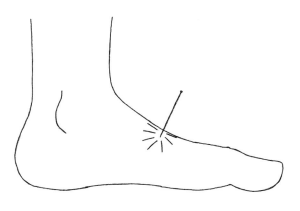

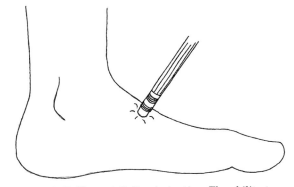

Figure 16–5. Sharp-dull discrimination. The ability to determine sharp vs. dull is used to assess nerve function in areas other than the hand.

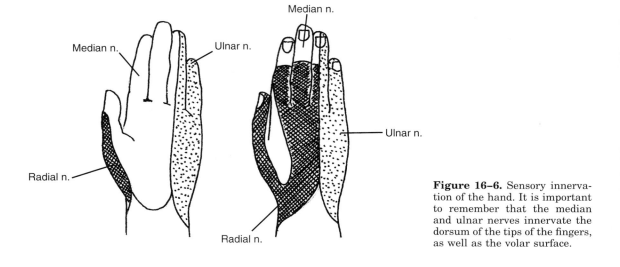

Figure 16–6. Sensory innervation of the hand. It is important to remember that the median and ulnar nerves innervate the dorsum of the tips of the fingers, as well as the volar surface.

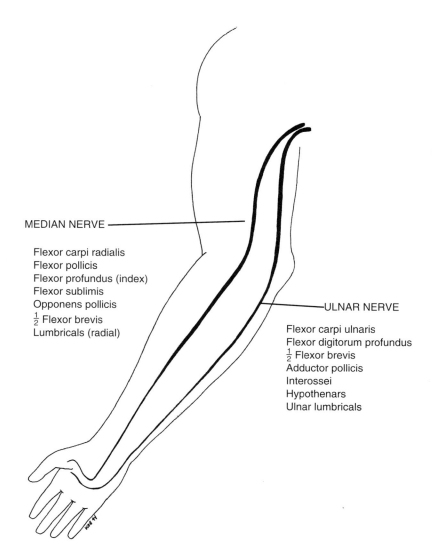

MEDIAN NERVE

Flexor carpi radialis
Flexor pollicis
Flexor profundus (index)
Flexor sublimis
Opponens pollicis
$\frac{1}{2}$ Flexor brevis
Lumbricals (radial)

ULNAR NERVE

Flexor carpi ulnaris
Flexor digitorum profundus
$\frac{1}{2}$ Flexor brevis
Adductor pollicis
Interossei
Hypothenars
Ulnar lumbricals

Figure 16–7. Motor innervation, upper extremity—anterior. The median nerve innervates the majority of muscles in the forearm, but also the opponens pollicis and part of the flexor brevis to the thumb. The ulnar nerve innervates the majority of muscles in the hand and the ulnar one half of the flexor profundus.

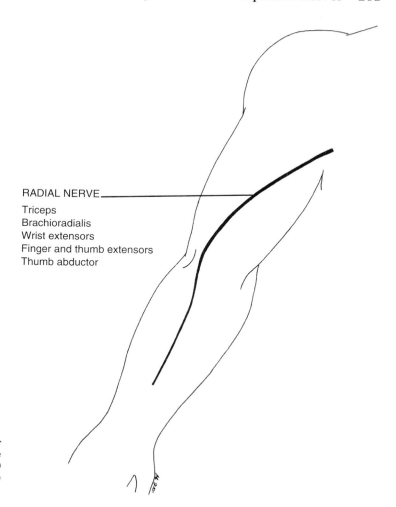

RADIAL NERVE
Triceps
Brachioradialis
Wrist extensors
Finger and thumb extensors
Thumb abductor

Figure 16–8. Motor innervation, upper extremity—posterior. The radial nerve innervates all posterior (or extension) musculature. It courses posterior to the humerus in the radial groove.

In the lower extremity, the femoral nerve supplies the muscles that extend the knee. The sciatic nerve supplies muscles that bend the knee, curl the toes, and plantarflex the toes and foot (posterior tibial branch of sciatic nerve) and dorsiflex and evert the foot (peroneal branch of sciatic nerve). Like the hand, areas on the foot correspond to particular nerves for sensation (Fig. 16–9).

After a good history and physical examination, the most important test for nerve function is nerve conduction (NC) velocity and electromyography (EMG). These are generally done by a neurologist. These tests can show a discrete area of injury and may predict the return of function. Nerve function returns in days to weeks after the majority of closed injuries. If it does not return in the expected time, then EMG and NC velocity may be helpful. These tests can be useful in

deciding when to intervene surgically in a nerve injury.

As the nerve regenerates, there should be a Tinel's sign (Fig. 16–10).[1] This is a sensation of shock felt by the patient when the area directly over the nerve in question is lightly tapped by the examiner's fingertip. The area where the tingling or electricity is felt represents the distalmost point of regeneration. The Tinel's sign should progress more distally over time as the nerve recovers. By following this sign, the progress of nerve return can be evaluated (Fig. 16–10).

Traction injuries occur to nerves whenever the normal length of the nerve has been rapidly exceeded. This may occur in a fracture or dislocation. In the neck, however, if the head is forced away from the shoulder at the same time the shoulder is markedly depressed, a traction injury to the brachial

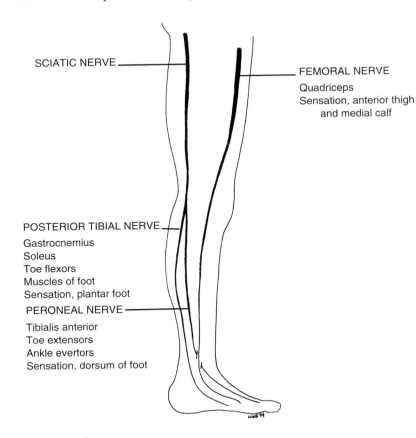

SCIATIC NERVE

FEMORAL NERVE
Quadriceps
Sensation, anterior thigh
and medial calf

POSTERIOR TIBIAL NERVE
Gastrocnemius
Soleus
Toe flexors
Muscles of foot
Sensation, plantar foot

PERONEAL NERVE
Tibialis anterior
Toe extensors
Ankle evertors
Sensation, dorsum of foot

Figure 16–9. Innervation of the lower extremity. The femoral nerve supplies motor fibers to the knee extensors (quadriceps), but it continues as a sensory nerve to the medial leg as far as the ankle. The sciatic nerve—largest nerve in the body—divides into the peroneal and posterior tibial nerve.

plexus may occur without skeletal changes (see Chapter 18).

The majority of traction injuries are Grade I or II injuries and require no intervention. As they are generally not associated with an open wound, treatment of the affected part should include protection or supportive splinting or both, with range of motion exercises until the nerve function returns. Between 10 and 20 percent of traction injuries, however, are Grade III lesions and require intervention by the appropriate specialist. This may be a retrospective diagnosis. If nerve recovery is not seen by return of muscle function or an advancing Tinel's sign at the rate of an inch per month or faster, then the injury to the nerve was probably complete.

A sudden nerve deficit that occurs with a laceration has a very high probability of being a Grade III injury and requires both prompt recognition and prompt treatment.[3] As with all penetrating injuries, wound care is paramount, and if necessary, repair of the nerve can be delayed a few days or a week. It is, however, very important to recognize

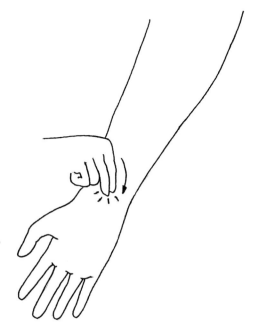

Figure 16–10. The proximal Tinel's sign indicates the area of injury; the distal sign indicates the point to which recovery has progressed.

that a nerve injury has occurred. If the injury goes unrecognized for a considerable time, then the nerves retract and nerve grafting becomes necessary. Results with grafting may not be as good as with primary repair.

Gunshot wounds are a cause of nerve injury.[2] In the low-velocity gunshot wound with an associated nerve deficit, there is a 60 percent chance the nerve will recover spontaneously.[3] Thus, the usual treatment regimen for the wound itself may be followed. If, after appropriate time and testing, it is seen that the nerve does not return, then secondary intervention is appropriate. In high-velocity injuries, nerve repair is secondary and wound care is the primary concern.

The last major category of nerve damage is blunt trauma. These injuries are primarily Grade I injuries, such as hitting the "funny bone" (blunt trauma to the ulnar nerve at the elbow), pressure on the radial nerve (the "Saturday night palsy;" see Chapter 19), injury to the peroneal nerve, ("suitcase" injury), and so on. Most patients recover in a short time, but some of the injuries take months. There is generally no acute treatment except for protecting the area supplied by the nerve and preventing stiffness. Bracing is sometimes warranted to aid in function (e.g., foot drop brace to aid walking, wrist drop brace to aid in hand grasp). Occasionally after blunt trauma to a superficial nerve, such as the radial nerve at the wrist, pain and numbness may persist even though the nerve is intact. Acutely the area should be padded or splinted until the local reaction settles down.

A transcutaneous electrical nerve stimulator often aids in pain relief. If the pain and numbness persist, referral to a specialist is warranted.

References

1. Henderson WR: Clinical assessment of peripheral nerve injuries; Tinel's test. Lancet 2:801, 1948.
2. Kline DG: Civilian gunshot wounds to the brachial plexus. J Neurosurg 70:166–174, 1989.
3. Omer GE Jr: Injuries to the nerves of the upper extremity. J Bone Joint Surg 56A:1615, 1974.
4. Seddon HJ: Three types of nerve injuries. Brain 66:237, 1943.

CHAPTER 17

Spinal Cord Injuries

John S. Kirkpatrick

Spinal cord injuries usually occur as the result of trauma, but they also may result from vascular or neoplastic conditions. Compression of the spinal cord from bone or disc fragments or from tumor is a potentially reversible cause of cord injury. Ischemia may result from trauma or compression and usually results in permanent damage. Contusion of the spinal cord results in functional disruption of the contused regions and may have a variable recovery pattern. Anatomic transection results in a permanent functional deficit without the potential for recovery.

The immediate resuscitation and evaluation of spine-injured patients are reviewed in Chapter 2 on orthopaedic emergencies. The initial resuscitation and secondary evaluation of these patients are guided by the Advanced Trauma Life Support protocols of the American College of Surgeons.[1] Once the spine is immobilized and any life-threatening conditions stabilized, documentation of spinal cord injury should be performed. Details of the examination are contained in Chapter 3.

Communication and documentation of the neurologic deficit are crucial to the care of the spine-injured patient. The American Spinal Injury Association (ASIA) has been instrumental in the development of standards for the classification of spinal cord injury. This chapter provides an overview of the classification scheme developed by ASIA.[3]

A commonly used grading scale originally described by Frankel describes the degree of impairment.[4] Grade A is complete neurologic injury. There is no sensory or motor function distal to the injury. Grade B is incomplete with sensory function preserved below the injury level but not motor function. Sensory function should be preserved through the sacral segments S4–S5. Grade C is incomplete with motor function preserved below the injury level, but the majority of the key muscles below the neurologic level are less than Grade 3. Grade D is incomplete; motor function is preserved below the injury site but is Grade 3 or 4. Grade E is normal for both sensory and motor function.

Review of some definitions will aid the physician in communication of neurologic deficits.

Tetraplegia is preferred to the term *quadriplegia*. This refers to impaired or absent motor or sensory function or both, resulting from damage to the cervical portion of the spinal cord. The reason tetraplegia is preferred to quadriplegia is that function of the trunk and pelvic organs is also impaired in these lesions. It is important to note that tetraplegia should be used only to describe lesions inside the spinal canal.

Paraplegia refers to impaired or absent function of motor and/or sensory function resulting from damage in the thoracic, lumbar, or sacral regions of the spinal cord. There may be variable involvement of the trunk and pelvic organs. Again, this term should only be used to describe lesions within the spinal canal.

Neurologic level refers to the most caudal bilaterally functional (motor and sensory) segment of the spinal cord. Sensory level and motor level may differ from the neurologic level in incomplete injuries and should be specified. For example, a patient with normal biceps and deltoid function but no other function on the right, but with biceps, triceps, wrist flexion and extension, and finger extension on the left but no other distal motor function, would be considered as having a C5 tetraplegic (the last normal bilateral segment is C5—biceps).

CLINICAL SYNDROMES OF CORD INJURY

Spinal shock frequently is encountered following spinal cord injury. This is defined by the absence of all spinal cord function, including reflexes. The return of sacral reflexes, in particular the bulbocavernosus reflex, signifies the recovery from spinal shock. This reflex is the contraction of the anal sphincter upon stimulation of the glans penis in men or the clitoris in women. This reflex also may be elicited by tugging on a Foley catheter, although care must be used to distinguish between the balloon pushing on the finger and the contraction of the sphincter. An additional reflex is the anal wink, or sphincter contraction following stimulation of the perianal region with a pin.

Central cord syndrome results from a lesion within the center of the spinal cord. This lesion occurs almost exclusively in the cervical region and is characterized by the sparing of sacral sensory function and greater weakness in the upper than in the lower extremities.

Anterior cord syndrome results from a lesion affecting the anterior portion of the spinal cord. The functional deficit involves a variable loss of motor and pinprick sensation, with preservation of proprioceptive sense.

Brown-Séquard syndrome results from a lesion affecting a lateral half of the spinal cord. The functional deficit involves ipsilateral proprioception and motor loss, with con-tralateral loss of pinprick and temperature sensation.

Conus medullaris syndrome involves lesions of the sacral cord. The functional deficit frequently involves an areflexic bladder (loss of micturition) and bowel (loss of defecation) and may include lower extremities (absence of deep tendon reflexes and plantar reflex).

Cauda equina syndrome results from injury to the lumbosacral nerve roots within the spinal canal. This may result in variable loss of motor and sensory function in the lower extremities. This is frequently difficult to distinguish from conus medullaris syndrome.

TREATMENT

Following the resuscitation of the patient and immobilization of the spine, the type of injury will dictate the treatment required. All patients with spinal cord injury less than 8 hours old should be considered for treatment with intravenous methylprednisolone, 30 mg/kg, administered over 15 minutes. Following a 45-minute pause, a maintenance dose of methylprednisolone should be administered at an infusion of 5.4 mg/kg/hr for 23 hours. Contraindications to this treatment are injury greater than 8 hours old and a spinal lesion below L2.[2] The efficacy of this treatment is still debated; however, the complications of the steroid administration are considered low. Prompt consultation of a specialist responsible for the treatment of spinal injuries is essential to provide provisional, if not permanent, stabilization and facilitate removal of emergency stabilization devices and the back board.

References

1. American College of Surgeons: Advanced Trauma Life Support Course. Student Manual. Chicago, 1993.
2. Bracken MB, Shepard MJ, Collins WF, et al: A randomized, controlled trial of methylprednisolone or naloxone in the treatment of acute spinal-cord injury: Results of the Second National Acute Spinal Cord Injury Study. N Engl J Med 322:1405, 1990.
3. Ditunno JF Jr (ed): Standard for Neurological and Functional Classification of Spinal Cord Injury, revised 1992. Chicago, American Spinal Injury Association, 1992.
4. Frankel HL, Hancock DO, Hyslop G, et al: The value of postural reduction in the initial management of closed injuries of the spine with paraplegia and tetraplegia. Paraplegia 7(3):179–192, 1969.

CHAPTER 18

Injuries to the Brachial Plexus

Richard D. Meyer

The brachial plexus is the collective nervous pathway through which the innervation of the shoulder and arm travels. Although the nerves that compose the plexus are actually peripheral nerves, injuries to this area can have devastating consequences. This, coupled with the complex anatomy of the plexus, makes it essential that injuries to the brachial plexus be diagnosed early and the appropriate referral be made.

The brachial plexus arises from the nerves of C5–T1 (Fig. 18–1). Occasionally C4 or T2 may contribute. The nerves from C5 and C6 combine to form the upper trunk (Fig. 18–2), the C7 nerve forms the middle trunk, and C8 and T1 combine to form the lower trunk. Two nerve branches commonly arise from the trunk level; the dorsal scapular and long thoracic nerves. The trunks then divide into anterior and posterior divisions. All the posterior divisions combine to form the posterior cord. The anterior divisions combine to form the lateral and medial cords. The cords are formed at the level of the clavicle and end in the various peripheral nerves. The lateral cord divides into the musculocutaneous and median nerves. The medial cord gives rise to the ulnar nerve and several cutaneous nerves. The posterior cord terminates in the axillary nerve and radial nerve.

All the roots are fixed at their exit from the spinal foramen; the peripheral nerves and cords are all fixed at various spots. Thus, anything that increases the distance between the neck and shoulder will put traction on the plexus and cause injury (Fig. 18–3). In adults, this most commonly occurs from motorcycle accidents, falls, and falling objects. Like other peripheral nerves, the plexus also may be injured from penetrating trauma, and, more frequently than other nerves, from irradiation. Because plexus injuries can be complete or partial, a thorough examination of the upper extremity needs to be done. A complete plexus injury involves all roots or nerves, and the extremity is flail; a partial injury may involve one or more roots or nerves, sparing the others. Since intervention is based on the rate and type of recovery, it is mandatory to know what levels are involved at the original injury.

Patients who complain of numbness in the arm or loss of function and burning pain after trauma to the shoulder or neck may have an injury to the brachial plexus. This is espe-

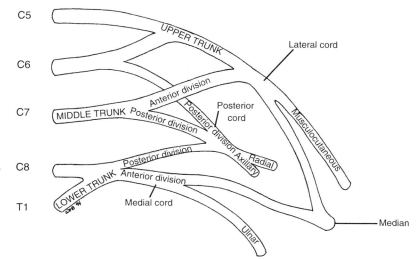

Figure 18–1. Diagram of the brachial plexus. The plexus arises from the nerve roots of C5–T1. These combine to form an upper, middle, and lower trunk. The trunks give rise to anterior and posterior divisions; these form lateral, posterior, and medial cords that terminate in the peripheral nerves.

cially true if the areas of numbness and weakness are supplied by multiple nerves. Acutely, there may be abrasions to the shoulder and swelling at the base of the neck, which is tender. Often, however, there is only tenderness at the base of the neck with profound loss of function in the arm.

The first area to examine is the vascular status of the arm; an absent pulse indicates a subclavian or axillary artery injury, and this should be referred immediately. Next,

examine the eyes; a drooped eyelid and constricted pupil (part of a Horner's syndrome) indicate a very proximal and severe plexus injury. The C8–T1 nerve roots are in close proximity to the stellate ganglia, so an injury involving these roots may disrupt the ganglia, resulting in a Horner's syndrome (Fig. 18–4).

Examination of the patient to determine scapular control should be done next. Loss of scapular control is also a sign of a very

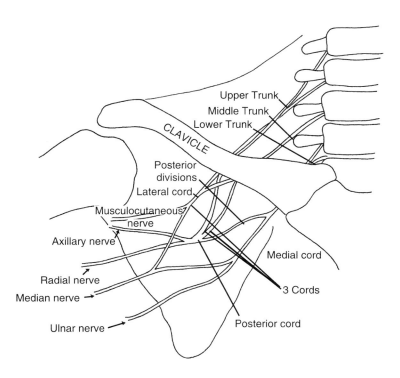

Figure 18–2. Relationships around the plexus. The trunks and roots are proximal to the clavicle. This is the upper plexus. The divisions are underneath the clavicle, and cords are distal.

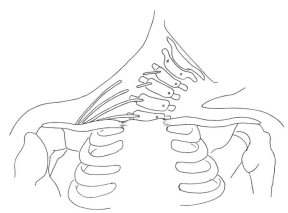

Figure 18–3. Mechanisms of injury to the brachial plexus. Any force that significantly increases the distance between the neck and shoulder will stretch or tear the plexus.

proximal and generally severe injury. This is because the nerves that help control the scapula (long thoracic and dorsal scapular) arise at a trunk or root level.

The physical examination should then continue in an orderly fashion, distally testing shoulder rotation, abduction, elbow flexion and extension, wrist flexion and extension, and so on. Each muscle in each area should be tested; it is easiest to do it by the various functional groups. After the muscles are examined, a sensory examination is done, including testing for two-point discrimination. By knowing the muscles affected and areas of sensory loss, one can diagnose the area(s) of injury.

After the history and physical examination, radiographs of the neck and shoulder should be obtained to rule out a dislocated shoulder, fractured clavicle or humerus, or cervical spine injury. A dislocated shoulder can cause a plexus injury, and the longer the dislocation is unreduced, the greater the likelihood of significant injury to the plexus. The fracture should be appropriately splinted to prevent further local injury.

Natural history studies show that function will recover spontaneously and almost completely in the vast majority of blunt trauma or traction injuries to the plexus.[5] In the remaining 10 to 20 percent, surgical intervention is necessary. If there has been no spontaneous recovery in the totally flail arm by 2 to 3 months and nerve conduction velocity and electromyographic studies show a severe injury, then an exploration should be done. In the partial injury, a slightly longer

time can be accepted before intervention, although waiting too long can diminish the amount of recovery. Since nerves recover at a rate of 1 mm per day, it may be 12 to 15 months before recovery in the forearm or hand is expected. The end organs begin to have irreversible changes by this time. Therefore, if repair is delayed, by the time the repaired nerve regenerates the motor endplates may be absent or in very poor condition, and no function returns.

Obstetric (birth) palsies are also a traction injury to the brachial plexus; most babies recover fully and have normal arms.[6] If biceps function does not appear by the third month, then the baby likely will have some degree of impairment and could be a candidate for surgical intervention.[2,4] For the first 3 weeks of life, no stretching exercises should be done in babies with birth palsies. The baby should be followed closely by a specialist in the field as soon after birth as practical. Of interest is that the severity of injury is related not only to the baby's weight but also to the mother's height and weight. Short, heavy-set mothers are at much greater risk of having babies with this complication.[4]

Open injuries to the plexus, either stab, puncture, or gunshot, should be handled expeditiously as there is a likelihood of major blood vessel damage. Appropriate studies should be done to determine the status of

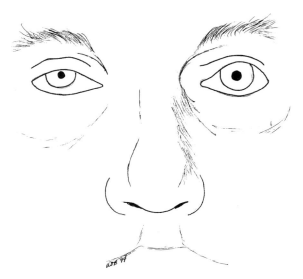

Figure 18–4. Horner's syndrome. A constricted pupil and drooping eyelid are visible signs. A dry mouth may also be included. Because of the close proximity of the lower trunk to the sympathetic chain, injuries to the area frequently affect both.

active bleeding. If the arm is viable and there is no expanding hematoma or evidence of active bleeding, no acute repair should be done. The patient should be stabilized and observed. Both nerve and vascular repair can then be electively done in a controlled environment with less chance of injury to other nerves and vessels.

The prognosis in plexus injuries depends largely on the nature of the injury and whether it is proximal or distal. The dividing line is generally felt to be the clavicle. Upper plexus injuries, that is, those injuries high in the neck, have a much poorer prognosis than those distal to the clavicle.[3] As mentioned earlier, this includes patients with loss of scapular control, a Horner's syndrome, and to a lesser extent loss of humeral control. As with peripheral nerves, gunshot wounds may recover to a significant degree, but injuries caused by a knife or other sharp object require immediate intervention.

There is no "acute" treatment for radiation injury. It is mentioned because many cancer patients (neck, breast, lung,) are just now beginning to present with symptoms of pain, numbness, and weakness of the arm many years after radiation therapy. Other than treatment with pain medication, nonsteroidal anti-inflammatory drugs, and transcutaneous electrical nerve stimulation, little can be done. A few series of surgically treated patients have reported some pain relief but no increase in function or recovery of the nerve.[1]

In summary, patients with open or closed injuries to the brachial plexus should be splinted and referred to a trauma center for treatment by a surgeon specializing in these injuries. If the patient is unstable because of vascular compromise even in the closed setting, stabilization and resuscitation should be done en route.

References

1. Brunelli G: Personal communication, December, 1993.
2. Gilbert A, Tassin JL: Obstetrical palsy. *In* Terzis JK (ed): Microreconstruction of Nerve Injuries. Philadelphia, WB Saunders, 1987, pp 529–553.
3. Leffert RD: Brachial Plexus Injuries. New York, Churchill Livingstone, 1985.
4. Meyer D: The treatment of adult and obstetrical brachial plexus injuries. Orthopaedics 9(6):889–903, 1986.
5. Narakas A: Brachial plexus surgery. Orthop Clin North Am 12:303–323, 1981.
6. Tassin JL: Paralysies obstetricals du plexus brachial: Evolution spontanee, resultats des interventions reparatrices precoces. Thesis, Universite de Paris VII, 1983.

CHAPTER 19

Nerve Entrapment

J. R. Tamarapalli

Richard D. Meyer

At the outset, it is important to realize that nerve entrapment is not a primary disease of the nerves. As the name implies, a peripheral nerve is "entrapped" by the pathologic changes in the tissues through which the nerve passes. Damage to the peripheral nerve results from localized pressure and inflammation caused by mechanical problems from an anatomic neighbor. Along the course of a peripheral nerve, there may be several narrow anatomic passages—e.g., a carpal tunnel. Because the nerve is always the softest structure in the area, entrapment of a nerve usually occurs at these vulnerable passages. Although every nerve is unique in its anatomy and hence in the ways it may be affected, the treatment is generally the same.

Nerve entrapment is not an uncommon problem.[1] It is generally a chronic condition, characterized by pain and paresthesias with or without variable degrees of sensory or motor loss or both.[2] Entrapment occurs more commonly in the upper than in the lower extremities. A common etiology is repeated microtrauma. This may be occupational, as in typists, poultry workers, assembly line workers, and so on, who do identical, repetitious movements all day. Other causes include long-standing compression from hypertrophied muscles, fibrous bands, gan-

glia, tumors, or bone prominences, resulting from injury or abnormal growth (e.g., osteoarthritis, fracture, hematoma). Acute swelling from burns or blunt trauma can cause an entrapment. Although causative factors can be identified for most nerve entrapments, some are idiopathic. The primary symptoms are pain, numbness, paresthesias, clumsiness, and muscle weakness in varying combinations. Other sensory symptoms include tingling, burning, and "pins and needles" or "electric shock" sensations.[3] Symptoms such as weakness, clumsiness, muscle wasting, or fasciculations without pain may represent entrapment, or they may be signs of a generalized neurologic problem.

Knowledge of the course of a peripheral nerve, coupled with suspicion of entrapment, is essential to make an accurate diagnosis. A complete present and past history should be taken. The insidious versus acute onset of the symptoms should be noted. Questions should be asked regarding occupation, old injuries, illnesses, and the presence of any chronic swelling. The distribution of the areas of sensory disturbance should be documented. Palpation along the course of the nerve may help identify any other abnormalities in the surrounding tissue. Provocative maneuvers should be performed to reproduce the symptoms of carpal tunnel syndrome and tenderness along the nerve. Phalen's test is performed by having the patient fully flex both wrists: within 60 seconds numbness appears in the median nerve distribution on the affected side). In reverse Phalen's sign, the wrists are fully extended to reproduce the numbness within 60 seconds on the affected side (Fig. 19–1). Tinel's (or percussion) sign (Fig. 19–2) is another provocative test. When positive, these signs help confirm the involvement of the suspected nerve and may lead to the site of the entrapped nerve. It is difficult to detect objective sensory loss and muscle weakness in the early stages of nerve compression, although pain and a feeling of numbness may be significant. Two-point sensory changes indicate a significant entrapment, probably of long duration. Radiographs are indicated for any patient

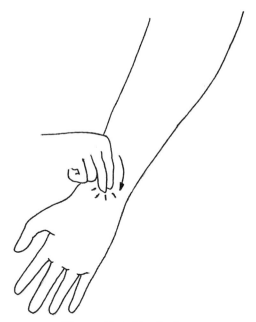

Figure 19–2. Tinel's sign.

with a history of trauma, or to rule out a mass or bone deformity.

Nerve conduction studies (NCS) and electromyography (EMG) are very useful.[4,5] In NCS, electrodes placed on the skin along the course of a nerve will evoke a response between them thus giving the speed of conduction. Conduction is slower across the suspected site of nerve entrapment. If the entire nerve conducts slowly, other pathology, such as a peripheral neuropathy, should be suspected. Electromyograms show electrical activity in the muscle. Abnormalities indicate the status of innervation of a muscle.

Many other conditions can mimic or predispose to nerve entrapment. In the differential diagnosis, the following conditions must be considered: diabetic neuropathy, radiculopathy (e.g., cervical spondylosis, sciatica), immunologic disorders (e.g., rheumatoid arthritis), and endocrine and metabolic disorders (e.g., hypothyroidism and vitamin B_{12} deficiency). When these are suspected, other laboratory investigations—rheumatoid factor determination, erythrocyte sedimentation rate, growth hormone levels, thyroid function tests, measurements of glucose metabolism—should also be performed.

The prevention of nerve entrapment is ideal. If the etiology is occupational, a change of work station, or arm positioning or tool modification might help. Sometimes a

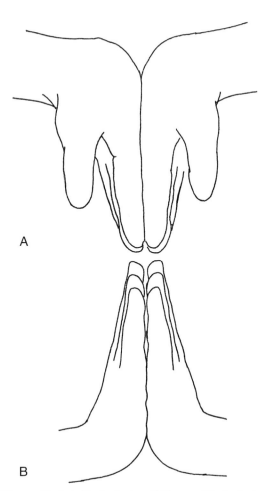

A

B

Figure 19–1. *A*, Phalen's sign. *B*, Reverse Phalen's sign.

change of job or occupation is necessary. A coexisting disease such as diabetes should be treated as well. Treatment usually includes activity modification, nonsteroidal anti-inflammatory drugs (NSAIDs), physical therapy (e.g., stretching and strengthening of muscles around the entrapment), and splints. Steroid injections may relieve symptoms temporarily and aid in confirming the diagnosis. Surgery to decompress the nerve is used when nonoperative measures fail.

NERVE ENTRAPMENT IN THE UPPER EXTREMITY

Thoracic Outlet Syndrome

Thoracic outlet syndrome (TOS) results from compression of the portions of the brachial plexus or the subclavian vessels or both at the thoracocervical junction. In this area, the great vessels leave the chest and the nerve roots leave the neck to enter the upper limb. Most commonly the compression results from a band of taut tissue pressing on the lower trunk of the brachial plexus. However, the entire plexus may be affected. This may be in the form of congenital bands or cervical ribs, or fibrosis in the scalene muscles.[6] Frequently it is the result of a hyperextension or hyperflexion injury of the neck caused by an accident or a body contact sport. Occasionally it is secondary to poor posture or may be work related (e.g., any activity that requires pressing hand controls, constantly working overhead, frequently turning the head).

The symptomatology of TOS varies as to the extent of involvement of the vascular and neurogenic structures. The symptoms may be bilateral and include pain, numbness, and weakness of the neck and upper extremities. Pain without significant neurologic findings is the hallmark of the condition. Neurologic changes may be seen in both the median and ulnar nerve distributions. Sensory loss may involve all the fingers, although primarily the ulnar fingers are affected. A positive Roos' sign (elevation of the arm to the shoulder level reproduces the patient's arm pain in less than 60 seconds) differentiates it from pure neurogenic compression.[7] Reproduction of pain is significant in TOS when the arm is elevated above the shoulder. Tinel's sign may be positive at the medial clavicle over the lower trunk. Electromyography and nerve conduction studies may be helpful but

are often normal. Radiography of the cervical spine and chest may identify a cervical rib, which may be compressing the brachial plexus.

In the differential diagnosis, carpal tunnel syndrome, C8 and T1 radiculopathy, and Pancoast tumor should be considered. The treatment of TOS should be scalene stretching and shoulder strengthening for 3 to 6 months; if this fails, then decompression of the plexus may be indicated.

Pronator Syndrome (Median Nerve)

The median nerve gives off no branches in the upper arm. It travels from the medial aspect of the arm, crossing the elbow anteriorly, to enter the forearm (Fig. 19–3). While crossing the elbow it passes below the lacertus fibrosis, between the two heads of the pronator teres, and under the fibrous arch of the flexor digitorum sublimis muscle. Pronator syndrome is the result of entrapment of the median nerve in one of these three areas.[8] Repeated movements of the elbow and forearm (e.g., in production or assembly line

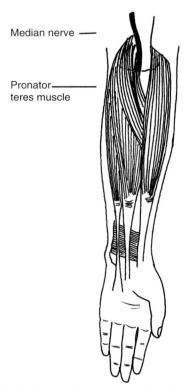

Median nerve ——

Pronator ——
teres muscle

Figure 9–3. The median nerve diving between two heads of pronator teres muscle just distal to the elbow.

workers) may produce or aggravate this syndrome.

The symptoms include pain in the volar aspect of the proximal forearm and, in some cases, numbness or paresthesias in the thumb, index, and long finger. Activity worsens the symptoms. There will be notable tenderness over the volar forearm, and there may be weakness in the muscles supplied by the median nerve. Weakness of DIP flexion at the thumb and index finger (e.g., the patient cannot make an "O" sign) is often present. A positive Tinel's sign is often elicited over the median nerve at the proximal border of the pronator teres muscle.

To identify the site of pathology, provocative tests may be performed. Resisting flexion of the PIP joint of the long finger puts pressure on the superficialis arch; resisting supination or pronation will put tension on the lacertus. Pressure is on the median nerve by the pronator teres with full passive supination and resisted pronation. Pain produced from these tests will not only confirm the diagnosis but also localize the entrapment site.

The initial treatment consists of activity modification and the avoidance of pronation and supination movements of the forearm. The application of a splint in 90° of elbow flexion and neutral forearm rotation and NSAIDs are helpful. If the site of compression is accurately identified, injection of hydrocortisone with a local anesthetic will usually give temporary relief. If no improvement is seen in 2 to 3 months, surgical intervention may be indicated.

It is important to distinguish this condition clinically from carpal tunnel syndrome. Pronator syndrome is frequently identified when symptoms persist after surgical release of the carpal tunnel.

Carpal Tunnel Syndrome

Carpal tunnel syndrome (CTS) is the most common nerve entrapment. It is caused by compression of the median nerve in the carpal tunnel (Fig. 19–4). The tunnel is volarly bordered by the thick transverse carpal ligament and dorsally by bones of the wrist. The carpal tunnel transmits the median nerve and the flexor tendons to the fingers. The median nerve gives motor branches to supply the thenar muscles and sensory branches to supply the thumb, index, long, and radial one-half of the ring finger.

Women are more commonly affected than men. The syndrome is often bilateral. The dominant hand is most commonly affected. Anything that takes up space within the carpal tunnel produces pressure on the median nerve. Carpal tunnel syndrome is most frequently associated with occupations involving repetitive movements of the wrist and hand.[2] It is seen in association with pregnancy, diabetes mellitus, synovitis of the wrist, flexor tenosynovitis, blunt trauma, thyroid disease, and any mass taking up space in the carpal tunnel. The condition may also be idiopathic.

The most common complaint is painful paresthesias in the wrist and hand, especially while sleeping. Patients usually get relief by shaking the hand, holding it in a dependent posture, or immersing it in warm water. Symptoms usually get worse by repeatedly using the hand, as in sewing, typing, and production work. Loss of dexterity and dropping things from the hand are frequent complaints. Symptoms are often brought about by sitting still, especially with the hand up, as in driving a car or holding a telephone. Some patients also have "pins and needles" in the fingers, or they may have profound numbness. Sometimes the pain spreads from the fingers to the arm and the shoulder.

On physical examination, sensory abnormalities may be found in the radial thumb, index, and long fingers, and the radial one half of the ring finger, but most commonly no objective sensory loss is present. Tinel's sign is frequently positive over the volar wrist, and the Phalen's test may be positive (see Fig. 19–1). Wasting and weakness of the thenar muscles occur only in advanced cases. Carpal tunnel syndrome can be distinguished from pronator syndrome by the area of tenderness, by Tinel's test, and by the fact that motor function to the thumb and index DIP flexion are not affected in CTS. Electromyography and nerve conduction studies[9] are helpful in reaching a diagnosis. Radiographs are rarely diagnostic.[10]

Treatment is to avoid the activity that is producing the symptoms. NSAIDs and a splint supporting the wrist in neutral position, especially at night, are helpful. Elastic splints should be avoided as these continue to compress the tunnel. If the patient shows no improvement in 3 to 4 weeks, a cortisone injection into the carpal tunnel may help temporarily. If no improvement is seen in

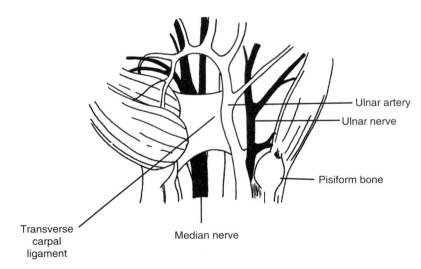

Ulnar artery

Ulnar nerve

Pisiform bone

Transverse carpal ligament

Median nerve

Figure 19–4. The relationship of the median and ulnar nerves to the transverse carpal ligament.

several months, division of the transverse carpal ligament may be indicated to relieve the compression. If persistent numbness or atrophy of the thenar muscles occurs, referral for surgical decompression should be made early. Carpal tunnel syndrome of pregnancy can almost always be treated nonoperatively since symptoms usually abate following delivery.

Cubital Tunnel Syndrome

The cubital tunnel is the groove around the medial side of the elbow through which the ulnar nerve passes. It is the "funny bone." The ulnar nerve may be compressed in this tunnel (Fig. 19–5) or at its exit into the flexor carpi ulnaris muscle.[11] Proximally, it may be entrapped by the medial intermuscular septum.

The symptoms are numbness and tingling in the ring and little fingers and along the ulnar border of the hand. There also may be numbness along the dorsum of the hand on the ulnar border. Clumsiness or weakness may be present. Flexion of the elbow tightens the aponeurosis of the flexor carpi ulnaris and may worsen the symptoms. This provocative maneuver helps locate the entrapment site. In severe cases, weakness may be found with pinching, gripping, spreading of the fingers against resistance, and flexion of the little finger DIP joint. Tinel's sign is positive over the cubital tunnel. Radiographs may be useful to rule out skeletal pathology. Electromyography and nerve conduction studies are often helpful in the diagnosis.

In the differential diagnosis, cubital tunnel syndrome should be distinguished from the radiculopathies and plexopathies involving the C8 and T1 nerve roots and entrapment at

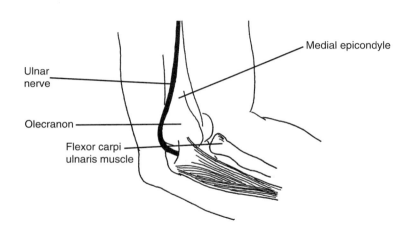

Medial epicondyle

Ulnar nerve

Olecranon

Flexor carpi ulnaris muscle

Figure 19–5. The ulnar nerve passing through the cubital tunnel at the elbow.

the wrist in Guyon's canal. For this, electrical studies may supplement the clinical examination.

The treatment is to avoid the cause (e.g., repetitive movements), modify activity, prescribe NSAIDs, and splint the elbow at 45° to 60° of flexion. If there is no relief in several months or if the condition is progressive, surgical decompression of the tunnel is considered.[12] If atrophy of ulnar innervated muscles or persistent (rather than intermittent) numbness occurs, surgical decompression should be performed early.

Guyon's Syndrome

Guyon's canal, through which the ulnar nerve passes (see Fig. 19–4), is situated between the pisiform bone and the hook of the hamate at the wrist. Guyon's syndrome is commonly seen in jackhammer workers, carpenters, and long distance cyclists, owing to constant pressure from handle bars.[13] Other causes are trauma, lipomas, ganglia, tumors, arthritis, and wrist fractures.

The symptoms include numbness of the ring and little fingers and weakness of grip. Examination confirms sensory loss and weakness of the ulnar-innervated intrinsic muscles. In contradistinction to cubital tunnel syndrome, the dorsum of the hand should not be numb, and the strength of flexion of the terminal phalanx of the little finger should not be affected in Guyon's syndrome. Nerve conduction velocity studies are helpful in the diagnosis.

This entrapment should be distinguished from cubital tunnel syndrome and C8/T1 radiculopathy. The treatment is splinting, avoiding exacerbating activity, and using well-padded gloves. If symptoms do not resolve, surgical decompression may be warranted.

Posterior Interosseous Nerve Entrapment

The radial nerve enters the forearm and in its upper part divides into the posterior interosseous nerve (PIN) (motor) and the superficial radial nerve (sensory). The PIN crosses over the anterior capsule of the radiocapitellar joint and passes under the arcade of Frohse (Fig. 19–6), going between the superficial and deep heads of the supinator.[14] As it travels down the forearm, it supplies the supinator, thumb and finger extensors, and extensor carpi ulnaris muscle.

PIN entrapment is also known as radial tunnel syndrome. The nerve may be compressed by the fibrous arcade of Frohse or by tightness within the supinator muscle. Workers using heavy tools and those sustaining blunt trauma and subsequent fibrosis are at risk.

Since the PIN is almost a pure motor nerve, it produces a different clinical picture. The patient complains of weakness in the wrist and some pain over the dorsum of the forearm. There will not be the characteristic wrist drop as seen in radial nerve neuropathy, because only some of the wrist extensors are involved in the PIN entrapment.

Weakness may be elicited in extension of wrist and fingers. Ulnar deviation of the wrist is weak. Attempted supination against resistance may reproduce the symptoms. The area is tender over the proximal border of

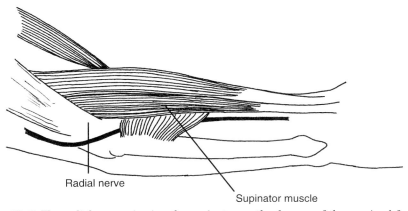

Radial nerve

Supinator muscle

Figure 19–6. The radial nerve piercing the supinator on the dorsum of the proximal forearm.

the supinator and usually over the lateral epicondyle, which sometimes confuses this syndrome with lateral epicondylitis (see Chapter 22). Electromyography helps confirm the diagnosis.[15]

NSAIDs, wrist and/or elbow splinting, and avoiding the inciting activity will usually lead to resolution of the symptoms. If not, surgical decompression may be warranted.

Radial Nerve Entrapment

The radial nerve may be compressed as it passes around the posterior border of the humerus. A common term for this is "Saturday night palsy," as from an inebriated person falling asleep with an arm against the chair. Pressure on the nerve results in a palsy. These conditions usually recover completely but may take 4 to 6 weeks. Less commonly, the nerve will be injured in this location as a result of blunt trauma or a fracture. Again, usual treatment is watchful waiting and splinting the wrist drop until motor function returns.

NERVE ENTRAPMENT IN THE LOWER EXTREMITY

Peroneal Nerve (Fibular Tunnel Syndrome)

The sciatic nerve divides into the common peroneal and the posterior tibial nerves in the upper popliteal fossa. The common peroneal nerve winds around the neck of the fibula and then passes through the superficial head of the peroneous longus (the fibular tunnel (Fig. 19–7). This segment of the common peroneal nerve is very superficial and is covered only by subcutaneous tissue and skin. The common peroneal nerve then enters the anterior compartment of the leg, where it divides into superficial and deep peroneal nerves. The superficial peroneal nerve supplies the peroneous longus and brevis muscles and provides sensation to the anterior and lateral aspect of the leg and dorsum of the foot. The deep peroneal nerve passes over the interosseous membrane and supplies the tibialis anterior and the toe extensors. The terminal branch supplies sensation to the web between the great and second toes.

The peroneal nerve is usually entrapped or compressed at the head and neck of the

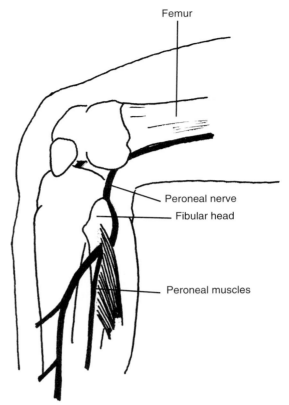

Figure 19–7. The peroneal nerve wrapping around the neck of the fibula and then piercing the peroneal musculature.

fibula or in the fibular tunnel. The compression may occur during sleep, from prolonged sitting with the legs crossed,[16] from tight bandages, or from blunt trauma. The complaint is that the foot is "asleep," and there is a foot drop.

The following conditions should be considered in the differential diagnosis: sciatic nerve compression or entrapment anywhere from its origin to the knee, lumbosacral plexus lesions, and L5 radiculopathy.

The treatment depends on the cause. If the symptoms are due to a temporary compression, then the patient should be advised to avoid pressure on the nerve while the progress is carefully monitored. If it is due to a sports injury, the initial treatment is rest, measures to reduce the swelling (elevation), and gentle physiotherapy (passive exercises). When the foot drop is moderate to severe, a brace in neutral position of the ankle is essential. Nerve conduction studies and electromyography should help in evaluating the progress. If no recovery is seen within a few months, surgical exploration and decompression of the nerve are indicated.

Tarsal Tunnel Syndrome

The posterior tibial nerve crosses behind the medial malleolus to enter the tarsal tunnel. The tunnel is a fibro-osseous canal similar to the carpal tunnel (Fig. 19–8).

In the tarsal tunnel, entrapment of the posterior tibial nerve or its branches is involved.[17] This may be the result of tight, ill-fitting footwear, tenosynovitis, osteophytes, ganglia, rheumatoid arthritis, or blunt trauma with swelling. Symptoms may appear many years after an injury around the ankle, the compression being caused by the chronic fibrosis around the nerve. A true entrapment from a thickened or tight flexor retinaculum is occasionally seen. Sometimes, as with carpal tunnel syndrome, no cause can be found.

Patients usually complain of pain or paresthesias in the sole. Sometimes there may be burning or sharp pains. The symptoms are intermittent and may get worse with walking or running. Tinel's sign is often positive. Radiographs are helpful to rule out skeletal lesions. Nerve conduction studies help in the diagnosis.

The treatment is usually rest, NSAIDs, loose-fitting shoes, and occasionally a steroid injection. If there is no improvement in about 2 to 3 months, surgical decompression may be indicated.

Lateral Femoral Cutaneous Nerve ("Meralgia Paresthetica")

The lateral femoral cutaneous nerve courses across the iliac crest and provides sensation to the lateral aspect of the thigh. Where it penetrates the fascia, it may become entrapped in scar resulting from blunt trauma. It is occasionally injured as a result of injections. Usually the pain and swelling will decrease with time and NSAIDs. Occasionally a steroid injection, TENS (transcutaneous electrical nerve stimulator) unit, and possibly decompression are necessary. If the pain is severe, excision of the nerve may be indicated.

Morton's Neuroma

Perhaps the most common entrapment in the lower extremity is Morton's neuroma. It is the result of compression or entrapment of a common digital nerve, usually the one to the third and fourth toes, at the level of the intermetatarsal ligament (metatarsal head). It is thought to be from microtrauma and repeated compression. Occasionally it occurs between the other toes. This is usually seen in people who wear high heels or shoes with a narrow toe box, and in dancers and runners. The common complaints are pain, numbness, and paresthesias in the adjacent toes. On examination, the affected web space is tender, and squeezing the metatarsal heads reproduces pain.

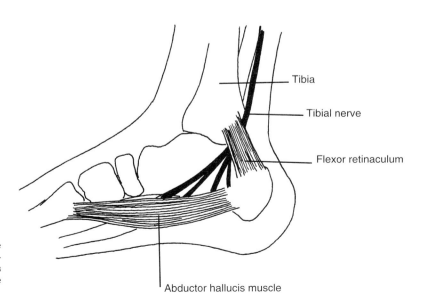

Figure 19–8. The tibial nerve traveling beneath the flexor retinaculum and abductor hallucis muscle on the medial side of the ankle and foot.

Tibia

Tibial nerve

Flexor retinaculum

Abductor hallucis muscle

The patient is advised to avoid pressure on the forefoot and to wear a shoe with a wide toe box and with an off-loading metatarsal pad. Often, injection of steroids into the tender area between the metatarsal heads gives relief. Excision of the neuroma is indicated when pain persists.

References

1. Kopell HP, Thompson WAL: Peripheral Entrapment Neuropathies, 2nd ed. New York, Robert E. Krieger, 1976.
2. Dyck PJ, Thomas PK, Griffin JW, et al. (eds.): Peripheral Neuropathy, 3rd ed. Vol. 2. Philadelphia, WB Saunders, 1991.
3. Bleeker ML: Medical surveillance for carpal tunnel syndrome in workers. J Hand Surg 12A:845, 1987.
4. Goodman HV, Gilliatt RW: The effect of treatment on median nerve conduction in patients with carpal tunnel syndrome. Ann Phys Med 6:137, 1961.
5. Johnson EW, Ortiz PR: Electrodiagnosis of the tarsal tunnel syndrome. Arch Phys Med Rehabil 47:776, 1966.
6. Roos DB: Congenital anomalies associated with thoracic outlet syndrome. Am J Surg 132:771, 1976.
7. Roos DB, Owens JC: Thoracic outlet syndrome. Arch Surg 93:71, 1966.
8. Johnson RK, Spinner M, Shrewsbury MM: Median nerve entrapment syndrome in the proximal forearm. J Hand Surg 4:48, 1979.
9. Kimura J: The carpal tunnel syndrome: Localisation of conduction abnormalities within the distal segment of the median nerve. Brain 102:619, 1979.
10. Middleton WD, Kneeland JB, Kellman GM, et al.: MR imaging of the carpal tunnel: Normal anatomy and preliminary findings in the carpal tunnel syndrome. AJR 148:307, 1987.
11. Miller RG: The cubital tunnel syndrome: Diagnosis and precise localisation. Ann Neurol 6:56, 1979.
12. Miller RG, Hummel EE: The cubital tunnel syndrome: Treatment with simple decompression. Ann Neurol 6:56, 1979.
13. Desai KM, Gingell JC: Hazards of long distance cycling. Br Med J 298:1072, 1989.
14. Hagert CG, Lundborg G, Hansen T: Entrapment of the posterior interosseous nerve. Scand J Plast Reconstr Surg 11:205, 1977.
15. Kaplan PE: Posterior interosseous neuropathies: Natural history. Arch Phys Med Rehabil 65:399, 1984.
16. Nagler SH, Rangell L: Peroneal palsy caused by crossing the legs. JAMA 133:755, 1947.
17. Mann RA: Tarsal tunnel syndrome. Orthop Clin North Am 5:109, 1974.

CHAPTER 20

Vascular Injuries

Ekkehard Bonatz

ARTERIAL INJURIES

Peripheral vascular injuries are most commonly caused by low-velocity gunshot wounds, followed in frequency by stab wounds. Injuries from fractures or dislocations are less frequent. There are well-known arterial complications following certain fracture-dislocations: in the upper extremity, the axillary artery may be injured by an anterior dislocation of the shoulder or fracture of the neck of the humerus. The brachial artery is in danger following supracondylar fractures of the humerus or dislocations of the elbow. In the lower extremity, a fracture of the middle one third of the femur may injure the superficial femoral artery, whereas a more distal fracture in the supracondylar area of the femur or a knee dislocation poses a risk to the popliteal artery. Fracture of the proximal tibia may injure the popliteal artery or the tibial/peroneal trunk or even the anterior tibial artery.

Diagnosis

Signs of arterial injury include massive external bleeding, a rapidly expanding hematoma, a palpable or audible bruit over a hematoma, distal pulselessness, pallor, paresthesias, pain, or paralysis. Other signs

are a history of arterial bleeding at the scene of the injury, proximity of a penetrating injury, a small nonpulsatile hematoma, or neurologic deficits.

Physical Examination

The presence of any obvious bone or joint deformities should be noted. The skin of the distal extremity is compared with that of the opposite side. Examination is made for the presence or absence of a hematoma, and whether or not it may be expanding. Any open wounds are noted. In the lower extremity, the knee joint should be carefully assessed, especially in closed injuries. Increased laxity of the knee ligaments suggests a dislocation that has spontaneously reduced. There is a known association between dislocation of the knee and injury to the popliteal artery (see Chapter 2). Distal arterial pulses in the injured extremity are then checked and compared with those in the opposite limb. The absence of palpable pulses in the distal extremity, skin temperature, and capillary refill should be noted. Blood pressure measurements of the ankle and upper arm can be performed. The antebrachial index can be calculated when the vascular status of the distal extremity is unclear. The Doppler flow meter may determine audibly the presence or absence of pulses in the distal extremity.

Early Management

The primary goal is to control hemorrhage in the patient with an extensive injury to the extremity. This is done by direct compression of the wound with a finger or by the application of a pressure dressing. A blood pressure cuff may be applied proximal to the area of the injury and inflated above systolic pressure for a short period of time, if the previous methods fail. In a fracture or dislocation, immediate reduction and appropriate splinting should be performed. If pulses do not return with reduction of the fracture or dislocation, an immediate vascular consultation must be obtained.[1] An arteriogram is ordered if it is unclear that the artery is actually severed. With a clear disruption of the artery, emergency surgery is needed.

Although the artery may be completely divided, exsanguinating hemorrhage is not necessarily a sequela, because the vessel ends retract. Arterial spasm and thrombosis often will seal the lumen (Fig. 20–1A,B). In a partial laceration, however, hemorrhage may be severe, and secondary hemorrhage is likely. Because the arterial ends cannot retract, a large hematoma will accumulate over the opening (Fig. 20–1C,D). The arterial pressure develops a cavity within the hematoma while the outer wall of the mass becomes organized, forming a so-called false (or pseudo-) aneurysm (Fig. 20–2). Simultaneous partial division of the accompanying vein will allow blood to re-enter the vein. An arteriovenous fistula is the result. A con-

tused vessel will go into spasm and also will involve its collaterals. Spasm alone does not necessarily result in thrombosis. This would require additional damage to the intimal layer of the artery, as well as slowed blood flow (Virchow's triad).

Early Management of Arterial Injuries in the Upper Extremity. Since unrepaired arterial injuries may cause persistent alteration of the hand vascularity with secondary signs of ischemia or cold intolerance, it is important to maintain repairability of vascular injuries. Initially, compression dressings should be applied, and no hemostats should be applied to any vascular ends in the emergency department. Nerve ends are sometimes mistaken for vascular endings (especially on the ulnar side of the wrist), and a superimposed hemostat crush injury to a damaged nerve may further hinder nerve repair and recovery. Definitive arterial repair or ligation should be performed in the operating room.

Direct compression of an artery usually occurs because of a bone fragment. The main complication of this is thrombosis. Vascular compression occurs where the vessels are held fixed closely to the bone, especially at the elbow or knee.

ANEURYSMS AND FISTULAS

An aneurysm is an abnormal outpouching from a vessel. If the wall of the aneurysm is made of the vessel structure itself, it is called a true aneurysm (Fig. 20–2A). If the vessel wall was penetrated and the wall of the sac is composed of a blood clot, fibrous tissue, and surrounding structures, it is termed a false aneurysm (Fig. 20–2B). A laceration of the vessel is caused from the outside by a penetrating wound or fracture. Only a portion of the circumference of the vessel is involved. With a laceration of the outer layers, the arterial pressure dilates the intact inner layer. The thin residual walls of the blood vessel are supported by surrounding tissue. Laminations of the blood clot enforce the wall, and eventually the distended clot will become endothelialized. The cavity will become part of the peripheral circulation.

Distally, the blood supply will be diminished. Often, there is a reflex spasm of the collateral vessels, or emboli are thrown into the distal smaller vessels, causing their occlusion.

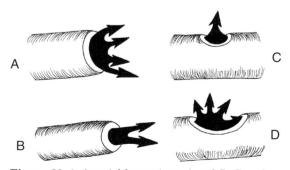

Figure 20–1. Arterial lacerations. *A* and *B,* Complete transection of an artery leads to spasm, with diminished arterial lumen and less bleeding. *C* and *D,* In a longitudinal laceration, spasm of the artery will increase the size of the laceration, making hemostasis difficult.

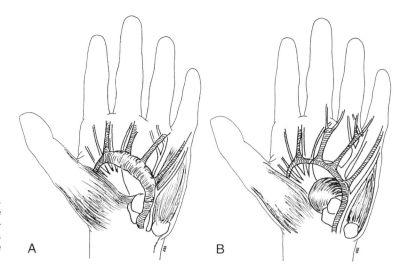

Figure 20–2. Arterial aneurysm. *A,* In a true aneurysm, the entire artery is involved. *B,* A false aneurysm originates from a small hole in the vascular wall and leads to the expanding, organized hematoma.

A

B

Symptoms will vary with the involved vessel. Since collateral circulation in the upper extremity is usually good, symptoms of peripheral ischemia are often absent. In the lower extremity, however, claudication or gangrene is possible. Sometimes a mass can be felt. Pain is usually localized in the area of the aneurysm owing to pressure on adjacent structures, because of nerve compression, or ischemic claudication. Paresthesias or paralysis may occur in addition to pain. Often, there will be signs of circulatory insufficiency, such as asymmetric pulses, decreased blood pressure, and diminished Doppler readings. Sometimes the skin temperature may be lower distal to the injury. Occasionally, a characteristic bruit may be heard over the aneurysm. In arterial aneurysms, the bruit is synchronous with systole, whereas in arteriovenous aneurysms there will be a to-and-fro murmur. When the extremity is compared with the contralateral one, trophic changes may also be seen. Treatment consists of resection of the aneurysm, with repair or interposition grafting of the artery.

Arteriovenous fistulas, while often presenting like false or true aneurysms, will show increased, not decreased, skin temperature. There may also be increased oxygenation of venous blood on venipuncture. Doppler readings will show decreased pressure distal to the arteriovenous communication. Pulses may be diminished or even absent. Surgical ligation of the abnormal arteriovenous connection and interposition grafting of one or both vessels are treatment options.

ARTERIAL THROMBOSIS IN THE UPPER EXTREMITY

Anatomy. The ulnar artery, which is larger than the radial artery, forms the primary arterial contribution to the hand. The radial artery passes deep to the abductor pollicis brevis and extensor pollicis longus tendons over the snuffbox area between the base of the thumb and index metacarpal to form the deep arch. The superficial palmar arch, which is distal to the deep palmar arch, is complete in only 34 percent of hands. The deep palmar arch is more proximal and is more consistent than the superficial arch (Fig. 20–3). In the fingers, the digital arteries are larger on the ulnar side than on the radial side, except for the small finger.

History. Exposure to vibrating tools or repetitive blunt trauma may cause the development of an aneurysm or thrombosis of the ulnar artery. With penetrating trauma (e.g., needle marks on the volar forearm), it is important to consider drug use or substance injections that might cause distal emboli. Pain with shoulder abduction might indicate a problem in the clavicular area. The most common vasoconstrictive drug is tobacco, and such history should be obtained. Occasionally, collagen diseases such as scleroderma or psoriatic arthritis can cause problems in the fingertips. Buerger's disease is usually seen in middle-aged men with a strong history of smoking. The history of blanched fingers with cold or emotional upset indicates Raynaud's phenomenon.

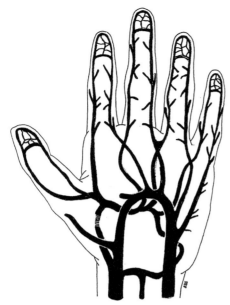

Figure 20-3. Arterial anatomy of the hand (palmar view). The superficial arch is complete in only 34 percent of people.

Physical Examination. Physical examination should include observation of the upper limb for any masses or discolorations. Peripheral pulses are recorded. Areas of tenderness may point to the location of the thrombosed vessel. The blood pressure should be taken bilaterally. Allen's test is obtained by obliterating both radial and ulnar arteries, and asking the patient to make a fist two or three times. He or she is then asked to relax the fingers. Either artery is released and blanching of the fingers observed. The average filling time through the radial or ulnar artery is slightly over 2 seconds. Rarely an ulnar or radial artery fails to fill the hand completely within 6 seconds. In an unconscious patient, the radial artery is located and marked. A blood pressure cuff is applied and the limb exsanguinated with a bandage. The cuff is inflated above systolic pressure and the bandage removed. The pre-marked radial artery is compressed digitally and the cuff deflated. The return of arterial fill in the hand shows the extent to which the ulnar artery supplies the hand.[2,3]

Thrombosis of the Ulnar Artery

Thrombosis in the upper extremity is most commonly seen in the ulnar artery secondary to repetitive trauma. It will present as a tender mass in the palm over the hypothenar eminence. There may be distal vascular insufficiency. It is usually seen in patients using power tools or using the hand as a hammer ("hypothenar hammer syndrome") but occasionally is seen following falls on the outstretched hand. Other arteries may be similarly involved.

Patients with ulnar artery thrombosis present with a tender, painful mass in the hypothenar area of the hand and will sometimes have ischemic symptoms with pallor or even early gangrene. Occasionally, there will be numbness or paresthesias secondary to nerve compression of one or more branches of the ulnar nerve. Cold sensitivity, cold intolerance, or Raynaud's phenomenon may be present. With unilateral Raynaud's phenomenon, only the ulnar two to three digits may be involved. Nerve involvement is usually ulnar sensory, but occasionally median motor nerve function will be affected. Most of the patients with ulnar artery thrombosis are working men subjected to blunt trauma in the hand. It may also occur in older people, e.g., it has been described in a 70-year-old woman using her cane. Normally, the radial artery is less involved but may be obliterated where it crosses beneath the extensor pollicis longus tendon. Systemic diseases such as temporal arteritis (giant cell inflammatory arterial disease) can cause similar symptoms.

The correct diagnosis is usually suspected from the history. An Allen's test, both by inspection and with a Doppler test, can further determine the site of injury: if the ulnar artery is thrombosed, compression of the radial artery will obliterate perfusion of the hand and fingers. Sometimes the artery is thrombosed in association with a fracture of the hook of the hamate. With vibratory tool exposure, the picture of Raynaud's phenomenon and cold intolerance often appears much later, even after cessation of working with the offending tool. Patients are usually forced to change jobs and to avoid cold temperatures. Symptomatic treatment is by cessation of smoking or the use of gloves to minimize cold exposure. Often, however, the aneurysm of the ulnar artery must be surgically resected in order to eliminate the source of distal emboli.

An embolic phenomenon can occur not only from a peripheral artery but also from the heart or from arteries in the neck. Referral to a vascular surgeon with the goal of embolectomy should be considered.

Cannulation and Injection Injuries

Acute injection trauma, such as the inadvertent cannulation or street drug injection of the artery instead of the vein in the cubital fossa, may lead to spasm and occlusion with major distal problems. This constitutes a vascular emergency. An attempt can be made to remove distal clots with a Fogarty catheter. Clot dissolvers, e.g., urokinase, may be helpful, as are alpha-receptor blocking agents (dibenzyline), myovascular relaxants such as nitroglycerine ointment, or catecholaminic antagonists such as reserpine administered via a Bier's block. A stellate ganglion block may increase collateral circulation.

Thoracic Outlet Syndrome

Compression of the subclavian and axillary arteries in the neck may result in pain and distal vascular occlusion. The occlusion may be venous or arterial. Provocative pulse obliteration may be positive with Adson's maneuver, the shoulder brace test, or abduction of the shoulder to 90 and 180 degrees. For Adson's maneuver, the arm of the side affected is placed on the sitting patient's thigh with the forearm supinated. The patient turns the head to the affected side and extends the neck while holding the breath. A positive test is the obliteration of the radial pulse (Fig. 20–4). In the hyperabduction maneuver, the patient places the extremity in full abduction and reaches back as far as possible. The test is done actively and passively. Radial pulse obliteration alone is not significant, but loss of the pulse with reproduction of symptoms is indicative (Fig. 20–5).

Thoracic outlet syndrome with vascular compression, as evidenced by gangrene of the fingers, can occur through bone or fibrous structures, such as the scalenus anterior muscle. A rudimentary first rib, linked to the second rib, may also cause compression of the vascular structures. Actions that precipitate this problem include prolonged abnormal hyperabduction of the arm (in painters, or in mechanics working under a car, or in persons holding the arm abducted while asleep).

A plain anteroposterior radiograph of the neck should be obtained to look for a cervical

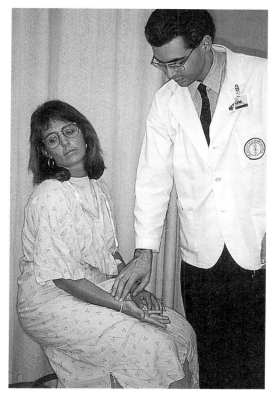

Figure 20–4. In the Adson maneuver, the arm of the affected side is placed on the sitting patient's thigh with the forearm supinated. The patient turns the head to the affected side and extends the neck while holding the breath. A positive test is the obliteration of the radial pulse.

rib. Arteriography or venography, however, often will be necessary to rule out vascular pathology.

The best treatment is behavior modification. Exercises to strengthen the shoulder girdle will improve posture and prevent drooping shoulders. Ultimately, surgical removal of any compressing structures may be considered.

Normal or at least asymptomatic persons may have their radial pulse obliterated by Adson's maneuver or hyperabduction of the arm. They should be cautioned about occupations that require raising the arms over the head or sleeping with the arms over the head. They should also be wary of placing unusual stress on the shoulder girdle (e.g., as may occur in carrying backpacks).

Primary Vasospastic Conditions

Raynaud's disease, or primary Raynaud's phenomenon, is known as pallor of the digits

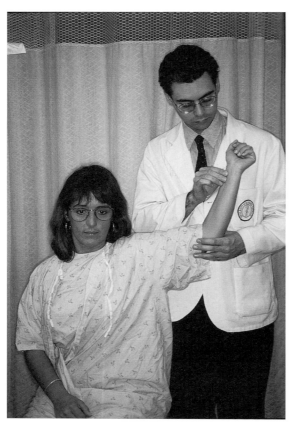

Figure 20–5. The hyperabduction maneuver. The patient places the arm in full abduction and reaches back as far as possible. Radial pulse obliteration with reproduction of symptoms indicates a positive test.

tive tissue, neurologic, or arterial occlusive disorders.

Treatment principles include protection from cold and trauma and cessation of smoking. Occasionally, pharmacologic treatment for alpha-receptor blockage—reserpine or nifedipine—can be used. If these fail, thermal biofeedback or surgical treatment, including digital or cervical sympathectomy, may be warranted. The patient must understand that without cessation of smoking, any other treatment will likely fail.

Cold Injury

Frostbite may be superficial or deep. If the entire layer of skin is involved, it is classified as deep. Two mechanisms involved are direct injury to the cells and vascular impairment. Vascular damage occurs through endothelial injury leading to thrombosis formation, hemoconcentration, and increased viscosity. Increased sympathetic tone will produce vasoconstriction and stasis with secondary pain. Treatment is rapid rewarming in a water bath to 40 degrees Celsius, local protection from further cold, and regional sympathectomy. At times distal amputations are needed following full demarcation of skin necrosis.

References

1. Feliciano DV: Evaluation and treatment of vascular injuries. *In* Browner BD (ed): Skeletal Trauma. Philadelphia, WB Saunders, 1992, pp 269–284.
2. Gelberman RH, Blasingame JP, Fronek A, et al: Forearm arterial injuries. J Hand Surg 4:401–408, 1979.
3. Newmeyer WL: Vascular disorders. *In* Green DP (ed): Operative Hand Surgery. New York, Churchill Livingstone, 1993, pp 2251–2308.

Suggested Reading

Coleman SS, Anson BJ: Arterial patterns in the hand based upon a study of 650 specimens. Surg Gynecol Obstet 113:409–424, 1961.
Koman LA, Urbaniak JR: Ulnar artery insufficiency—a guide to treatment. Proceedings of the American Society for Surgery of the Hand, J Hand Surg, January 1981.
Wilgis EFS: The evaluation and treatment of chronic digital ischemia. Ann Surg 193:693–698, 1981.

with or without cyanosis on exposure to cold. On rewarming, an intense hyperemia is seen. The color changes classically occur in three phases: digital pallor is followed by cyanosis and hyperemia. The hands are normal between these episodes. Raynaud's disease has no demonstrable associated disease. It will occur mostly in young women and is often bilateral. Attacks are precipitated by cold or emotional upset. There is no clinical occlusion of peripheral arteries, and no organic disease can be found. Gangrene or trophic changes are usually limited to the distal skin. Raynaud's syndrome, also known as secondary Raynaud's phenomenon, is present when the phenomenon is associated with or caused by a disease, such as connec-

CHAPTER 21

Injuries to Muscles and Tendons

Jean E. Oakes

Donald H. Lee

Muscle contusions are a result of blunt trauma. This results in a hematoma and an inflammatory reaction. The hematoma usually resolves, with replacement of the muscle by connective tissue scar. Occasionally, myositis ossificans develops. In this condition, heterotopic bone formation results from a muscle hematoma. Clinically, pain, swelling, and impairment of muscle function are seen. Heterotopic bone can be seen radiographically within 3 to 4 weeks from injury. The trabecular bone can be seen within the muscle belly. Treatment consists of restricting use of the muscle, light compressive dressings, ice, elevation of the extremity to reduce the size of the developing hematoma, and use of nonsteroidal anti-inflammatory medications. This is followed by gradual rehabilitation to regain range of motion as pain allows, usually within a few days. Surgical excision of the hematoma is contraindicated.[4,19]

Ruptures of muscles and tendons occur when the muscle tendon unit is subjected to excessive stretch or tension. A muscle strain or pull usually refers to an incomplete rupture of the muscle. The rupture, whether incomplete or complete, usually occurs at the muscle tendon junction. The injury can occur during a muscle contraction, but it can also occur when the muscle is inactive. Most are incomplete tears. The muscles most susceptible to strain and rupture are those that cross two joints. Other predisposing factors to muscle injury are fatigue and intrinsic tightness of the muscle.[4]

Tendon ruptures may be complete or incomplete. They occur in areas of weakness in the tendon substance that develop from either repetitive microtrauma or from an injury to a poorly healed area of previous trauma. They are most commonly seen in middle-aged or elderly people. Predisposing conditions include rheumatoid arthritis, systemic lupus erythematosus, hyperparathyroidism, xanthoma, renal failure, use of systemic steroids, and local injection of steroids into a tendon.[17]

Patients with muscle strains are found clinically to have a painful, functional muscle-tendon unit. Local tenderness and pain upon active contraction or passive stretch of the muscle are noted. A history of a stretch injury or pain with a strong muscle contraction is usually found. Patients may note an immediate onset of pain with a strong muscle contraction. Muscle strains are treated with rest, ice, and nonsteroidal anti-inflammatory drugs, followed by a rehabilitation period of stretching and progressive strengthening when the discomfort diminishes (1 to 2 weeks). A return to full use of the muscle prior to regaining full range of motion and strength may result in a recurrent injury.[17]

Complete muscle and tendon ruptures are associated with the clinical findings of pain, loss of function, and often proximal migration of the muscle mass. The most common areas of complete rupture are the achilles tendon, plantaris tendon, posterior tibial tendon, finger flexor and extensor tendons, biceps, rotator cuff, and quadriceps tendons. Complete ruptures may be treated with surgical repair if a functional loss is noted.

Lacerations of muscles and tendons are associated with penetrating injuries. The injury can be located anywhere along the muscle-tendon unit. The diagnosis is made by a physical examination demonstrating a loss of function or by direct inspection of the wound. Most open injuries usually require prompt wound debridement and surgical repair of the damaged structures.

ACHILLES TENDON

The Achilles tendon, located in the posterior calf, is formed by the union of the tendons of the gastrocnemius and soleus muscles. The tendon inserts into the posterior aspect of the calcaneus. The Achilles tendon is one of the more frequently ruptured tendons. The mechanism of injury is often from a forced dorsiflexion of the foot or during push-off while the knee is extended. A laceration or direct blow to the contracting muscle can also result in a ruptured Achilles tendon. The tendon has a relatively hypovascular area 2 to 6 cm proximal to its insertion on the calcaneus. Repetitive microtrauma or a supraphysiologic load placed on the tendon may result in a tendon rupture.[8]

A history of a sudden popping sound or sensation may be given. Clinically, a ruptured Achilles tendon is demonstrated by Thompson's test (Fig. 21–1). The test is performed with the patient in a supine position or kneeling on a chair. By squeezing the calf muscles firmly, the foot should plantar flex. If the foot fails to plantar flex, rupture is

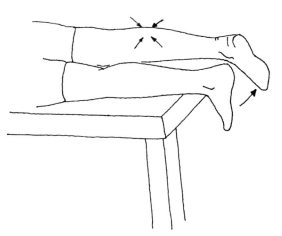

Figure 21–1. The Thompson test is performed with the patient in a supine position or in a kneeling position. The calf is manually compressed and plantar flexion of the foot should occur if the Achilles tendon is intact.

likely. A palpable tendon defect and inability to raise up on one's toes will also help confirm the diagnosis.

Treatment can include either long leg casting or operative repair followed by casting.[2] For the patient treated with casting alone, a splint or cast is used with the ankle placed in a plantar flexed position. The cast is worn for a minimum of 6 to 8 weeks. During this period the foot is gradually dorsiflexed so that a neutral position is reached by 6 to 8 weeks. At this time, the patient is allowed to bear weight on the cast. A short leg cast can be used at approximately 3 to 4 weeks following initial casting. Full activity is limited until full motion is obtained, usually 3 to 6 months. Operative treatment, usually in the younger, more athletic population, is followed with a similar casting regimen.

PLANTARIS TENDON

The plantaris muscle, when present, originates from the lower lateral supracondylar ridge of the femur. It travels obliquely between the gastrocnemius and soleus muscles to insert onto the calcaneus medial to the Achilles tendon. The plantaris functions in assisting plantarflexion of the foot and flexion of the knee.

Rupture of the plantaris tendon occurs with forced ankle dorsiflexion during attempted active plantar flexion of the ankle. It can cause marked swelling and disabling pain in the upper middle calf near its musculotendinous junction. Its diagnosis can be confused with a medial gastrocnemius muscle rupture. The diagnosis is made by the history of an injury and with calf pain and swelling. A history of a popping sensation may be present. The treatment includes rest, immobilization for comfort if needed, and nonsteroidal anti-inflammatory medications. No repair is needed, since usually there is no functional deficit. A gradual return to full activities depends on the patient's level of discomfort.

GASTROCNEMIUS MUSCLE

The gastrocnemius muscle is the most superficial calf muscle. It is composed of two heads of origin. The lateral head originates from the lateral femoral condyle and the medial head from the femur above the medial condyle. They insert into a broad aponeurosis, which joins the tendon of the soleus muscle to form the Achilles tendon. The function of the gastrocnemius is to plantar flex the foot and flex the knee.

Rupture of the medial head of the gastrocnemius can be confused with a rupture of the plantaris tendon or with thrombophlebitis.[15] Frequently, these injuries cannot be distinguished. However, the care of these conditions is the same. The injury occurs most commonly in middle-aged male athletes, during activities such as jogging or playing tennis.[17] Overload of the muscle causes a rupture at the insertion of the medial head into the soleus aponeuroses. This usually occurs when the knee is extended and the ankle is dorsiflexed. Examination of a ruptured medial gastrocnemius muscle reveals pain and swelling in the medial calf area. A mass may be palpable in this area. Treatment includes rest, ice, elevation, and nonsteroidal anti-inflammatory medications. Activity is limited by the patient's level of discomfort. One can usually distinguish between gastrocnemius and plantaris rupture by the presence of a change in the symmetry of the calf musculature with a gastrocnemius rupture. Treatment is the same for either injury.

PERONEAL TENDONS

The peroneal muscles are located on the lateral side of the leg. The peroneus longus and brevis originate from the upper two thirds of the fibula and the lower two thirds of the fibula, respectively. The peroneal tendons pass behind the fibula and posterior to the lateral malleolus in a groove. They are held in place by the superior peroneal retinaculum. The peroneus longus then enters a groove on the plantar side of the cuboid and inserts on the medial cuneiform and the base of the first metatarsal. The peroneus brevis remains on the lateral side of the foot and inserts onto the base of the fifth metatarsal. Their action is to plantar flex and evert the foot.

The peroneal tendons may become painful without rupturing secondary to tendinitis, tenosynovitis, and subluxation. The tendons become tender behind the fibula and under the lateral malleolus. With subluxation of the tendons, a popping or clicking may be palpable along the posterior lateral malleolus where the superior peroneal retinaculum may be insufficient.

Clinically, there is localized tenderness on palpation. This can be demonstrated with either active motion (active eversion against an inversion force) or attempted subluxation of the tendons out of their groove by the examiner's finger. The mechanism of injury is usually of forced ankle dorsiflexion during strong peroneal contraction. Provocative testing is performed by having the patient actively dorsiflex, evert, and externally rotate the foot while an inversion and plantar flexion force is applied by the examiner.[17] Tenderness, pain, or subluxation of the peroneal tendons may be noted.

The treatment of peroneal tendinitis and tenosynovitis includes rest, immobilization, and nonsteroidal anti-inflammatory medications. Judicious use of local steroid injections (less than three injections per year) may be warranted to treat recalcitrant tendinitis. Painful acute and chronic tendon dislocations frequently need surgical correction.

Ruptures of the peroneal tendons occur with contraction of the peroneal muscles and simultaneous forced inversion and dorsiflexion of the foot. Clinically, tenderness is along the course of the tendon from the level of the musculotendinous junction to an area under the superior peroneal retinaculum. Radiographs may show an os peroneum (sesamoid of the peroneal tendon) displaced from its normal position near the cuboid.[18] Attempted active eversion of the foot is usually painful. Ruptures of the peroneal tendons are usually surgically repaired within the first week or two. The initial treatment should include a posterior short leg splint, elevation, and non-steroidal anti-inflammatory medications.

POSTERIOR TIBIAL TENDON

The tibialis posterior muscle originates from the posterolateral tibia, the interosseous membrane, and the proximal posterior fibula. Its insertion is into the navicular bone after it passes behind the medial malleolus. Its action is to plantar flex and invert the foot. It also helps maintain the medial longitudinal arch of the foot.

A rupture of the posterior tibial tendon is not likely to occur as an acute event, although occasionally a patient may note a sudden loss of the medial arch of the foot. Tendon ruptures usually develop as a result of chronic tenosynovitis. Symptoms are episodic medial ankle pain with tenderness along the tendon, followed by the gradual development of lateral foot pain when the lateral talus impinges on the sinus tarsi. A flat foot deformity develops. Physical findings include a unilateral flat foot with loss of the medial longitudinal arch upon weight bearing, a hindfoot valgus, and forefoot pronation deformity.[18] When both feet are viewed from behind, a "too many toes" sign may be present on the lateral side of the involved foot, compared with the normal foot (Fig. 21–2). More toes may be seen on the lateral aspect of the foot due to the foot deformities. Treatment consists of a double upright brace or ankle foot orthosis (University of California, Berkley). Operative treatment may be indicated for the relatively

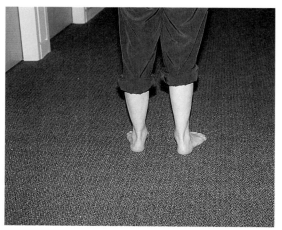

Figure 21–2. "Too many toes" sign on patient's right foot.

acute injury or for the treatment of long-standing painful deformities of the foot that are unresponsive to bracing.

KNEE EXTENSOR MECHANISM— PATELLAR AND QUADRICEPS TENDON

The quadriceps femoris muscle is composed of four muscles: the rectus femoris, vastus lateralis, vastus medialis, and vastus intermedius. The rectus muscle originates from the anterior inferior iliac spine and the ilium; the vasti originate from the proximal femur. All four muscles unite to form the quadriceps tendon which inserts on the medial, superior, and lateral surfaces of the patella. The patella is actually a large sesamoid bone within the quadriceps tendon. The patellar tendon is the ligament attaching the lower pole of the patella to the tibial tubercle.

The most common cause for disruption of the extensor mechanism is a fracture of the patella, followed by disruption of the quadriceps and patellar tendons. The injury usually occurs when the knee is forcibly flexed as the quadriceps muscle is contracting. Stumbling is a common method of generating this force. In patients less than 40 years of age, patellar tendon rupture is common, whereas quadriceps rupture is seen more frequently in the older population. Conditions associated with quadriceps rupture include diabetes mellitus, lupus, gout, hyperparathyroidism, uremia, and obesity.[17] A radiograph should be taken to exclude patellar fracture. Pain, swelling, and inability to extend the knee is the usual history. The patient may have a palpable defect in the patellar tendon just distal to the patella and proximal migration of the patella associated with a patellar tendon rupture. With a rupture of the quadriceps tendon, the patella may be displaced inferiorly. A palpable defect may be present at the superior border of the patella. Treatment of a traumatic rupture is a bulky compressive dressing with a knee immobilizer, and referral for surgical repair.

POPLITEUS TENDON

The popliteus muscle arises from the lateral surface of the lateral femoral condyle within the knee joint. It inserts on the posterior proximal tibia. It acts to rotate the tibia medially during flexion of the knee and to stabilize the lateral meniscus. Isolated injuries to the popliteus tendon have been reported from nonspecific twisting injuries and blows to the lateral knee. An injury is suspected with an otherwise unexplained hemarthrosis or knee effusion and associated tenderness following a popping sensation in the posterior or lateral knee. A radiograph occasionally may demonstrate an osteochondral fragment near the nonweight-bearing portion of the lateral femoral condyle. The initial treatment includes the use of a bulky dressing with a knee immobilizer, rest and elevation. Surgical repair of a large osteochondral fragment may be indicated.[5]

ROTATOR CUFF TENDINITIS

The rotator cuff of the shoulder is composed of the tendons of the subscapularis, supraspinatus, infraspinatus, and teres minor muscles. These muscles arise from the scapula and insert on the lateral humeral head. Impingement of these tendons as they pass between the humeral head and the coracoacromial arch (coracoid, acromion, and coracoacromial ligament) causes rotator cuff tendinitis. Impingement is found in three groups of patients: one third result from occupations with overhead lifting activities; one third occur in athletes with overhead throwing, swinging, or swimming motions; and one third have no specific activity related to their impingement but tend to occur in people with an average age of approximately 60 years.[14]

Patients present with pain, stiffness, symptoms of catching or popping, and problems sleeping on the involved shoulder. The symptoms are reproduced with forward flexion and internal rotation of the shoulder. Treatment consists of avoiding aggravating activities, strengthening exercises for the rotator cuff muscles, nonsteroidal anti-inflammatory medications, and occasionally subacromial steroid injections. See Chapter 22 for more details on the impingement syndrome.

BICEPS

The biceps brachii has two heads, a long head originating from the supraglenoid tubercle on the scapula and a short head originating from the coracoid process. The muscle inserts on the radial tuberosity. The biceps acts to flex the elbow and supinate the forearm. The biceps can rupture either proximally or distally. Proximal ruptures are usually ruptures of the long head of the biceps tendon. They can be acute ruptures associated with a history of heavy lifting[6] or with tears of the rotator cuff muscles. With acute injuries, patients may experience pain and occasionally a sudden snap or pop. A mass representing the retracted muscle belly appears in the midarm. The size of the mass may increase with active supination of the forearm or flexion of the elbow against resistance.[22] Initially there may be weakness of forearm supination and elbow flexion. Treatment is usually a shoulder sling for comfort. Loss of function is frequently minimal, with only a 10 percent loss of supination strength.[21] Surgery may be indicated in the treatment of young, active patients, such as carpenters or mechanics needing full supination strength.

Rupture of the distal biceps with avulsion off the radial tuberosity occurs in only 3 percent of biceps ruptures.[1] The mechanism is lifting a heavy load or contracting the elbow against an unexpected resistance. Rupture of the biceps at its radial insertion frequently results in a significant loss of flexion and supination strength.[16] Treatment includes resting the arm in a sling with referral for surgical repair.

TRIGGER FINGER

The flexor tendons of the hand travel through a pulley system that keeps the tendon approximated to the bone and prevents bowstringing of the tendons. The first annular ligament or pulley (A1) is located at the level of the metacarpophalangeal (MP) joint. The flexor digitorum profundus and flexor digitorum superficialis tendons enter the narrow fibro-osseous tunnel at the A1 pulley.

A trigger finger can develop, with a nodularity or thickening of the flexor tendons. The normal gliding motion of the tendon(s) at the A1 pulley is restricted. Tendon enlargement can occur from a variety of causes, including a congenital predisposition (congenital trigger finger), trauma or repetitive microtrauma, synovitis of rheumatoid arthritis, in association with diabetes, or without any etiology (idiopathic).[9]

With finger flexion, the nodule is pulled through the A1 pulley.[10] The finger extensor muscles, being relatively weak compared with finger flexors, cannot easily pull the nodule or thickening back through the pulley. The nodule "jams" in the pulley until it suddenly pops through when additional extensor force is applied. The catching observed is known as triggering.[11]

The diagnosis is made through the presence of the triggering phenomenon in association with tenderness over the pulley (palmar side of the MP joint), and a palpable nodule in the tendon. Treatment consists of the judicious use of steroid injections (three injections or less per year) into the tendon sheath, splinting of the digit in extension at night, and use of nonsteroidal anti-inflammatory medications. Surgery is indicated in those patients not responding to nonoperative treatment.[10] With congenital trigger fingers, splinting without injection may be effective. Surgical release is required early before progressive deformities develop.

FLEXOR TENDONS OF THE HAND

Two flexor tendons are present in each finger, the flexor digitorum superficialis (FDS) and the flexor digitorum profundus (FDP). The thumb has only a single tendon, the flexor pollicis longus (FPL).

The FDS muscle originates from the medial epicondyle of the humerus, the coronoid process of the ulna, and the anterior surface of the radius. The FDS tendon attaches to the medial and lateral aspects of the middle phalanx.

The FDP muscle originates from the proximal ulna and the interosseous membrane. The FDP tendons lie deep to the FDS tendons until they reach the level of the proximal phalanx, where they pass through the split in the FDS tendon and insert onto the base of the distal phalanx. The FDS muscle is innervated by the median nerve. The radial half of the FDP muscle is innervated by the median nerve and the ulnar half by the ulnar nerve. The FDS flexes the proximal interphalangeal (PIP) joint, and the FDP flexes the distal interphalangeal (DIP) joint. The FPL tendon originates from the radial shaft and interosseous membrane. It inserts onto the distal phalanx of the thumb. It is innervated by the median nerve and acts to flex the distal phalanx of the thumb.

Ruptures of the flexor tendons are most often due to sharp lacerations. They can also be associated with flexor tenosynovitis in rheumatoid arthritis, fractures of the distal radius, and osseous prominences. The diagnosis is made by physical examination. With open wounds, the cut end of the tendons may or may not be seen. The level of the tendon injury may not be at the level of the skin wound. If the tendon has been cut with the finger in a flexed position, the proximal tendon stump is usually retracted proximally, and the distal portion is pulled distally when the digit is extended for examination. Inspection of the hand should reveal a normal resting attitude to the digits. The normal attitude or posture of the hand reveals a cascade of finger flexion that is greatest in the little finger and least in the index finger. A digit out of sequence, i.e., more extension than expected, is suspected of having a flexor tendon laceration.

Testing of finger flexion at the PIP joint and DIP joint individually will diagnose a FDS or FDP laceration, respectively. To test the status of the FDS tendon, all digits, except the one being examined, are held in extension. The patient should be able to flex the PIP joint of the tested finger. The FDP tendon is assessed by holding the PIP joint of the digit being tested in an extended position. The patient should be able to flex the DIP joint actively. In the thumb, to test the FPL tendon, the MP joint is held in extension while the patient attempts to flex the interphalangeal joint of the thumb. The distal phalanx of the thumb should flex if the FPL is intact.[12]

The fingers should be examined for associated neurovascular injuries. The neurovascular bundles lie on either side of the digit and are often lacerated with the tendon. Wound inspection is important to determine whether there is communication into the joint space. Radiographs should be taken to rule out associated fractures and dislocations. With a clean wound not associated with an exposed joint, fracture, or dislocation, soft tissue injuries can be repaired on a semi-elective basis, preferably within a week. The wound should be irrigated and cleaned and the skin closed if delayed repair is planned. The hand should be placed in a bulky soft dressing, with a dorsal splint with the wrist in a neutral to slightly flexed position and MP joints flexed 60 to 70 degrees.

JERSEY FINGER

Avulsion of the flexor digitorum profundus insertion into the distal phalanx is an injury that often occurs in young men playing football and rugby. When the patient grabs at the jersey or clothing of another player, the ring finger is the most likely to be caught in the cloth, and an avulsion injury occurs as the person tries to flex his digits as the other player breaks away (jersey finger). Often there is a delay in diagnosis; the patient may continue to play and be told he simply "jammed" his finger.[10]

Examination shows an inability actively to flex the DIP joint, tenderness along the volar surface of the finger, and perhaps a palpable painful mass in the finger or palm. Radiographs may show a variably sized avulsed bone fragment. Surgical repair is best performed within 10 days of the injury. The immediate treatment includes the use of a dorsal hand splint.

EXTENSOR TENDONS OF THE HAND

The extensor muscles of the fingers include the extensor pollicis longus (EPL), the extensor digitorum communis (EDC), the extensor indicis proprius (EIP), and the extensor digiti quinti (EDQ). The EPL originates from the ulna and interosseous membrane and inserts on the distal phalanx of the thumb. It acts to extend the distal phalanx of the thumb. The EDC originates from the lateral condyle of the humerus and inserts, after dividing into four tendons, into the extensor mechanism. Here it splits into three parts: a central portion (central slip) that inserts onto the middle phalanx, and two lateral parts that converge distally to insert on the distal phalanx. It acts to extend the MP joint and assists in the extension of the PIP and DIP joints.[20]

The EIP originates from the ulna and inserts by a mechanism similar to that of the EDC onto the index finger. It acts primarily to extend the index MP joint. The EDQ originates from the lateral epicondyle of the humerus and inserts onto the extensor mechanism of the little finger. It acts primarily to extend the MP joint of the small finger.

All extensors are innervated by the radial nerve. Tendinous interconnections, known as junctura tendinum, exist between the extensor tendons and act to limit independent extension of all but the index finger. The extensor tendons are most often injured by sharp lacerations but also may be injured by chronic synovitis, as in rheumatoid arthri-

tis, following distal radius fractures (EPL rupture), or with forced flexion of the actively extended digit (as with being hit on the end of the finger by a ball). Clinically, the resting attitude of the relaxed hand may be altered. With an extensor tendon rupture, there may be slightly more flexion of the injured digit relative to the other digits. Normally a tenodesis of the digits is seen when the wrist is moved passively from extension to flexion. All digits should extend passively as the wrist is flexed. With wrist extension, the digits should flex. A normal cascade of all the digits should be maintained.

The EPL is tested by assessing active extension of the interphalangeal joint of the thumb. The MP joint of the thumb should be held in extension to limit the effect of the short thumb extensors. Active extension of the MP, PIP, and DIP joints of the digits also should be individually tested. With an extensor tendon laceration, an extensor lag (passive extension is present but active extension is limited or absent) and pain at the site of the tendon laceration will be present.[12] Radiographs should be taken to rule out fractures. Open wounds should be cleaned and irrigated. If the laceration is simple and clean and does not enter the joint space, the wounds can be closed and the tendons repaired on a semielective basis within 1 to 2 weeks.

The hand should be immobilized in a volar splint with the wrist in about 30 to 40 degrees of extension and the MP joints and the interphalangeal joints in about 0 to 20 degrees of flexion.[3]

MALLET FINGER

A mallet finger is a traumatic rupture of the extensor mechanism at the level of the distal phalanx. This may be caused by blunt trauma, by a laceration or deep abrasion, or by a hyperflexion or hyperextension injury. A fracture may be associated with the injury. Clinically, an extensor lag of the DIP joint is noted (Fig. 21–3). Radiographs are taken to assess the presence of an avulsed fragment, an intra-articular fracture, or subluxation of the DIP joint. The treatment for closed mallet injuries with a small avulsion fracture or fractures involving less than one third of the articular surface and not associated with joint subluxation, includes immobilization by splint. An aluminum foam splint or com-

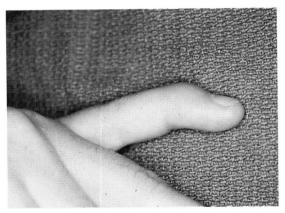

Figure 21–3. An example of a mallet deformity with an extensor lag at the distal interphalangeal joint.

mercially available (STACK) splint to hold the DIP joint in extension is used. The PIP joint is not immobilized. The splint is worn continuously for 6 weeks and then at night for 2 more weeks. Longer periods of immobilization may be needed if an extensor lag remains. Indications for surgery include the debridement of open injuries; reducing large, displaced intra-articular fractures; and reducing subluxed DIP joints or displaced physeal injuries in children.[3]

SWAN NECK DEFORMITY

A swan neck deformity of the finger consists of a hyperextension deformity of the PIP joint and flexion deformity of the DIP joint (Fig. 21–4).[10] The causes of a swan neck deformity include traumatic or acute injuries of the PIP joint with hyperextension. The mechanism of

the formation of this deformity is disruption, either partial or complete, of the volar plate structures supporting the volar PIP joint or sublimus tendon during a hyperextension force. Swan neck deformities frequently require operative treatment. A swan neck deformity tends to occur or develop in association with a mallet finger deformity. An imbalance of flexor and extensor forces causes the dynamic deformity, which may be initially present during active extension only; however, progression to a fixed deformity can occur. This deformity does not respond to splinting and needs to be referred for surgical correction.[10]

BOUTONNIÈRE DEFORMITY

A boutonnière deformity of a digit is a posture of PIP flexion associated with DIP, and later MP, hyperextension (Fig. 21–5). As with swan neck deformity, there are many causes. Traumatic boutonnière may occur about 10 days to 3 weeks following an injury that disrupts the central slip of the extensor mechanism at or proximal to the PIP joint. This can occur with a dorsal laceration over the middle phalanx or by acute forceful flexion of the PIP joint and avulsion of the central slip. Radiographs may or may not demonstrate an avulsion fracture. Closed deformities are treated with PIP extension splinting and simultaneous active and passive flexion exercises to the DIP joint. Splinting is continued until full passive extension of the PIP and full active flexion of the DIP can be achieved.[3] Open lacerations over the PIP joint need surgical intervention. Since

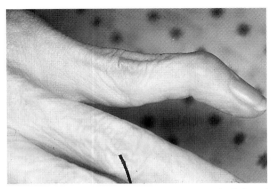

Figure 21–4. An example of a swan neck deformity with hyperextension deformity of the proximal interphalangeal joint and flexion deformity of the distal interphalangeal joint.

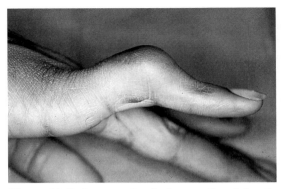

Figure 21–5. An example of a boutonnière deformity with a flexion deformity of the proximal interphalangeal joint, which can be associated with a hyperextension deformity of the distal interphalangeal joint.

these lacerations are likely to enter the joint space, an emergency referral is the rule.

FLEXOR AND EXTENSOR TENDONS OF THE TOES

The tendon most commonly ruptured or lacerated in the foot is the flexor hallucis longus (FHL). The muscle originates from the lower two thirds of the fibula and inserts into the distal phalanx of the great toe. It is innervated by the tibial nerve. Its action is flexion of the great toe. Injuries to the plantar foot occur most commonly by laceration or penetrating injury, as when stepping on a sharp object. Closed ruptures of the FHL have been described infrequently in football players and ballet dancers.[7] The mechanism is a forced extension during active flexion.

The diagnosis is made from a history of an extension injury or of stepping on a sharp object in association with the inability to flex the great toe. Injuries to the flexor hallucis tendon in the foot do not require repair. A professional athlete or dancer may elect to have a surgical repair. In most individuals, there is not a functional loss.[18] If there is an extensive proximal or hindfoot laceration on the plantar surface of the foot, wound exploration and repair of any lacerated structures are recommended on an emergency basis. Immediate management consists of radiographs to reveal foreign bodies, cleaning and irrigating the wound, skin closure, and a posterior splint.

Injuries to the extensor tendons on the dorsum of the foot are usually to the long toe extensors. These tendons are frequently used for tendon graft and are not essential for normal foot function.[13] Routine wound care is all that is usually needed. Exceptions are dancers and other professionals or athletes who depend on maximal foot function for their careers. These tendons can be repaired on an elective basis by a surgeon within a few days of injury.

References

1. Agins HJ, et al: Rupture of the distal insertion of the biceps brachii tendon. Clin Orthop 234:34–38, 1989.

2. Carden DG, et al: Rupture of the calcaneal tendon; The early and late management. J Bone Joint Surg 69B:416, 1987.

3. Doyle JR: Extensor tendons—acute injuries. *In* Green DP (ed): Operative Hand Surgery, 2nd ed. New York, Churchill Livingstone, 1988, pp 2045–2072.

4. Garrett WE Jr: Injuries to the muscle tendon unit. *In* American Academy of Orthopaedic Surgeons Institute: Course Lectures. 1988, pp 275–282.

5. Garth WP, et al: Isolated avulsion of the popliteus tendon: Operative repair. J Bone Joint Surg 74A:130–132, 1992.

6. Gilcreest EL: The common syndrome of rupture, dislocation and elongation of the long head of the biceps brachii. Surg Gynecol Obstet 58:322, 1934.

7. Jahss MH: Tendon disorders of the foot and ankle. *In* Jahss MH (ed): Disorders of the Foot and Ankle, Philadelphia, WB Saunders, 1991, pp 1461–1513.

8. Lagergren C, Lindholm A: Vascular distribution in the Achilles tendon: An angiographic and microangiographic study. Acta Chir Scand 116:491, 1958–1959.

9. Lapidus PW: Stenosing tendovaginitis. Surg Clinics North Am 33:1312–1347, 1953.

10. Leddy JP: Flexor tendons—acute injuries. *In* Green DP (ed): Operative Hand Surgery. New York, Churchill Livingstone, 1988, pp 1935–1968.

11. Lister G: Inflamation. *In* Lister G (ed): The Hand: Diagnosis and Indications. London, Churchill Livingstone, 1993, pp 323–354.

12. Lister G: Injury. *In* Lister G (ed): The Hand: Diagnosis and Indications. London, Churchill Livingstone, 1993, pp 1–154.

13. Mann RA: Traumatic injuries to the soft tissues of the foot and ankle; Tendon injuries. *In* Mann RA (ed): Surgery of the Foot. St. Louis, CV Mosby, 1986, pp 456–501.

14. Matsen FA, Arnte CT: Subacromial impingement. *In* Rockwood CA, Matsen F (eds): The Shoulder. Philadelphia, WB Saunders, 1990, pp 647–677.

15. McClure JG: Gastrocnemius musculotendinous rupture: A condition confused with thrombophlebitis. South Med J 77:1143, 1984.

16. Morrey BF, et al: Rupture of the distal tendon of the biceps brachii: A biomechanical study. J Bone Joint Surg 67A:418–421, 1985.

17. Phillips BB: Nontraumatic disorders. *In* Crenshaw AH (ed): Campbell's Operative Orthopaedics. St. Louis, Mosby Yearbook, 1992, pp 1895–1938.

18. Richardson EG: Disorders of tendons. *In* Crenshaw AH (ed): Campbell's Operative Orthopaedics. St. Louis, Mosby Yearbook, 1992, pp 2851–2874.

19. Rothwell AG: Quadriceps hematoma: A prospective clinical study. Clin Orthop 171:97–103, 1982.

20. Snell RS: The upper limb. *In* Snell RS (ed): Clinical Anatomy for Medical Students. Boston, Little, Brown, 1979, pp 359–488.

21. Warren RF: Lesions of the long head of the biceps tendon. *In* American Academy of Orthopaedic Surgeons Instructional Course Lectures. 34:204–209, 1985.

22. Watson-Jones R: Injuries of the shoulder. *In* Watson-Jones R (ed): Fractures and Joint Injuries. Baltimore, Williams & Wilkins, 1960, pp 445–502.

CHAPTER 22

Overuse Syndromes

- ## PART I

Overuse Syndromes of the Upper and Lower Extremities

William P. Garth, Jr.

Overuse syndromes show symptoms of pain, tenderness, and sometimes swelling resulting from musculoskeletal structures being subjected to repetitive forces until failure occurs secondary to fatigue or erosion. The pathology resulting in overuse syndromes may involve any of the structures in the musculoskeletal system or the nerves that pass through the structures.

The fatigue failure mode of bone, ligaments, muscles, tendons, and fascia is predominately that of repetitive tensile load that results in microscopic fracture of the tissues. In contrast, joint cartilage may fatigue and fracture under concentrated compressive loads. Excessive friction may erode tendons and result in tenosynovitis in tendon sheaths or in tendinitis and secondary bursitis in extra-articular spaces.

An understanding of how the musculoskeletal system reacts to forces is necessary to understand both the etiology of an injury and the recommended treatment. Segmental rigidity of the musculoskeletal system provided by the bones allows support and locomotion as forces act through these rigid levers and stable joints. Static strength of bones, cartilage, ligaments, tendons, and fascia, along with the contractile strength of muscle, must be sufficient to provide structural support and allow efficient locomotion.

However, in addition to strength, segmental rigidity, and stability, there also must be an element of flexibility. Flexibility of the muscles and joints allows the dampening of compressive forces by joint flexion or of tensile forces through physiologic strain. Inadequate strength or flexibility will lead to structural failure in individuals who subject their bodies to forces for which they lack the strength to withstand or the flexibility to dampen these forces.

By understanding the physical definition of stress as force per unit area, one gains insight into the biomechanical factors that may lead to stress injuries and result in overuse syndromes.

Stress on a musculoskeletal structure may become excessive by way of training errors, such as excessive exercise too soon, prior to physiologic adaptation to gradually increasing work loads; training under conditions of functional malalignment that concentrate tensile forces on one side and compressive forces on the opposite side, such as occurs at the ankle when one runs constantly on one side of a slanted road; or failing to use proper equipment, such as appropriate shoes, or to run on a soft surface which dampens impact loads transmitted to the musculoskeletal system. In addition to training errors, anatomic malalignments such as pronated or flat feet, cavus feet with rigid arches, lateral sub-luxation of the patella, genu varus or genu valgus, and leg length discrepancies may lead to increased stress by concentrating forces in smaller areas of musculoskeletal structures than occurs with normal alignment or by failing to dampen forces to which the musculoskeletal structures are subjected. As a result, secondary fatigue failure of the musculoskeletal structures experiencing this concentration of force may occur.

MECHANISM OF FAILURE

The prototypical stress injury is the common stress fracture that occurs in bone. Structural failure of bone due to accumulated stress occurs most readily secondary to tension associated with repetitive bending or spiral forces occurring with twisting motions. Bone strength is greatest in resisting compressive loads, and, therefore, unless bone is pathologically weak, failure in compression except under acute traumatic loads is rare. A stress fracture in bone is analogous to the fracture that we commonly witness when one bends a wire coat hanger repeatedly until it snaps. Stress fractures commonly present prior to a stage in which an actual fracture is visible by x-ray, but more commonly at that stage analogous to the wire which is becoming easier to bend prior to its complete fracture. Therefore a stress fracture is commonly diagnosed clinically by tenderness and swelling isolated over a bone which by history has been subjected to repetitive activity. When the diagnosis is not obvious, bone scan will confirm the presence of a stress fracture.[18]

Bone subjected to repetitive stress will hypertrophy and become capable over time of carrying heavier loads. Stress fractures occur when a bone is subjected to repetitive activity over a concentrated period of time to such an extent that physiologic bone hypertrophy does not keep pace with accumulative microscopic fractures of the bone trabeculae.

The basic principles of stress injury as just described can be applied to all musculoskeletal structures, although a definitive diagnostic test as accurate as a nuclear bone scan is not available for soft tissue structures. The fatigue failure of tendons and muscles occurs when repetitive, active tensile forces exceed the strength or flexibility (physiologic strain capability) of these structures, resulting in gross fracture (tear) of the structures. Ligaments and fascia, being static restraints, are prone to failure when subjected to excessive accumulative passive tensile forces that may result from doing too much before adequate physical conditioning or from functional or anatomic malalignment during repetitive activities. Malalignment of joints will concentrate compressive and frictional forces on limited areas of articular cartilage, which can result in fatigue failure and chondromalacia.

The physician who cares for active people should be thoroughly familiar with the palpation of topical anatomy and with the optimal alignment and function of musculoskeletal structures. This knowledge is necessary to diagnose overuse injuries accurately and to prescribe stress-reducing alignment correction and appropriate modification of activities.

Nonoperative treatment for stress injuries always includes relative but not absolute rest. The runner may be taken off impact loading activities but be allowed to cycle or run in the buoyancy of a pool. The tennis player with shoulder problems may be restricted from overhead serving but allowed to work on ground strokes. Ice, compression (when swelling occurs), and nonsteroidal anti-inflammatory drugs are used routinely to reduce the vascular dilatation of inflammation. The judicious use of corticosteroid local injections for soft tissue injuries also can be helpful in some cases. Corticosteroids should never be injected directly into a tendon, however. Functional or anatomic malalignment and strength and flexibility deficits must be corrected during convalescence and rehabilitation, or recurrent injury will occur upon return to activity.

THE FOOT

Since in most people the lower extremities are subjected to more repetitive forces, overuse syndromes involving the lower extremities are more common than any other location. Forces acting on the lower extremity at heel contact during running a mile are three to eight times the body weight (450 to 1200 lb) repeated up to 2000 times.[2] It is no wonder that fatigue or erosion from this repetitive activity commonly presents as pain and swelling.

The frequency of stress fracture is directly proportional to the proximity of the bone and contact reactive forces with the ground. Therefore, the most common stress fracture occurs in the foot, whereas the least common stress fractures occur in the hip or pelvis. The classic march fracture, named so because of its frequency of occurrence in poorly conditioned new military recruits subjected to prolonged marching, is the stress fracture that occurs in the diaphysis of the second, third, or, less frequently, fourth metatarsal. Fortunately, this classic stress fracture generally heals uneventfully and does not require casting but may be treated simply with reduction in impact activity. Exercise such as bicycling and other low-impact activity can be substituted to maintain physical conditioning until tenderness resolves.

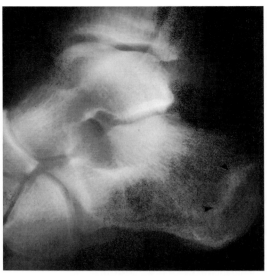

Figure 22–2. An actual fracture may never be seen in cases of some stress fractures, particularly of the os calcis, but several weeks later evidence of sclerosis indicates reactive healing and confirms the diagnosis.

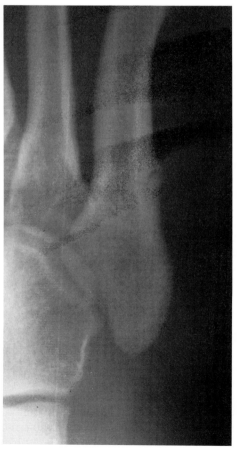

Figure 22–1. The Jones' fracture, a stress fracture of the proximal shaft of the fifth metatarsal, is prone to delayed union or nonunion. In the competitive athlete, strong consideration should be given to intramedullary screw fixation as primary treatment to facilitate union, rehabilitation, and return to competition.

The stress fracture on the lateral border of the proximal shaft of the fifth metatarsal, commonly known as a Jones' fracture, is particularly prone to delayed union or nonunion (Fig. 22–1). In the athlete, it can be a particularly troublesome fracture and in fact has ruined the hopes for the Heisman Trophy of two leading candidates within the last 10 years. Management of the acute fracture can be either an initial short leg cast with non-weight-bearing, or, in an athlete who has little time before competition is to begin, surgical management with intramedullary screw fixation.[21] The Jones' fracture in the proximal shaft of the fifth metatarsal must be distinguished from the more proximal fracture of the base of the fifth metatarsal tuberosity, which usually heals without difficulty.

Another troublesome fracture is an occult intra-articular fracture of the base of the second metatarsal, most commonly seen in ballerinas, which can be troublesome and sometimes needs surgical treatment.[14]

Stress fractures commonly occur in the tarsal bones. Occult calcaneal fractures can result in diagnostic dilemmas but usually heal uneventfully (Fig. 22–2). Tarsal navicular stress fractures are relatively common in jumping athletes, but frequently there is a delay in recognition.[22] Oblique x-ray views of the foot, nuclear bone scan, and CT scan of the foot can be helpful in recognizing this injury. Tarsal navicular fractures commonly require bone grafting and screw fixation to obtain healing.

A stress fracture also may occur in one of the two sesamoid bones found in the flexor brevis tendons plantar to the first metatarsal head. A fracture of the sesamoid may be distinguished from an incidental bipartite sesamoid by use of a nuclear bone scan. Ununited symptomatic stress fractures of the sesamoid require excision or bone grafting to promote healing and resolution of symptoms.[20]

In the skeletally immature patient, pain frequently occurs at sites of the apophyses. Most common is traction apophysitis of the calcaneus (Sever's disease), resulting in posterior heel pain in those between the ages of 12 and 15 years. Treatment consists of reassurance that the pain will resolve with maturity and symptomatic treatment with acetaminophen or ibuprofen, Achilles stretching, soft heel cups, and rest when pain is severe.

The most common overuse syndrome involving the articular cartilage of the foot presents with degenerative changes of the first metatarsophalangeal joint. As a result of repetitive activity or traumatic hyperextension injuries of the great toe, chondromalacia may present in the first metatarsophalangeal joint. Pain with motion in and about the first metatarsophalangeal joint is best treated by a rigid insert placed in the shoe to reduce the motion of the first metatarsophalangeal joint. In more severe cases in which osteophytes form, resulting in significant limitation of motion and pain—a condition called hallux rigidus—surgical resection of the osteophytes and debridement of the joint may be necessary.[13]

Attritional ligament sprain about the foot usually results from either an anatomic malalignment of the foot, such as pes planus, or functional malalignments such as occur with prolonged running on a slanted surface, which places repetitive varus or valgus stress on the foot and ankle. As a result of foot pronation, the ligaments about the medial aspect of the ankle, as well as the posterior tibial tendon, are subjected to significant accumulative stress, resulting in sprain of the deltoid ligament, or excessive strain of the posterior tibial tendon, resulting in tendinitis. Correction of the malalignment with an arch support and medial heel wedge or, in cases of functional malalignment, by restricting the patient from running on a slanted surface is required to allow healing and the prevention of recurrence of the syndrome.

Tendinitis is common about the foot and ankle. In addition to posterior tibial tendinitis, Achilles tendinitis and less frequently peroneal or toe flexor tendinitis will be seen in active people. Tendinitis is characterized by tenderness and nodular or diffuse swelling of the involved tendon. For cases not responding to routine anti-inflammatory management, correction of foot malalignment, and rehabilitation to improve strength and flexibility, immobilization for several weeks in a removable cast boot with a rocker bottom sole is necessary. Following immobilization, predisposing malalignment and strength and flexibility deficits must be corrected prior to resumption of activities, or symptoms will recur. Cases resistant to conservative measures require surgical debridement of central tendinous degeneration, repair of longitudinal splits, or release of stenotic tendon sheaths that cause tendon erosion (Fig. 22–3).[4]

One of the most common overuse disorders of the foot results from repetitive strain to the plantar fascia. This results in the so-called "heel spur" syndrome in which pain is present on the plantar aspect of the heel. At times a bone spur is seen on radiographs at the plantar origin of the fascia as new bone forms due to the repetitive tearing of the origin of the plantar fascia from the os calcis. Plantar fasciitis can be a very difficult disorder to correct. Routine management includes the use of heel cups. At times, arch supports with metatarsal pads, used to reduce hyperextension of the second and third metatarsophalangeal joints, will be useful. These orthotics are useful because the plantar fascia arises from the plantar aspect of the os calcis and inserts on the base of the proximal phalanges. Hyperextension of the second and third toes, as occurs with claw toes, will cause bowstringing and tension on the plantar fascia as it crosses the arch from the os calcis to the toes. By preventing the hyperextension of the second and third toes, tension can be reduced on the plantar fascia. Standard modalities such as ice, ultrasound with hydrocortisone cream, and, in resistant cases, direct injections of corticosteroid preparations can at times relieve pain. Recalcitrant cases are managed with release of the plantar fascia and, if present, resection of the heel spur.[23]

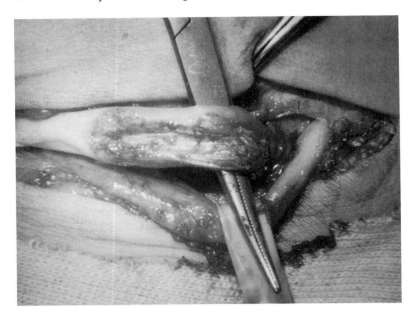

Figure 22–3. The flexor hallucis tendon at the posterior medial ankle of a professional ballerina. After symptoms of tendinitis at this location for 2 years, she finally became incapacitated and required surgical management. Notice the significant erosive lesion in the tendon, which occurred deep to the flexor retinaculum.

Retrocalcaneal bursitis is a common cause of posterior heel pain at the insertion of the Achilles tendon on the os calcis. The bone prominence of the posterior aspect of the os calcis just proximal to the insertion of the Achilles tendon may predispose patients to this disorder when the Achilles tendon is subjected to friction against the bone prominence by a shoe. The resulting swollen area has been referred to as a "pump bump," since it can commonly be seen in women who wear pumps that strike the heel at that level. Retrocalcaneal bursitis can be a particularly bothersome problem to the athlete. Management is similar to that of plantar fasciitis, with a stepwise progression of management of rest, shoe modification with a softer heel counter or none, corticosteroid injection of the bursa, and, as a last resort, surgical resection of the bone prominence and inflamed bursa, which occurs between the os calcis and the Achilles tendon.[17]

THE LEG

Stress fractures of the tibia and fibula are less commonly seen than stress fractures in the foot. Although stress fractures of the fibula are generally benign, a stress fracture in the anterior tibial cortex is a particularly frustrating problem for the athlete. Anterior unicortical fractures of the tibia commonly progress to delayed union or nonunion and predispose to displaced fractures.[19] In addition to prolonged low-impact activities, additional treatment by stimulation with an electromagnetic field or by bone grafting may be required. A newly described modality that may promote bone union in these difficult cases is the use of ultrasound to stimulate bone union.[7]

Pes planus, or the pronated foot, may result not only in posterior tibial tendinitis beneath the medial malleolus but also in pain at the origin of the posterior tibial muscle from the posterior medial aspect of the distal tibia. The medial tibial stress syndrome that results from excessive strain of the posterior tibial muscle origin is commonly referred to as shin splints. Shin splints are characterized by pain with activity and residual tenderness at periosteal muscle origins for days following running or other repetitive activity. Shin splints respond to strengthening of the posterior tibial muscle and passive correction of the malalignment with the use of a semirigid arch support. More proximal posteromedial shin splints in the middle and proximal third of the tibia are commonly associated with weakness of the foot intrinsic muscles or claw toes, which results in overuse of the origin of the flexor digitorum longus muscle arising from the proximal two thirds of the tibia.

Shin splints are best treated with strengthening of the muscles involved and orthotic correction of malalignment of the feet to reduce strain on the injured muscle. While arch supports with a medial heel wedge correcting the pronated foot are necessary for the distal posterior tibial shin splints, the proximal tibial shin splints frequently respond to an orthotic device with a metatarsal pad added to the arch support. The reduction of the claw toes with use of the metatarsal pad reduces the strain in the flexor digitorum longus, and symptoms frequently abate.[6]

A second disorder associated with the muscles in the leg is that of a chronic compartment syndrome. In these individuals, the fascial envelope incorporating a muscular compartment of the leg is taut and has a reduced volume. The vascular engorgement of muscle, or "pump-up," normally occurring with exercise, results in an elevated intracompartmental pressure if there is a tight unyielding fascia preventing expansion of the muscle compartment. This increased compartmental pressure results in increasing pain with prolonged activity, which is relieved by rest as pressure subsides. Symptomatic numbness may occur in the distribution of the cutaneous nerves that pass through these compartments. These symptoms of pain and numbness differ from chronically recurring shin splint symptoms in that pain is relieved in a matter of hours without the prolonged tenderness that characterizes shin splints. Relieving the intracompartmental pressure (after documentation by intracompartmental pressure measurements) by fasciotomy is the treatment of choice.[12]

THE KNEE

Overuse syndromes of the knee include jumper's knee, Osgood-Schlatter disease or Sindig-Larsen-Johannsen-disease, and iliotibial band syndrome.

Jumper's knee syndromes result from repetitive tensile loads placed on the extensor mechanism through participating in sports that require repetitive jumping, e.g., basketball and volleyball. The patients present with pain, tenderness, and sometimes swelling at the inferior or superior pole of the patella. Pain and tenderness are aggravated by activities, particularly by jumping. The infrapatellar or quadriceps tendinitis resulting in this syndrome is secondary to microscopic disruption of the attachment of these tendons to the patella. These microscopic disruptions are usually unilateral and rarely progress to complete rupture. Bilateral cases that may progress to complete rupture should be evaluated for pathologic disorders resulting in abnormal weakness of the tendons or the bone to which they are attached.[11]

Treatment consists of nonsteroidal anti-inflammatory drugs, reduction in provocative activities, and improvement in flexibility of the hamstrings and rectus femoris to improve efficiency of knee flexion and extension. Corticosteroid injections should be used rarely and, if used, should be injected into the fat pad adjacent to the tendon and not the tendon itself. A neoprene knee sleeve with a felt pad positioned superior to the patella also gives some symptomatic relief during activity.

Osgood-Schlatter's disease and Sindig-Larsen-Johannsen disease, traction apophysitis of the tibial tubercle or inferior pole of the ossifying patella, respectively, are preadolescent or early adolescent conditions analogous to the soft tissue forms of jumper's knee. During the growth spurt, these apophyses are the weak link of the extensor mechanism exposed to the tensile forces experienced during repetitive activity. Displaced avulsion fractures of the tibial tubercle or the inferior pole of the patella also may occur in this age group, but, in our experience, Osgood-Schlatter or Sindig-Larsen-Johanssen disease is usually not a prodrome to displaced fracture. Therefore, in addition to therapy as prescribed for jumper's knee, reassurance should be given that symptoms usually resolve with maturation and leave only a residual harmless protuberance of the tibial tubercle. Activities may be continued as tolerated. Rare cases will have symptoms that persist through skeletal maturity and result from ectopic ossicles that fail to attach to the tibia. Occasionally, excision of these ossicles is required when symptoms are severe enough in the mature patient.

Iliotibial band syndrome consists of inflammatory symptoms of pain and tenderness at the lateral femoral epicondyle, usually in runners with tibia vara. The syndrome is traditionally believed to be due to friction occurring as the iliotibial tract rubs repetitively over the lateral femoral epicondyle. However, the lateral femoral epicondyle is the origin of the lateral collateral ligament. By placing the knee in the figure four position, the lateral collateral ligament becomes taut and easily palpable. The tenderness is then frequently discovered to involve specifically the proximal one half of the lateral collateral ligament. Since the syndrome occurs commonly in varus knees and improves with replacement of laterally worn shoes and avoidance of running with the injured knee on the down side of a slanted road surface, which are measures that reduce varus tensile stress on the lateral collateral ligament, an alternate hypothesis for the source of this syndrome is overuse sprain of the lateral collateral ligament. Regardless of the exact biomechanical source of this syndrome, appropriate treatment consists of oral or local anti-inflammatory measures, rest, and reduction of varus stress on the knee and stretching of the iliotibial tract. If necessary, local corticosteroid injections at the most tender spot are frequently helpful.

THE HIP

The most serious stress fracture occurring in an adult involves the femoral neck. Groin pain radiating to the knee, which can be reproduced with internal and external rotation of the hip, in an individual with a recently increased level of activities, should be considered a stress fracture of the femoral neck until proved otherwise. If radiographs are negative, a bone scan should be performed to establish the diagnosis.

It is extremely important to recognize an occult stress fracture of the femoral neck. A displaced fracture of the femoral neck occurring through a stress fracture is a very serious condition that can result in avascular necrosis of the femoral head and the eventual need for total hip replacement. Therefore, the recognition of stress fracture of the femoral neck is of paramount importance over any other overuse disorder. If stress fracture of the femoral neck is suspected, the patient must be treated with crutches for nonweight-bearing on the involved extremity. A prophylactic pinning may be indicated, particularly if the stress fracture is on the superior aspect of the femoral neck where tensile forces may lead to a displaced fracture. Stress fractures on the compression side of the femoral neck, that is, the inferior calcar region, are more commonly treated nonoperatively since they are less likely to displace.

In the prepubescent child, a serious condition analogous to the stress fracture of the femoral neck in the adult is a slipped capital femoral epiphysis. Groin, anterior thigh pain, or knee pain in the prepubescent child, particularly in the obese boy, should be evaluated thoroughly. Pain with hip rotation, particularly if internal rotation is limited and even if the pain is referred to the knee, always should lead to a radiograph of the hip. Widening of the femoral capital epiphysis or any displacement of the femoral head on the neck of the femur requires fixation of the femoral head on the neck with a single screw inserted percutaneously. A delay in treatment can result in further displacement with secondary avascular necrosis or chondrolysis of the femoral head and permanent impairment.

The most common overuse syndrome about the hip is that of tendinitis at the greater trochanter. Microscopic failure of the hip abductors as they insert on the greater trochanter, or of the origin of the vastus lateralis as it arises on the inferior aspect of the greater trochanter, is the culprit in this disorder. For athletes such as distance runners, care must be taken to ensure that there is no pelvic obliquity resulting from even subtle leg length discrepancy. In an individual who has as little as one half an inch of leg length discrepancy and who is subjected to repetitive force loads associated with running, the pelvic tilt resulting from the longer leg results in a varus stress about the hip and increases the concentration of stress on the hip abductor. Therefore, in addition to the usual modalities for tendinitis, care must be taken to recognize leg length discrepancy and correct this with shoe inserts. A common training error that may result in this greater trochanteric tendinitis is running frequently on the same side of a slanted road. This results in a pelvic obliquity and increased tension on the hip abductors of the extremity on the lower side of the slanted road. Therefore it is important for road runners to change directions and sides of the roads every other workout to prevent excessive wear on the abductors of one hip.[10]

THE PELVIS

Stress fractures of the pubic rami and osteitis pubis, i.e., inflammation of the pubic symphysis, can be seen in mature athletes. Management is rest and, in the case of osteitis pubis, local corticosteroid injection of the pubic symphysis.

In the adolescent athlete, traction apophysitis of the iliac crest or ischial tuberosity is common. The diagnosis is made by tenderness of the apophysis and pain elicited with stretching or contraction of muscle arising from these apophyses, e.g., ischial pain elicited with straight leg raising, which tenses the hamstrings arising from the ischium.

Apophyseal avulsion fractures of the anterior superior iliac spine by the sartorius, the anterior inferior iliac spine by the rectus femoris, or the ischial tuberosity by the hamstrings is common in these athletes. A sudden pop and pain in the pelvic region that occurs during running warrants x-ray examination for these fractures in adolescents. These fractures typically respond to a few weeks of rest and rehabilitation of the muscle involved. Open reduction and internal fixation should be considered for ischial avulsion with more than 1.5 cm displacement, since these displaced ischial fractures can result in delayed union or nonunion. The return to activities is exceedingly prolonged, and the result is often a significant mass in the buttocks causing sitting discomfort.

THE UPPER EXTREMITY

Although less common in the upper extremity, stress fractures do occur, most commonly in poorly conditioned athletes who attempt stressful activities prior to a gradual conditioning program. For example, a spiral fracture of the humerus, sustained while throwing, is relatively common.[5] Baseball for weekend athletes (in less than optimal physical condition) has resulted in numerous spiral fractures of the humerus as a result of the twisting movement placed across the humerus in the act of throwing. Most of these individuals have experienced a prodrome of pain in the arm but unfortunately have dismissed it as muscle soreness, only to discover that the pain was due to a stress fracture. Then a displaced spiral fracture occurs with a hard throw. These fractures are seldom identified prior to displacement. Fortunately, they can be managed with a simple U-splint extending from the lateral aspect of the deltoid distally around the elbow and extending medially up to the axilla. They are held in compression with cast padding and an ace bandage. Less common stress fractures of the ulna have occurred in athletes, but fortunately these generally present as pain and localized tenderness and without displacement of the fracture.[15] Usually these can be treated with a splint or functional brace.

THE SHOULDER

Little League shoulder is the common term for epiphysiolysis (x-ray evidence of widening of the epiphysis compared with the nondominant shoulder) of the proximal humerus. It is the result of the repetitive traction on the epiphysis that occurs with excessive throwing. Preventive measures in Little League play have been instituted in the form of rules that limit the amount of pitches the young athlete can perform on a weekly basis. Although these rules help, the condition still occurs relatively commonly and requires avoidance of hard throwing until all symptoms and x-ray signs have abated. Usually it means there will be no hard throwing until the next season.[1]

Another relatively common bone stress injury seen on the radiographs of active people with shoulder pain is osteolysis of the distal clavicle. Usually this occurs in weightlifters or as a late sequela of Grade I acromioclavicular (AC) separations. The erosive changes seen in the distal articular end of the clavicle result from degenerative changes of the AC cartilage. Tenderness is noted at the AC joint, pain and weakness are demonstrated with resistance to forward flexion of the arm, and pain can be elicited by adduction of the flexed arm across the torso. The flexion-adduction maneuver reproduces compressive forces across the joints that simulate the activity that led to the condition. The treatment is permanent restriction of activities, but there is a good prognosis following surgical resection of the distal clavicle in those unwilling to modify their activities.[3]

In the adult who is active in overhead activities, the most common source of pain and impairment is impingement of the rotator cuff or biceps long tendon or both. Late sequela of the impingement syndrome is complete tear or rupture of the rotator cuff or biceps tendon.

Impingement syndrome is one of the most common problems encountered in the athlete involved in repetitive overhead activity. This is a complex of symptoms of pain and weakness associated with forward flexion or lateral abduction of the shoulder above 70 degrees. Specifically, the range of motion from 70 to 120 degrees is referred to as the "painful arc." During this motion, the undersurface of the anterior acromion and the proximal humerus are in closest proximity. As a result, the soft tissue structures that reside in this "impingement interval" (subacromial bursa, long head of the biceps, and rotator cuff) are subject to compressive and frictional forces from any conditions that further narrow the space. A hooked acromion, calcium deposits, bone spurs, or soft tissue inflammation can compromise this area and lead to impingement.

The patient/athlete generally will present with a complaint of pain with a specific, usually overhead, activity. Occasionally, there will be a baseline dull ache in the affected shoulder. On exmination, tenderness of the supraspinatus and biceps tendon may be present. Evaluation of motion often reveals the "painful arc." Muscle testing may reveal weakness of the supraspinatus or external rotator muscles. A positive impingement sign supports the diagnosis. This is solicited by forcibly forward elevating the affected arm while stabilizing the scapula.[16] Pain with this maneuver is considered a positive finding. The impingement injection can also help confirm the diagnosis:[16] A local anesthetic agent is injected into the subacromial bursa and if alleviation or reduction of pain occurs, then the test is deemed positive. Roentgenograms can be performed but are often normal in the early stages.

Treatment initially involves relative rest, i.e., avoiding the offending activity. Nonsteroidal anti-inflammatory medications are typically used to help decrease inflammation. A subacromial injection with a mixture of anesthetic and cortisone derivative to decrease inflammation in the bursa is also acceptable. A major portion of the recovery phase focuses on physical therapy. Pain-free range of motion is the initial goal, with strengthening exercises for the supporting soft tissue structures of the shoulder girdle added as tolerated. Return to athletic activity should be a slow, progressive process, with special attention given to abnormal mechanics and technique.

It is fairly common that patients experience chronic impingement syndrome resistant to conservative treatment. In those instances, shaving of the inferior surface of the acromion and AC joint, with resection of the coracoacromial ligament to allow more room for the rotator cuff to glide beneath the acromial arch, can be performed.

In the adolescent or young adult athlete, symptoms of impingement must make one suspicious of instability problems. Impingement symptoms in this age group are most commonly associated with occult instability allowing anterior and perhaps superior migration of the humeral head, with resulting pinching of the rotator cuff. Surgical management of impingement syndromes in the young athlete frequently results in failure to relieve the symptoms, because the underlying instability may not be addressed.

THE ELBOW

Bone stress injuries are rare about the elbow of the adult but are relatively common in late childhood and early adolescence. "Little League elbow" refers to avulsion or epiphysiolysis of the medial humeral epicondyle as a result of valgus stress occurring with excessive baseball throwing. The Little League's rules that require limitation of the number of pitches thrown per week are as much for prevention of this Little League elbow as they are for Little League shoulder.

The young ballplayer will present often with a complaint of acute onset of pain at the elbow with throwing. Tenderness will be localized to the medial humeral epicondyle. Radiographs frequently will demonstrate widening of the apophyses of the medial humeral epicondyle.

Fortunately, when these injuries do occur, they rarely result in significant displacement of the medial epicondyle and heal with abstinence from throwing until the patient is symptom-free. Since this condition rarely results in a displaced fracture, generally surgical management or casting is not required.

The baseball pitcher may develop fatigue, sprain, or tear of the ulnar collateral ligament, the primary restraint to valgus instability. In younger athletes, an ulnar collateral ligament sprain usually will heal with rest. Failure of the ulnar collateral ligament and the need for reconstruction are more common in the experienced pitcher.[9]

Perhaps because of subtle laxity of the ulnar collateral ligament, osteophytes frequently will form on the posterior medial olecranon of the experienced pitcher. The valgus extension overload resulting from excessive throwing leads to impingement of the posterior medial olecranon against the posterior medial humeral condyle. This chronic recurring impingement leads to osteophyte formation and loose bodies, both of which can lead to posterior medial pain and limited extension. Arthroscopic debridement of the posterior elbow is commonly needed. These osteophytes will probably recur with continued pitching, and it is important to rule out significant ulnar collateral ligament deficiency in these individuals prior to any initial surgical management, as surgical reconstruction of the ulnar collateral ligament may be the procedure needed primarily.[24]

The terms *tennis* and *golfer's elbow* are commonly used to refer to lateral and medial humeral epicondylitis, respectively. Despite these common terms, the disorders are seen not only in tennis players and golfers but also in anyone involved in activities in which repetitive use of the wrist extensors or flexors is necessary. Most commonly, these patients are 30 to 45 years old. The disorders are actually a tendinitis of the origin of the wrist extensors laterally or of the common origin of the wrist flexors and pronator teres medially. Nonoperative treatment to reduce inflammation is followed by careful rehabilitation while using a counterforce brace. Rehabilitation includes gradual stretching of the wrist extensors in lateral cases and of the wrist flexors and pronator in medial cases. Isometric exercises are utilized to gain strength. If symptoms have not recurred, then gradual eccentric exercises, i.e., contraction of the muscle as it elongates as do the wrist flexors when slowly resisting wrist extension, are begun. Once the patient is pain-free and full active motion and strength are present, a return to full activity can be allowed while using the counterforce brace. The counterforce brace is a strap worn circumferentially about the forearm just distal to the site of pain. Pressure from the strap inhibits full muscle expansion and decreases tension on the injured tissue. Another important part of treatment includes modifying the activity that originally led to the symptoms, in order to prevent recurrence. For example, the tennis player may benefit from professional instruction in proper stroke technique to prevent recurrent overload of the previously injured tissue. Corticosteroid injections and, as a last resort surgical release, are sometimes necessary for recalcitrant cases.[8]

THE HAND AND WRIST

See Part II for discussion of overuse syndromes of the hand and wrist.

References

1. Barnett LS: Little League shoulder syndrome: Proximal humeral epiphysiolysis in adolescent baseball pitcher. J Bone Joint Surg 67A:495–496, 1985.
2. Browdy DM: Running injuries. Clin Symp 32(4):P3, 1980.
3. Cahill BR: Osteolysis of the distal part of the clavicle in male athletes. J Bone Joint Surg 64A:1053–1058, 1982.
4. Garth WP: Flexor hallucis tendinitis in a ballet dancer. J Bone Joint Surg 63A:1489, 1981.
5. Garth WP, LeBerte MA, Cool TA: Recurrent fractures of the humerus in a baseball pitcher. J Bone Joint Surg 70A:305–306, 1988.
6. Garth WP, Miller ST: Evaluation of claw toe deformity, weakness of the foot intrinsics, and posteromedial shin. Am J Sports Med 17(6):821–827, 1989.
7. Heckman JD, Ryaby JP, McCabe J, Frey JJ, et al: Acceleration of tibial fracture-healing by noninvasive low-intensity pulsed ultrasound. J Bone Joint Surg 76A:26–34, 1994.
8. Jobe FW, Ciccotti MG: Lateral and medial epicondylitis of the elbow. J Am Acad Orthop Surg 2:1–8, 1994.
9. Jobe FW, Stark H, Lombardo SJ: Reconstruction of the ulnar collateral ligament in athletes. J Bone Joint Surg 68A:1158–1163, 1986.
10. Lloyd-Smith R, Clement DB, McKenzie DC, Tauton JE: A survey of overuse and traumatic hip and pelvic injuries in athletes. Physicians Sports Med 13(10):131–141, 1985.
11. Maddox PA, Garth WP: Tendinitis of the patellar ligament and quadriceps (jumper's knee) as an initial presentation of hyperparathyroidism. J Bone Joint Surg 68A:288–292, 1986.
12. Martens MA, Backaert M, Vermaut G, Mulier JC: Chronic leg pain in athletes due to a recurrent compartment syndrome. Am J Sports Med 12:148–151, 1984.
13. McMaster MJ: The pathogenesis of hallux rigidus. J Bone Joint Surg 60B:82–87, 1978.
14. Micheli LJ, Sohn RS, Solomon R: Stress fractures of the second metatarsal involving Lisfranc's joint in ballet dancers. A new overuse injury of the foot. J Bone Joint Surg 67A:1372–1375, 1985.
15. Mutoh Y, Takemi M, Suzuki Y, Sugiura Y: Stress fractures of the ulna in athletes. Am J Sports Med 10:365–367, 1982.
16. Neer CS II: Impingement lesions. Clin Orthop 173:70, 1983.

17. Pavlov H, Heneghan MA, Hersh A, et al: The Haglund syndrome: Initial and differential diagnosis. Radiology 144:93–98, 1982.
18. Prather JL, Nusynowitz ML, Snowdy HA, et al: Scintigraphic findings in stress fractures. J Bone Joint Surg 59A:869–874, 1977.
19. Redig AC, Shelbourne DK, McCarroll JR, Bisesi M, et al: The natural history and treatment of delayed union stress fractures of the anterior cortex of the tibia. Am J Sports Med 16(3):250–255, 1988.
20. Richardson EG: Injuries to the hallucal sesamoids in the athlete. Foot Ankle 7:229–244, 1987.
21. Torq JS, Balduini FC, Zeeks RR, Pavlov H, et al: Fractures of the base of the metatarsal distal to the tuberosity. J Bone Joint Surg 66A:209–214, 1984.
22. Torq JS, Pavlov H, Cooley LH, Bryant MH, et al: Stress fractures of the tarsal navicular. A retrospective review of twenty-one cases. J Bone Joint Surg 64A:700–712, 1982.
23. Torq JS, Pavlov H, Torq E: Overuse injuries in sport: The foot. Clin Sports Med 6(2):291–319, 1987.
24. Wilson FD, Andrews JR, Blackburn TA, McCluskey G: Valgus extension overload in the pitching elbow. Am J Sports Med 11:83–88, 1983.

- PART II

Overuse Syndromes of the Hand and Wrist

Ekkehard Bonatz

TENDINITIS

Tendinitis involving the hand and wrist is quite common. It is usually transitory, but, when persistent, it may impair the patient's ability to work. Early nonsurgical treatment offers the best chance for a good result. It is important to determine accurately the origin and severity of symptoms. It is no longer sufficient to label wrist pain just as "tendinitis." Histologic changes in tendinitis include thickening, fibrocytic proliferation, adhesions, and amyloid depositions. Because tendons are the mechanical link between muscle and bone, they are exposed to considerable stresses. These stresses, especially when cumulative, may exceed the limit of the tendons. Tendinitis has been linked to a stress fracture of bone, when repetitive loading produces microfractures and adequate physiologic repair can no longer take place.

Motion of the tendons requires gliding, sometimes crossing joints at angles of up to 105 degrees. Osteophytes, fractures, or malunion also can cause mechanical irritation, leading to tendinitis or eventual rupture. Occasionally, trigger digits may have a history of previous laceration, and may be caused by an unrecognized retained foreign body. Anatomic variations, such as multiple tendon slips or a separate sheath within the first dorsal compartment of the wrist extensors (extensor pollicis brevis, abductor pollicis longus), may predispose to tendinitis. Systemic factors, such as diabetes, rheumatoid arthritis, or hypothyroidism, are associated with a higher incidence of carpal tunnel syndrome, DeQuervain's disease, and trigger digits; they may also be seen in association with shoulder bursitis and tennis elbow. Pregnancy may aggravate conditions such as carpal tunnel syndrome and DeQuervain's disease.

People at risk for tendinitis are those who engage in activities requiring repetitive gripping, pinching, pulling, or lifting with repetitive wrist motion. Sharp edges on tool handles also may cause mechanical irritations.

Diagnosis

A careful history should inquire into both work and recreational activities. The physical examination may reveal a nerve compression syndrome rather than tendinitis, based on anatomic pain distribution. Tendinitis should be described according to its location and the affected muscle-tendon unit. One should look for scars, swelling, erythema, warmth, crepitus, snapping, pain, and numbness. Roentgenograms are obtained to rule out foreign bodies, arthritis, calcifications, fractures, or other abnormalities.

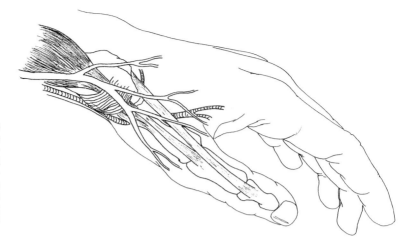

Figure 22–4. In DeQuervain's tenosynovitis, the tendons of the abductor pollicis longus and extensor pollicis brevis become inflamed within their retinaculum. Occasionally the radial sensory nerve becomes irritated in the same area, leading to paresthesias on the dorsal aspect of the thumb and first web space.

DeQuervain's Tendinitis

Tendinitis of the abductor pollicis longus and extensor pollicis brevis at the wrist is known as DeQuervain's tendinitis.[1] Pain, swelling, and tenderness over the radial styloid are the presenting symptoms (Fig. 22–4). The pain may radiate proximally and distally. It is aggravated with wrist ulnar deviation and thumb flexion and adduction, and resisted thumb extension. There may be a palpable swelling and thickening of the tendon sheath of the extensor pollicis brevis and abductor pollicis longus. There may even be palpable nodules in these tendons, causing triggering in the area of the radial styloid. Finkelstein's test places the wrist into ulnar deviation while the thumb is clenched under the fingers (Fig. 22–5). The test occasionally will be positive bilaterally, making its usefulness somewhat limited. A modification of the test uses acute wrist flexion to 80 degrees or more, with the thumb metacarpophalangeal joint extended. In this position, active flexion and extension of the thumb interphalangeal joint is an alternative provocative maneuver and will reproduce the patient's pain at the wrist.

Occasionally, DeQuervain's tenosynovitis is confused with nerve entrapment of the superficial branch of the radial sensory nerve at the area of the radial styloid (see Fig. 22–4). If there is a history of paresthesias over the dorsum of the hand, this diagnosis should be considered. Percussion or pressure over the radial nerve at the level of the radial styloid may reproduce the patient's symptoms and indicates nerve, rather than tendon, entrapment.

The initial treatment for DeQuervain's tendinitis includes splinting with a thumb spica splint or cast, or a cortisone injection into the tendon sheath. Surgical release is considered if this fails (Fig. 22–6).

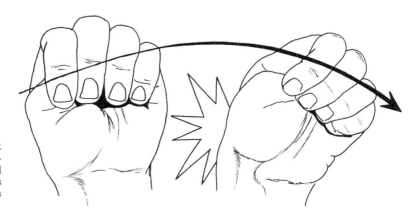

Figure 22–5. Finkelstein's test places the wrist into ulnar deviation while the thumb is adducted into the palm. To be positive, this should reproduce the patient's pain.

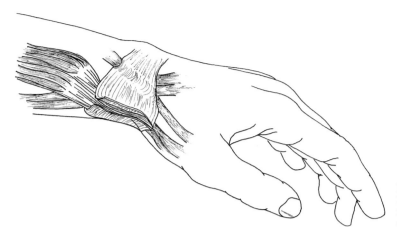

Figure 22–6. Surgical treatment of DeQuervain's tendinitis involves release of the thickened and inflamed extensor retinaculum at the wrist.

Intersection Syndrome

Pain, swelling, and crepitus over the dorsal portion of the distal forearm, approximately 6 cm proximal to Lister's tubercle, are caused by inflammation of the radial wrist extensor tendons, where they cross beneath the abductor pollicis longus and extensor pollicis brevis tendons. Irritation of the tendons at this location may result from direct trauma or from repetitive wrist flexion and extension, especially when associated with heavy gripping. It is sometimes seen in rowers, weight lifters, canoeists, motorcycle riders, or workers whose jobs require repetitive wrist motion.

Splinting of the wrist, nonsteroidal anti-inflammatory medication, or an injection of 3 ml of lidocaine (with or without 0.5 ml of a cortisone solution) into the inflamed area will alleviate symptoms. Care should be taken not to inject cortisone directly into the tendons.

Extensor Pollicis Longus Tendinitis

Extensor pollicis longus tendinitis is sometimes seen in recreational or professional athletes, especially in patients involved in racquet sports. It is otherwise associated with rheumatoid arthritis or repetitive motion. It presents with pain, swelling, and occasional crepitus at Lister's tubercle. Sometimes it is seen after nondisplaced distal radius fractures. Attrition of the extensor pollicis longus tendon may even lead to tendon rupture. A thumb spica, splint, or cast is applied early if this condition is suspected.

If symptoms persist, surgical release may be warranted.

Extensor Carpi Ulnaris Tendinitis

The extensor carpi ulnaris tendon may sublux due to a tear in its retinaculum. Repetitive subluxation will cause tendinitis. To reproduce this subluxation, the patient is asked to supinate the wrist while the hand is held in ulnar deviation. The tendon should be palpated during this motion, and occasionally a snap can be felt. Treatment is by limitation of wrist pronation and supination if possible. A splint must be applied to extend from the wrist to above the elbow in order to limit wrist rotation effectively. Nonsteroidal anti-inflammatory medication or a brief course of physical therapy, including ultrasound treatments, often affords significant relief.

Flexor Carpi Ulnaris Tendinitis

The flexor carpi ulnaris is the most common of the flexor tendons to become involved with tendinitis. It is sometimes bilateral and is seen in racquet sports. Pain and swelling are usually localized just proximal to the pisiform. Pain is aggravated by wrist flexion and ulnar deviation. Radiographs may show calcific deposits and are best seen on an oblique roentgenogram of the wrist. Splinting; physical therapy including cold application, ultrasound, isometrics, and stretching exercises; and nonsteroidal medication are usually effective.[2]

Carpal Tunnel Syndrome

Carpal tunnel syndrome is the most frequently encountered peripheral compression neuropathy associated with repetitive manual work. The diagnosis continues to increase in frequency.

Carpal tunnel syndrome typically affects women more than men. Symptoms consist of pain and paresthesias in the thumb, index, and long fingers, as well as the radial half of the ring finger, often worse at night. As an overuse disorder it is seen in younger workers of both sexes who experience these symptoms during the course of repetitive manual labor. The symptoms usually will improve with rest from manual work. Particularly at risk are meat packers, supermarket checkout clerks, seamstresses, assembly line workers, and others engaged in repetitive tasks involving flexion and extension of the wrist, a strong grip, or even exposure to vibratory tools.

Other nerve compression syndromes are frequently associated with repetitive manual work. These include compression of the ulnar nerve at the elbow, the radial nerve at the wrist or elbow, or the median nerve in the forearm. For a more detailed discussion of peripheral nerve compression, see Chapter 19.

References

1. Froimson AI: Tenosynovitis and tennis elbow. *In* Green DP (ed): Operative Hand Surgery. New York, Churchill Livingstone, 1993, pp 1989–2006.
2. Taylor Mullins PA: Use of therapeutic modalities in upper extremity rehabilitation. *In* Hunter JM, et al (eds): Rehabilitation of the Hand. St. Louis, CV Mosby, 1990, pp 195–220.

Suggested Reading

Thorson E, Szabo RM: Common tendinitis problems in the hand and forearm. Orthop Clin North Am 32(1): 65–74, 1992.

CHAPTER 23

Bite Injuries and Infections in the Hand and Foot

Ekkehard Bonatz

Microbiology

Improper treatment of infections in the hand or delay of therapy can result in a disastrous outcome. Antibiotics alone are rarely helpful. For example, they may be used early in high doses against a low-virulence organism. Soon, however, because of thrombosis of the small vessels, antibiotics will be unable to reach the area of infection.

Cultures should be taken when the patient is seen and drainage can be observed. The most common organism is *Staphylococcus aureus*. The choice of antibiotic is determined by the results of these cultures (first-generation cephalosporin or oral synthetic penicillin). Other organisms that may not respond to these antibiotics are also found, such as streptococci, enterobacteria, pseudomonads, and so on. *Pasteurella multocida* infection may follow a dog or cat bite, and *Eikenella corrodens* is commonly cultured after a human bite. In the 2-month to 3-year age group, *Haemophilus influenzae* is common. Various anaerobes are also found.

Herpes simplex infections have a characteristic vesical formation. Herpes zoster and even rabies have been described in the hand. Fungal infections, although rare, may be present in the immunocompromised patient or when a long-standing systemic antibiotic is given. These may consist of sporotrichosis, *Histoplasma* infections, *Candida* infections, or tinea pedia cutis (ringworm). Mycobacterial infections also can be confused with synovitis caused by rheumatoid arthritis or other chronic inflammatory conditions (gout, pseudogout).

History and Physical Examination

A penetrating injury often will precede an infection and should always be considered in the history. Diabetes mellitus, rheumatoid arthritis, chemotherapy, or other conditions compromising the patient's immune status are important factors, as they will aggravate any infectious process. Prior antibiotic treatment may influence further management decisions—e.g., a 2-day history of worsening pain and redness despite oral antibiotics most likely requires intravenous administration of antibiotics and serious consideration of surgical drainage. Painful blisters on the fingertips of a dental hygienist are almost always due to herpes simplex. A several-day or weeks-old injury in a farm environment with indolent joint swelling of a finger raises the suspicion of a mycobacterial infection.

On examination, the extent of any erythema should be noted. Active and passive range of motion of any affected joints should be evaluated and the degree of pain noted. Axial compression of a joint suggests purulent arthritis, whereas pain on passive extension of a digit may indicate septic flexor tenosynovitis. Local or regional lymphadenopathy indicates a more cellulitis-type of presentation rather than intra-articular infection. Fine vesicles about the fingertip are characteristic of herpes infections.

Treatment Principles

The initial treatment should include rest and splinting in a position of function (Fig. 23–1). Bacterial identification is important in order to treat an infection specifically and efficiently. Incision and drainage frequently will become necessary for abscesses or delayed presentations. Occasionally, surgical treatment can be rendered sufficiently in the emergency room, but hospitalization for intravenous antibiotics may be necessary. Antibiotics like penicillins or cephalosporins are directed toward gram-positive organisms. Infections following home or industrial injuries are usually caused by gram-positive organisms. Prophylaxis for these injuries may consist of intramuscular or intravenous oxacillin or cephazolin.[4]

Prophylaxis has not been shown to prevent infections in mutilating or farm injuries, because these are commonly contaminated with a mixed flora. However, after initial culture, parenteral antibiotic administration,

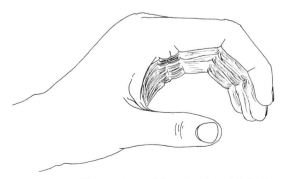

Figure 23–1. The position of function (partial flexion of the fingers with the wrist straight) is most appropriate for immobilization in the early stages of hand infections.

such as a first-generation cephalosporin, to cover the gram-positive organisms may still be useful.

PULP ABSCESS (FELON)

A felon is a subcutaneous abscess in the area of the distal pulp of the finger or thumb. *Staphylococcus aureus* is the most common organism. It presents with erythema and throbbing pain and occasionally with early abscess formation. The pain is due to the increased pressure, contained by the fibrous septa in the pulp.

Radiographs are usually negative or at most may show a small accumulation of subcutaneous air in the fingertip. Soft tissue swelling is usually evident on roentgenograms. Any bone involvement of the distal phalanx reflects osteomyelitis and indicates a poor prognosis.

At times, spontaneous decompression of the pulp may occur. If the abscess is superficial, the thin layer of tissue over the abscess should be opened with a sharp blade, and the adjacent fibrous septa spread and disrupted with a hemostat. A good rule of thumb is to incise the felon over the point of maximal swelling. The wound cavity is cultured and irrigated, and packed with a wick, and appropriate antibiotics are given.

Frequently, the sinus or abscess will not be evident. In this case, a medial or lateral incision of the pulp should be undertaken under digital block anesthesia. Incisions used for this purpose should be longitudinal to the long axis of the finger to avoid injuries to the digital nerves, and care should be taken to stay at least 2 mm away from the nail and nail bed. A fish-mouth type of incision around the entire fingertip will destabilize the pulp and should be avoided (Fig. 23–2). Lateral incisions should be placed on the ulnar side in the index, middle, and ring fingers and radially on the thumb and small finger.

Antibiotics are given for 5 to 10 days, according to severity and resolution of symptoms. For more severe presentations, such as erythema of the entire distal tip of the finger, referral for further surgical treatment and possible hospitalization for continuous irrigation and intravenous antibiotics may be necessary.

Some skin loss is often seen immediately over the abscess, but it will heal with good

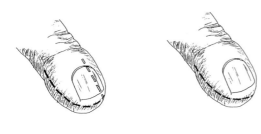

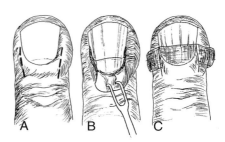

Figure 23–4. *A* to *C,* Drainage of a nail bed infection can be performed by incising the nail fold on both sides and placing a wick into the resulting wound.

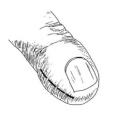
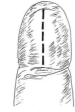

Figure 23–2. Incisions used to drain a pulp abscess of the finger (felon). Fish-mouth type incisions should be avoided, because they destabilize the fingertip.

wound care. Complications resulting from felons are osteomyelitis of the distal phalanx and septic flexor tenosynovitis following spread of the infection to the flexor tendon sheath. Secondary violation of the flexor tendon sheath may occur iatrogenically.

PARONYCHIA

A paronychia is an infection of the soft tissue fold around the fingernail. The most common organism involved is *Staphylococcus aureus.* It often begins as a cellulitis and erythema around the nail. There may be a history of trauma, such as by a hangnail, a manicure instrument, or a tooth. One should also keep

the possibility of herpes simplex infection in mind, especially in children or dental personnel. The characteristic painful blisters are the clue for this type of infection, which will usually resolve without manipulation of the tissues (see herpes simplex infections next).

Early treatment of paronychia with soaking and oral antibiotics may be sufficient. Gently pulling the paronychial fold away from the nail plate several times a day after soaking often will produce a drop of pus and decompress the paronychia. If no improvement is seen after 48 hours, debridement and irrigation become necessary. Under digital block anesthesia, the eponychial fold is opened after removal of only one fourth of the nail. If the abscess is still not drained, further incision of the nail fold with a scalpel blade directed away from the nail bed may effect drainage (Fig. 23–3). This may be performed on both sides of the fingernail. The resulting cavity must be irrigated and packed with a wick, which is removed after 48 hours (Fig. 23–4). Soaks are then insti-

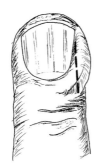

Figure 23–3. Drainage of a paronychium involves incision of the nail fold with a scalpel blade directed away from the nail bed.

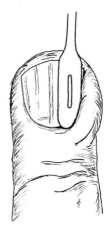

Figure 23–5. If the entire nail fold is involved with an infection, elevation with a probe may suffice.

tuted. When pain and redness subside, soaks and antibiotics can be discontinued.

Occasionally, the entire nail fold is involved. One must resist the temptation to remove the entire nail. Elevation of the nail fold with a probe usually will suffice (Fig. 23–5). Antibiotics are generally not necessary.

HERPES SIMPLEX (HERPETIC WHITLOW)

Vesicles on the fingertips are usually due to herpes simplex Type I infections (Fig. 23–6). They are most commonly seen in medical personnel who care for orotracheal areas but also in children with a history of finger or thumb sucking. In medical personnel, the diagnosis can be confirmed by the increased complement-fixing antibody titers against herpes simplex.

No surgical treatment is needed. The patient is advised to splint and elevate the hand for 10 to 14 days. The disease usually resolves in 3 to 4 weeks. Topical agents such as idoxuridine or acyclovir cream are sometimes effective. Gentle cleansing with soap and water is recommended, but this sometimes aggravates the inflammation or delays healing. In children, occasionally a *Staphylococcus aureus* superinfection occurs when the blisters rupture, and a brief course (2 to 5 days) of topical or oral antibiotics may be given.

FURUNCLE

A furuncle is an abscess on the dorsal aspect on the hand in the hair-bearing areas. Treat-

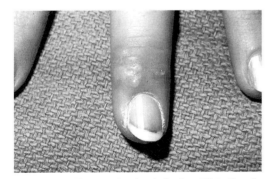

Figure 23–6. Herpes simplex infection. Note the characteristic vesicles. (Courtesy of W. Mitchell Sams, Jr., MD.)

ment consists of antibiotics and soaks. If there is a definitive abscess, debridement and irrigation with packing and immobilization are necessary.

WEB SPACE ABSCESS

An abscess in the soft cutaneous tissue of the palm will cause palmar *and* dorsal swelling. There will be swelling, pain, and erythema about the web space. There is usually a history of a penetrating wound. The erythrocyte sedimentation rate and white cell count may be elevated. Treatment consists of surgical debridement and irrigation, cultures, and appropriate antibiotics.

ACUTE SUPPURATIVE TENOSYNOVITIS

Pain on passive extension of the finger, a flexed position of the digit, and swelling and tenderness along the tendon sheath extending proximally into the palm and more proximal than any erythema may signal acute purulent tenosynovitis.

Because of the proximal extent of the flexor tendon sheaths, acute suppurative tenosynovitis may extend to the thenar area or into the midpalm or to the distal forearm. There may be a history of fever, or fever may be present on the initial visit. The erythrocyte sedimentation rate and white cell count are characteristically elevated.

Radiographs usually show only soft tissue swelling of the entire digit. One should look for any foreign body or a minimally displaced fracture.

If the patient is seen within 24 to 48 hours of the onset of the infection, parenteral antibiotics in high doses, elevation of the entire hand and forearm, and splinting in a functional position (see Figure 23–1) may control the process. The patient should be seen frequently, as often as twice a day, to assure improvement. After 48 hours, there must be definitive improvement. If there is no improvement, or the patient is seen later than 48 hours after the onset of the infection, surgical referral is mandatory.

PYOGENIC ARTHRITIS

Erythema, tenderness, and swelling of the involved joint are usually seen in pyogenic arthritis. There is loss of active motion. Increased pain on axial compression is characteristic. Compression of the joint from either side between the examiner's fingers reveals tenderness. This will usually aid in distinguishing septic arthritis from flexor tenosynovitis (in which the tenderness is on the palmar side). There is often a history of a penetrating injury or immune compromise. The white cell count and erythrocyte sedimentation rate will be elevated.

Treatment consists of surgical debridement and irrigation, open wound management, obtaining cultures and sensitivity studies, and immobilization. Suspected pyogenic arthritis should be referred for definitive surgical treatment. It may spread to flexor tendon sheaths, complicating its clinical presentation.

BITE INJURIES

An infection following a bite injury may progress rapidly after initial inoculation. Suspicion should be high in patients with metacarpal fractures, especially with metacarpal neck fractures (boxer's fractures). A puncture wound over the dorsum of the metacarpal head is always suspicious for a human bite injury. Because of the movement of the extensor tendon as the metacarpophalangeal (MP) joint is brought from a position of flexion to one of extension, a penetrating injury into the joint may not be immediately obvious. The portion of the tendon overlying the joint in MP flexion will move proximal to the skin wound when the MP joint is extended, thus being hidden (Fig. 23–7). Any remote possibility of penetrating joint injury must be ruled out by probing the laceration for any further extension into the MP joints. Any injury to the extensor tendon or extensor hood lends credence to the injury being in an open joint. In this instance, referral for irrigation in the operating room is indicated. Tooth marks or even fragments of teeth should be sought and ruled out roentgenographically.

Animal Bites

Cat and dog bites can introduce *Pasteurella multocida,* causing cellulitis, synovitis, and abscesses. These wounds are best treated by debridement and irrigation. Penicillin, ampi-

cillin, or cephalosporins will cover *Pasteurella,* as well as most *Staphylococcus* species. Infection may be persistent despite adequate debridement and antibiotics.

Organisms are usually of a mixed flora, commonly *Pasteurella multocida* (especially in cats and dogs). If only the early stage of cellulitis is present and no evidence of penetration into extensor tendon sheath or joint is seen, treatment is with ampicillin, penicillin, or a first-generation cephalosporin. However, deeper infections of the joint or tendon sheath are notorious for causing a very indolent infection requiring surgical debridement and long-term antibiotics.[1]

Human Bites

A mixed flora is common in human bites. This consists of *Bacteroides* species, *Staphylococcus* species, and others and will require treatment with a broad-spectrum antibiotic. *Eikenella corrodens* species are frequently present and are identified only with specific cultures. Treatment is with penicillin or ampicillin. Cephalexin may be given if the injury is seen within 24 hours; other antibiotics with gram-negative coverage (e.g., ticarcillin with clavulanic acid) may become necessary if the infection presents later or there is evidence of tendon or joint involvement.

The erythrocyte sedimentation rate and white cell count with a differential can give additional information about the severity of the infection. If there is evidence of penetration of a human or animal bite into the bone, joint, or tendon sheath, surgical consultation must be obtained.

MYCOBACTERIAL INFECTIONS

Mycobacterial infections are often seen in a farming or water environment and present days or weeks after an initially minor injury. Typically, acid-fast bacteria will cause an indolent joint swelling and pain with few other signs of inflammation. A history of minor injury followed days or weeks later by joint swelling is often the only clue. Radiographs will show joint erosions after 2 to 3 weeks. Characteristically, no improvement is seen with oral antibiotics. Further consultation should be obtained, since surgical synovectomy and treatment with antituber-

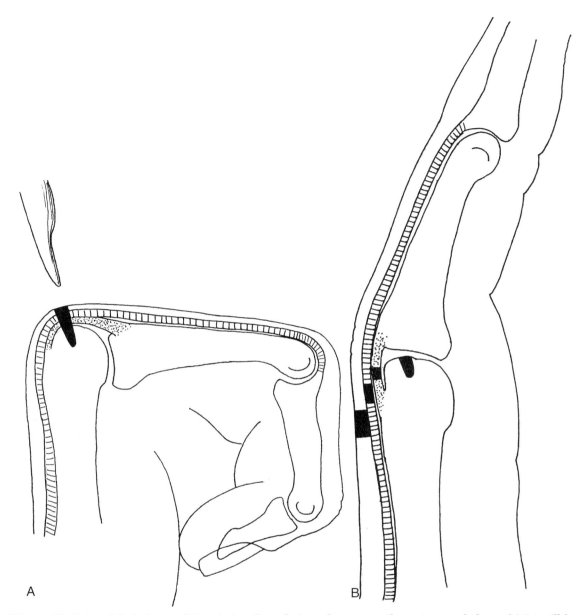

Figure 23–7. *A* and *B,* In human bite injuries, the soft tissue layers over the metacarpophalangeal joint will be aligned differently at the time of injury than at presentation to the physician.

culosis agents (isoniazid, rifampin, ethambutol, and so on) may become necessary.[3]

Miscellaneous Infections

Gram-negative infections are often seen following mutilating farm injuries and will be resistant to the usual antibiotics. Gas gangrene due to *Clostridium perfringens* does

occur in hand wounds and requires immediate surgical attention for fasciotomy, treatment with hyperbaric oxygen, and possibly amputation. Tetanus infections (*Clostridium tetani*) carry a death rate of up to 50 percent. It is rarely seen today. However, tetanus prophylaxis, as with any other open wound, should be performed in hand injuries.

Gonorrhea presents as a septic arthritis or tenosynovitis and is often seen in adolescents. Although usually seen in larger joints, such as ankles or knees, it may occur in the wrist and fingers. With an appropriate history, penicillin or tetracycline may suffice as an oral antibiotic for 2 weeks.

SPIDER BITES

The spider bite most frequently seen in the emergency department is that of the brown recluse. The spider is found in domestic areas that have been left undisturbed for a time (sheds, barns, garages, gutters), and the bite will not always be evident by history. A characteristic central area of necrosis surrounded by a halo of erythema will be present. This is often exquisitely painful and may be accompanied by local lymphadenopathy. Treatment is by infection prevention (first-generation cephalosporin) and prevention of further necrosis. Dapsone, a powerful antibacterial drug, is given orally and requires frequent monitoring of the peripheral blood count. A brief hospitalization may be appropriate. If necrosis or a subsequent bacterial infection occurs, surgical debridement may be needed.

PUNCTURE WOUNDS TO THE FOOT

Puncture wounds to the foot are most common in children. They are often due to injuries with penetrating objects, such as splinters, thorns, glass, or nails. Early sequelae are cellulitis and abscess formation. More serious and late consequences are osteomyelitis and septic arthritis. The offending organism is often *Pseudomonas aeruginosa,* especially if a sneaker was being worn at the time of the puncture. Infection and abscess formation are usually due to retained foreign material.

If the patient is seen within 48 hours of the injury, the wound should be cleansed and irrigated. It is paramount that joint penetration or bone injury is ruled out by radiograph. Large foreign bodies may be seen with x-rays using a soft tissue technique. If the wound is contaminated or deep or suspicion of a joint violation exists, oral antibiotics such as first-generation cephalosporins or semisynthetic penicillins are appropriate.[2] It is important to observe these patients carefully and obtain cultures early, especially if a deep infection is suspected. Tetanus prophylaxis should be

given for all but the most superficial wounds. Prophylaxis against *Pseudomonas* has not been studied, although suspicion of *Pseudomonas* exists when early cellulitis does not subside with cephalosporins or penicillins. If an abscess forms, surgical debridement may be needed.

INFECTIONS IN THE DIABETIC FOOT

In diabetics, foot problems are common reasons for hospital admissions and account for significant hospital stays. There is a high risk of eventual amputation. Because of their peripheral neuropathy, diabetic patients do not feel pain, and ulcers often have been present for a long time before medical advice is sought. Additionally, arterial and renal insufficiency as well as malnutrition with immunocompromise will impair healing. *Staphylococcus aureus* is the most frequent organism, but almost half the patients will have a mixed infection. A foul smell suggests anaerobes. Gas in the tissues indicates a mixed infection with gram-negative or anaerobic organisms and does not necessarily indicate necrotizing fasciitis. *Pseudomonas* is often seen in patients recently treated with oral antibiotics.

Radiographs are obtained to rule out neuropathic fractures, osteomyelitis, or gas in the soft tissues. To obtain cultures, aspiration is preferred over wound swab. Aspiration, however, should be done under sterile conditions to avoid secondary infection following violation of ischemic tissue.

After cultures have been obtained, empiric antibiotics are started. In mild or superficial infection, a first-generation cephalosporin or semisynthetic penicillin may be used. For suspicion of a more complex infection, a broad-spectrum antibiotic should be initiated, usually parenterally. Preferred choices are imipenem or ticarcillin with clavulanic acid. It is important to rule out necrosis or to evaluate the foot for possible debridement, as infections will not heal in the presence of necrotic tissue. The circulatory status must be carefully assessed, since vascular impairment carries a worse prognosis. Surgical evaluation is necessary in all but the most superficial infections. Necrotizing fasciitis can progress dramatically, and surgery may be necessary to save a limb or a life.

Prevention of Diabetic Foot Infections

Prophylactic foot care is of paramount importance in preventing recurrent foot infections in diabetic patients. Toenails should be trimmed square and not too close to the skin. The feet should be checked every night for blisters, if necessary with the help of a hand-held mirror to inspect the sole. Before stepping into water, its temperature should be tested with one's hand, since the neuropathic foot lacks temperature sensibility. Orthopaedic shoes with special inserts (e.g., total contact inserts) are helpful in preventing pressure ulcers. Use of these shoes should be considered once an infected pressure ulcer has healed.

References

1. Arons MS, Fernando L, Polyaes IM: *Pasteurella multocida:* The major cause of hand infections following domestic animal bites. J Hand Surg 7:47–52, 1982.
2. Frierson JG, Pfeffinger LL: Infections of the foot. *In* Mann RA (ed): Surgery of the Foot and Ankle. St. Louis, Mosby-Yearbook, 1992, pp 859–876.
3. Linscheid RL, Dobyns JH: Common and uncommon infections of the hand. Orthop Clin North Am 6:1063–1104, 1975.
4. Neviaser RJ: Infections. *In* Green DP (ed): Operative Hand Surgery. New York, Churchill Livingstone, pp 1021–1039, 1993.

Suggested Reading

Harrelson JM: Management of the diabetic foot. Orthop Clin North Am 20:4, 605–620, 1989.
Louis DS, Sylva J Jr: Herpetic whitlow: Herpetic infections of the digits. J Hand Surg 4:90–94, 1979.
Maggiore P, Echols RM: Infections in the diabetic foot. *In* Jahss MH (ed): Disorders of the Foot and Ankle. Philadelphia, WB Saunders, 1991, pp 1937–1957.
Neviaser RJ, Butterfield WC, Wieche DR: The puffy hand of drug addiction. J Bone Joint Surg 54A: 629–633, 1972.
Williams CS, Riordan DC: *Mycobacterium marinum* (atypical acid-fast bacillus) infections of the hand: A report of six cases. J Bone Joint Surg 55A:1042–1050, 1973.

CHAPTER 24

Chronic Pain Syndromes

Victoria Masear

Chronic pain disorders are one of the most difficult management problems in medicine. The experience is often filled with frustration for the patients, their families, third-party payers, and health care workers involved in their treatment. After months or even years of intensive treatment, the patient is often left with some residual degree of permanent pain. This chapter outlines the most common conditions causing chronic pain in the musculoskeletal system and the treatments for these that have helped the most.

REFLEX SYMPATHETIC DYSTROPHY (SHOULDER/HAND SYNDROME)

Reflex sympathetic dystrophy (RSD) results from vasomotor dysfunction of the sympathetic nervous system. The vasomotor dysfunction follows an inciting incident such as trauma or surgery to the involved extremity, or certain systemic diseases.[5,9,13,19,22,26,30] The hallmark findings of RSD include pain and swelling, both of which are out of proportion to the initial insult to the extremity. Both the pain and swelling continue to increase with time rather than decrease as would be expected following trauma. Due to the vasomotor instability there is often discoloration of the skin. The color combinations range from cyanosis to erythematous to a pale

color.[14] The redness is often localized around the joints, especially the proximal interphalangeal and metacarpophalangeal (MP) joints.

In the first several months, pain is the most notable symptom. The pain continues to increase for several months before reaching a plateau. The initial edema is a pitting type and is often quite massive (Fig. 24–1). Secondary to the vasoconstriction, the skin temperature is often much cooler than that of the opposite extremity. Increased sweating is usually prevalent early. Later in the disease process the skin may become dry, but it may take several months to a year before the hyperhidrosis gives way to dry skin. Near the end of the first year, the swelling often turns to a brawny edema, and stiffness in the joints becomes much more pronounced. Eventually the swelling and pain will subside, but the patient is often left with residual contractures of the MP and interphalangeal joints of the fingers and often the wrist. The skin may become shiny and have a pale appearance secondary to subcutaneous and dermal atrophy.

Dermineralization of bone in the involved extremity is usually apparent by x-ray by the end of the first month and becomes more severe throughout the first year. The demineralization usually begins near the joints and eventually involves the entire bone (Fig.

258

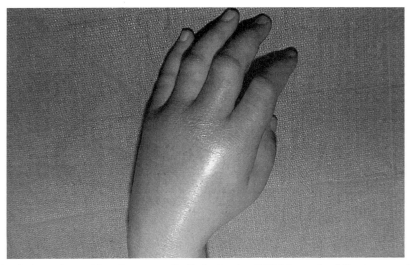

Figure 24–1. Hand of a patient with reflex sympathetic dystrophy (RSD) 4 months following carpal tunnel release. Marked edema and shiny skin are demonstrated.

24–2). Sudeck's atrophy has been described as spotty areas of demineralization in the carpal bones.[30] [99m]Tc bone scintigraphy has been one of the most frequently used diagnostic tests for RSD (Fig. 24–3). Typically, increased uptake in all three phases of the bone scan has been felt to be diagnostic of RSD. However, more recently controversy about the specificity and sensitivity of bone scans in RSD has increased.[8,12,25]

Other diagnostic tests have been used for RSD. Most of these deal with the evaluation of vascularity and sudomotor changes. Thermography has been heavily used but it is not specific for RSD. Thermography is accurate in evaluating skin temperature but probably no more accurate than either a skin thermometer or the examiner's hands. There is quite a bit of debate among reports as to what constitutes a positive thermogram for RSD.[2,4,6,15,23,24] Several other sudomotor tests, such as laser doppler velocimetry and cold stress tests, incur the same problems as thermography. They may accurately record the temperature or abnormal vasomotor changes, but they are not specific for RSD since other vasospastic vascular diseases cannot be excluded.

The single most definitive diagnostic test for RSD remains the response to sympathetic or adrenergic blocks. This includes either a stellate or brachial plexus block or an intravenous regional block with bretylium.* With

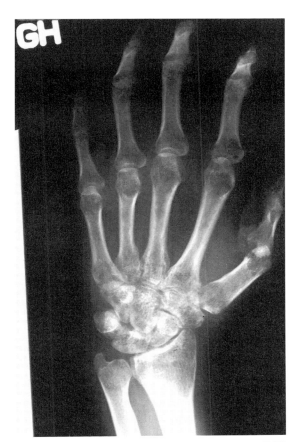

Figure 24–2. Hand radiograph of a patient with RSD showing periarticular demineralization.

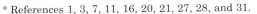
* References 1, 3, 7, 11, 16, 20, 21, 27, 28, and 31.

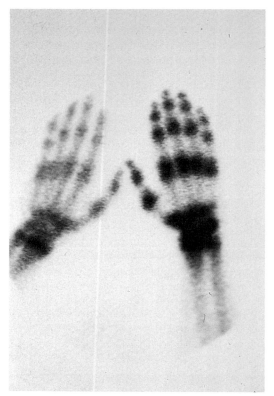

Figure 24-3. Bone scan showing increased uptake of isotope in periarticular regions of a patient with RSD.

therapy. Application of a transcutaneous electrical nerve stimulator (TENS) unit for control of a localized nerve irritation is often of significant benefit. Hand therapy must be instituted immediately for control of the edema and regaining motion. Passive motion is never used with reflex sympathetic dystrophy as this serves only to increase the pain and swelling.

Before any therapy can be successful, the pain must be reduced or eliminated by blocks. Active exercises and light use of the hand are the main treatment, and the patient needs to be encouraged to use the hand as much as possible within pain tolerance. Heat and elevation, as well as splinting to prevent contractures or regain motion, are needed. Stress loading, which constitutes light activities within the patient's pain tolerance, and no passive motion are the mainstays of hand therapy.[33] Once the pain is under control and the edema has subsided, then hand surgery for relief of joint contractures may be indicated. The success rate of this, however, is limited. No surgery for regaining motion should be performed prior to the quiescence of symptoms of the RSD.

The multidisciplinary approach continues with the help of a psychologist or psychiatrist. Usually patients with an RSD have a dependent personality that predisposes to this type of problem. The problem, however, is real and cannot be treated by the psychologist. The psychologist does aid in helping the patient cope, and at times biofeedback measures have been successful. Although the pain of RSD is constant, it is aggravated by emotional factors and upsets. For these aggravations of symptoms, the psychologist can play an important role.[18]

Medications for RSD include sympatholytic drugs, especially alpha-blockers and calcium channel blockers. Local control of pain with topical analgesics or transdermal patches has also shown some success. Narcotic prescriptions should be avoided, as this is a long-term ongoing problem and addiction to prescription drugs can easily occur.

Unfortunately, the diagnosis of RSD seems to be made too frequently. Often a patient with pain of unexplained origin is given a diagnosis of RSD when none of the other factors of RSD are present. RSD may occur in varying proportions, but pain out of proportion to what is expected should not be the only factor considered when a diagnosis of RSD is made.

either of these blocks, the original pain is not necessarily relieved, but the dysesthesias and hyperalgesias usually are.[13] The pain relief may be only for several days, and the blocks often need to be repeated several times before a more permanent effect is seen. The advantage of either sympathetic or adrenergic blocks as diagnostic tools is that they also serve as the best form of treatment.

The treatment of RSD is served best by early diagnosis and the institution of appropriate blocks and therapy. The earlier the institution of treatment, the more relief from symptoms is expected. The patient is often referred to a pain center for multidisciplinary treatment. Usually an anesthesiologist is recommended for performing either stellate ganglion or intravenous regional blocks. If after several sympathetic blocks, the patient's symptoms persist, then referral for a sympathectomy may be indicated. The success rate of sympathectomy in the treatment of RSD has been quite high, especially in patients who responded with improvement from sympathetic blocks.[20,21,32] The services of a hand surgeon are often needed to direct

PAIN OF NERVE ORIGIN

Causalgia (Mitchell's causalgia[19]) has been described as a form of RSD. The difference from the typical RSD is that there has been a nerve injury, and the continued pain and pain syndrome stem from this fact. The patient presentation may be similar to that with RSD, and indeed autonomic dysfunction of the sympathetic nervous system may be present, but there also will be a more severe localized pain and a Tinel's sign over the injured nerve. With a distinct nerve injury, the diagnosis often can be aided by a peripheral nerve block, in which a local anesthetic is injected directly around the nerve in question. If this relieves a significant proportion of or all the pain, then that lends credence to the fact that nerve is the problem. Also, nerve conduction studies often will show slowing of conduction or absent conduction across the nerve in question.

The nerve injury may be secondary to a laceration, blunt trauma, traction injury, or scarring around the nerve, usually secondary to a previous surgical procedure or radiation in that area. The diagnosis and treatment will be similar to those of RSD, but additional treatment should be directed toward the nerve injury itself. Often, a scarred nerve may undergo neurolysis, be moved to another area out of the bed of scar, or wrapped with a substance to prevent future scarring.[17] If the nerve is injured to the point of no longer functioning or it has been transected, then either resection of the neuroma with repair or nerve grafting, resection of the neuroma and burying the end of the nerve more deeply into muscle or bone, or surgically capping the nerve may be warranted. A transcutaneous electrical nerve stimulator is often of significant benefit when placed directly over the injured nerve proximal to the level of injury.

FACTITIOUS PAIN SYNDROMES

Patients will often present with marked edema of unexplained origin in a hand, forearm, or both. There may or may not be an associated history of injury. The edema is usually a boggy type of soft edema but over months may become a brawny, hard edema. It is important to examine the entire upper extremity with any history or signs of swelling. If the edema stops abruptly and circumferentially (usually just below or just above the elbow), then a self-inflicted edema secondary to the repeated application of a tourniquet should be suspected. It is not helpful to confront the patient with this fact, as the patient usually will not return and the problem continues. It is important to get psychologic help for these patients; often, sending them to a psychologist for the stated reason of helping them cope with the situation will serve patients best. These are some of the most difficult treatment problems in hand surgery as there is often hostility toward the physician from both the patient and the patient's family.

In 1901, Secretan described a woody, hard edema over the dorsum of the hand.[29] Patients with this symptom normally have a history of a work-related injury from a contusion to the dorsum of the hand. However, the edema and ecchymosis persist. Ultimately, a peritendinous fibrosis with stiffness in the fingers and a brawny edema over the dorsum of the hand develop. The diagnosis can usually be made by placing the patient in a short arm cast. The edema and ecchymosis subside, but as soon as the cast is removed they usually recur. Again, psychologic assistance is needed, because repeated, self-inflicted blows to the dorsum of the hand are most likely the cause.

Unexplained infections or blistering of the hand that fail to resolve with antibiotics and local wound care are often self-induced. Many instances have been identified with repeated burns or injection of materials (e.g., feces) as self-inflicted conditions.

Another psychologic problem that often presents in the hand is an apparent contracture of the fingers. Usually the ulnar digits are most involved, and often the ring or little finger or both are flexed into the hand and the patient states that they cannot be moved. If the patient is distracted while the examiner is talking, the fingers often can be gently manipulated into extension and they will then stay there. At times the patient will allow the examiner to bring the fingers into extension and then hold them in extension. However, as soon as the hand is flexed, the fingers will again stay in flexion. There is no anatomic reason for the patient to be capable of holding the fingers in extension but to be unable actively to extend them. The diagnosis is, again, one of psychologic origin.

Patients often complain of numbness in an extremity or the entire side of the body that may be feigned. These are very difficult diagnostic dilemmas, but some basic tests can determine whether the nerves are actually funtioning. The skin of fingers or toes will wrinkle like a prune if immersed in water for 10 to 15 minutes. This indicates that the nerves are functioning. If a nerve is not functioning to a given part, then no wrinkling of skin will occur. Also, any sweating pattern that is noted in the fingers or toes indicates that the nerves are indeed functioning, and there should at least be some sensibility to the part. Reflexes and muscle tone will be normal. There is no muscle atrophy. Nerve conduction studies can aid equivocal cases.

One must remember that although many of these conditions are not related to anatomic abnormalities, they may be real to the patient. Confronting the patient is often the worst thing that can occur, since strong denial exists, and to the patient the problem may be quite real. Enlisting psychologic support and therapy when necessary are the mainstays of treatment.

References

1. Bonica JJ (ed): The Management of Pain, 2nd ed. Philadelphia, Lea & Febiger, 1990, pp 220–243.
2. Bryan AS, Klenerman L, Bowsher D: Measurement of somatic sensory modalities in reflex sympathetic dystrophy (abstract). J Bone Joint Surg 72B:1106, 1990.
3. Cooper DE, DeLee JC, Ramamurthy S: Reflex sympathetic dystrophy of the knee. Treatment using continuous epidural anesthesia. J Bone Joint Surg 71A:365–369, 1989.
4. Coughlan RJ, Hazleman BL, Page-Thomas DP, Sattelle L, Crisp AJ, Jenner JR, Dandy DJ: Algodystrophy: A common unrecognized cause of chronic knee pain. Br J Rheumatol 26:270–274, 1987.
5. deTakats G: Causalgic states in peace and war. JAMA 128:699–704, 1945.
6. Ecker A: Contact thermography in diagnosis of reflex sympathetic dystrophy: A new look at pathogenesis. Thermology 1:106–109, 1985.
7. Hanowell LH, Kanefield JD, Soriano SG III: A recommendation for reduced lidocaine dosage during intravenous regional bretylium treatment of reflex sympathetic dystrophy (letter). Anesthesiology 71:811–812, 1989.
8. Hoffman J, Phillips W, Blum M, Barohn R, Ramamurthy S: Effect of sympathetic block demonstrated by triple-phase bone scan. J Hand Surg 18A:860–864, 1993.
9. Homans J: Minor causalgia: A hyperesthetic neurovascular syndrome. N Engl J Med 222:870–874, 1940.
10. Hord AT, Rooks MD, Stephens BO, Rogers HG, Fleming LL: Intravenous regional bretylium and lidocaine for treatment of reflex sympathetic dystrophy: A randomized, double-blind study. Anesth Analg 74:818–821, 1992.
11. Kettler RE, Abram SE: Intravenous regional droperidol in the management of reflex sympathetic dys-

trophy: A double-blind, placebo-controlled, crossover study. Anesthesiology 69:933–936, 1988.
12. Kline SC, Holder LE: Segmental reflex sympathetic dystrophy: Clinical and scintigraphic criteria. J Hand Surg 18A:853–859, 1993.
13. Lankford LL: Reflex sympathetic dystrophy. *In* Green DP (ed): Operative Hand Surgery, 3rd ed. New York, Churchill Livingstone, 1993, pp 627–660.
14. Lankford LL: Reflex sympathetic dystrophy. *In* Omer GE Jr, Spinner M (eds): Management of Peripheral Nerve Problems. Philadelphia, WB Saunders, 1980, pp 216–244.
15. Lightman HI, Pochaczersky R, Aprin H, Ilowite NT: Thermography in childhood reflex sympathetic dystrophy. J Pediatr III: 551–555, 1987.
16. Manchikanti L: Role of intravenous regional bretylium in reflex sympathetic dystrophy (letter). Anesthesiology 73:585–586, 1990.
17. Masear VR: Venous wrapping of nerves to prevent scarring. American Society for Surgery of the Hand, 44th Annual Meeting, Seattle, September 15, 1989.
18. Mitchell SW: Injuries of Nerves and Their Consequences. Philadelphia, JB Lippincott, 1872.
19. Mitchell SW: On the diseases of nerves resulting from injuries in contributions relating to the causation and prevention of disease, and to camp disease. *In* Flint A (ed): United States Sanitary Commission Memoirs. New York, Hurd & Haughton, 1867.
20. Mockus MB, Rutherford RB, Rosales C, Pearce WH: Sympathectomy for causalgia. Patient selection and long-term results. Arch Surg 122:668–672, 1987.
21. Olcott C IV, Eltherington LG, Wilcosky BR, Shour PM, Zimmerman JJ, Fogarty TJ: Reflex sympathetic dystrophy—the surgeon's role in management. J Vasc Surg 14:488–495, 1991.
22. Patman RD, Thompson JE, Persson AV: Management of post-traumatic pain syndromes. Report of 113 cases. Ann Surg 177:780–787, 1973.
23. Perelman RB, Adler D, Humphreys M: Reflex sympathetic dystrophy: Electronic thermography as an aid in diagnosis. Orthop Rev 16:561–566, 1987.
24. Pochaczersky R: Thermography in post-traumatic pain. Am J Sports Med 15:243–250, 1987.
25. Pollock FE Jr, Koman LA, Smith BP, Poehling GG: Patterns of microvascular response associated with reflex sympathetic dystrophy of the hand and wrist. J Hand Surg 18A:847–852, 1993.
26. Richards RL: Causalgia. A centennial review. Arch Neurol 16:339–350, 1967.
27. Roberts WJ: A hypothesis on the physiological basis for causalgia and related pains. Pain 24:297–311, 1986.
28. Schwartzman RJ, McLellan TL: Reflex sympathetic dystrophy. A review. Arch Neurol 44:555–561, 1987.
29. Secretan H: Oedeme dur et hyperplasie traumatique du metacarpe dorsal. Rev Med Suisse Romande 21:409, 1901.
30. Sudeck PHM: Ueber die acute entzundliche Knochenatrophie. Arch Klin Chir 62:147–156, 1900.
31. Vanos DN, Ramamurthy S, Hoffman J: Intravenous regional block using ketorolac: Preliminary results in the treatment of reflex sympathetic dystrophy. Anesth Analg 74:139–141, 1992.
32. Walsh JA, Glynn CJ, Cousins MJ, Basedow RW: Blood flow, sympathetic activity and pain relief following lumbar sympathetic blockade or surgical sympathectomy. Anesth Interns Care 13:18–24, 1984.
33. Watson HK, Carlson L: Treatment of reflex sympathetic dystrophy of the hand with an active "stress loading" program. J Hand Surg 12A:779–785, 1987.

Tumors of the Musculoskeletal System

Kenneth Jaffe

Although musculoskeletal neoplasms are rare, a working knowledge of these tumors and masses is of great practical importance to the primary care physician. The key to successful management of any tumor or reactive process is a thorough understanding of its biologic behavior and natural history (Table 25–1). This knowledge is based on accurate physical, diagnostic, radiographic, and histologic evaluation.[50] The method of treatment depends on the neoplastic nature of the lesion as well as its actual anatomic location and involvement with local structures. Clinical factors such as patient age, tumor size, occupation, lifestyle, and expectations also play key roles. The treatment of these tumors also requires both a consideration of their possible life-threatening nature and an understanding of the principles of orthopaedic surgery.

GENERAL WORK-UP FOR BONE TUMORS AND SOFT TISSUE TUMORS

To evaluate patients with bone or soft tissue tumors fully, the physician must undertake a systematic approach to avoid any pitfalls.

These lesions can be quite misleading; many nontumorous conditions can present like tumors and can appear to be quite aggressive. For these reasons, the work-up is divided into four categories: (1) complete history and physical examination, (2) radiographic staging, (3) diagnosis, and (4) treatment.

History and Physical Examination

Patient evaluation includes taking a history and performing a detailed physical examination. Patients usually present with a mass, a lesion incidentally discovered when a radiograph is made for other reasons, or a pathologic fracture. Pertinent points to be addressed are the manner of onset, duration, rate of growth, evidence of inflammatory signs, and whether or not there has been any change. When the facts about the local lesion have been ascertained, questions concerning systemic manifestations should be entertained. Weight loss, fever, chills, pulmonary status, smoking history, and past medical management are all important points that may shed light on the possibility of metastasis of a sarcoma or the existence of a primary carcinoma.

TABLE 25–1.
Musculoskeletal Neoplasms

Tissue type	Benign	Malignant
Tumors of Bone		
Osseous	Osteoid osteoma	Classic osteosarcoma
	Osteoblastoma	Parosteal osteosarcoma
	Osteoma	Periosteal osteosarcoma
Cartilaginous	Enchondroma	Primary chondrosarcoma
	Exostosis	Secondary chondrosarcoma
	Periosteal chondroma	
	Chondroblastoma	
	Chondromyxoid fibroma	
Fibrous	Nonossifying fibroma	Fibrosarcoma of bone
	Desmoplastic fibroma	Malignant fibrous histiocytoma
	Fibrous dysplasia	
	Ossifying fibroma	
Reticuloendothelial	Eosinophilic granuloma	Ewing's sarcoma
	Hand-Schüller-Christian disease	Reticulum cell sarcoma
	Letterer-Siwe disease	Myeloma
Vascular	Aneurysmal bone cyst	Angiosarcoma
	Hemangioma of bone	Hemangioendothelioma
		Hemangiopericytoma
Unknown origin	Simple bone cyst (unicameral)	Giant cell sarcoma
	Giant cell tumor of bone	Chordoma
		Adamantinoma
Tumors of Soft Tissue		
Osseous	Myositis ossificans	Extraosseous osteosarcoma
Cartilaginous	Chondroma	Extraosseous chondrosarcoma
	Synovial chondromatosis	
Fibrous	Fibroma	Fibrosarcoma
	Fibromatosis	Malignant fibrous histiocytoma
Synovial	Pigmented villonodular synovitis	Synovial sarcoma
	Ganglion cyst	
Vascular	Hemangioma	Angiosarcoma
		Hemangioendothelioma
		Hemangiopericytoma
Fatty	Lipoma	Liposarcoma
	Angiolipoma	
Neural	Neurilemmoma	Neurosarcoma
	Neurofibroma	Neurofibrosarcoma
Muscular	Leiomyoma	Leiomyosarcoma
	Rhabdomyoma	Rhabdomyosarcoma
Unknown origin	Giant cell tumor or tendon sheath	Epithelioid sarcoma
		Clear cell sarcoma
		Mesenchymoma
		Undifferentiated sarcoma

Physical examination is guided by the history; the clinical situation, the exact location of the lesion, size, consistency, mobility, tenderness, and the reaction of the surrounding tissues should be documented. The mobility of the lesion is important because superficial lesions that can be moved about usually have not invaded the deep fascia and have a high probability of being benign. Large, firm, fixed lesions are much more likely to be malignant. Tenderness to palpation is another helpful point. It may be due to infection or an active neoplastic process. Range of motion of the joints in proximity to the lesion should be documented, as well as the neurologic status of the extremity.

The laboratory evaluation may help differentiate an infectious versus a malignant process. A complete blood count with differential and sedimentation rate should be obtained. Other tests should aim at finding a primary cause if one is trying to rule out a metastatic process. These include thyroid function studies, urinalysis, acid phosphatase, liver function test, and serum immunoelectrophoresis. Alkaline phosphatase, calcium, and phosphorus are usually elevated in destructive bone lesions.

Staging Techniques

As stated, the purpose of radiographic staging of tumors is twofold. The first reason is to obtain information concerning the probable diagnosis, and the second is to define the anatomic extent of the lesion.[24] The extent of the necessary work-up depends on the expected diagnosis.

Plain Radiography

The first study obtained in most instances is a plain radiograph. Plain radiographs provide the most general diagnostic information. This information, in combination with the clinical presentation, gives some indication as to whether the tumor is malignant or benign and determines the extent and type of the subsequent staging studies.[24] Plain radiographs demonstrate which bone is involved, which region of the bone is involved, the extent and type of destruction, and the amount of reactive bone formed (Fig. 25–1). Radiographs also may give some clue about the type of matrix being formed by the lesion.[31] The pattern of bone destruction and the reaction to that destruction have been well described and can be used to place the lesion in one of a few major categories.[56] These categories are based on biologic aggressiveness of the lesion and are used to direct the remainder of the diagnostic work-up.

Radioisotope Scanning

Skeletal scintigraphy is most commonly performed using ^{99m}Tc-labeled phosphonates. ^{99m}Tc is incorporated into sites of tumor, bone growth repair, and reactive bone.[1,5,33] Increased isotope uptake also occurs in areas of increased vascularity seen in the flow phase of the three-phase bone scan. The two major functions of this study are to provide an estimation of the local intramedullary extent of the tumor and to screen for other areas of skeletal involvement.[24] To accomplish these goals, it is necessary to obtain anterior and posterior views of the entire skeleton, with toned-down views in two planes of the involved bone, and of any other areas of increased uptake. The extent and intensity of increased uptake may give information about the biologic aggressiveness of the tumor.

Computed Tomography

Once a lesion is identified on plain radiographs, further information can be obtained with computed tomography. This enables the diagnostician to view a lesion and the surrounding anatomic structures in an axial plane. New programs can also offer three-dimensional reconstruction, as well as the ability to view structures from different angles, to remove certain structures (disarticulate joints), or to eliminate the soft tissue. Computed tomography is the best study for evaluating cortical penetration and osseous detail. It is also valuable in the assessment of matrix calcification or ossification.[64] Adding contrast aids in the identification of vascular structures, as well as in the enhancement of well-vascularized lesions.

Magnetic Resonance Imaging

Magnetic resonance imaging is being increasingly used for the evaluation of musculoskeletal tumors.[64] These studies include axial images with T1 and T2 weighting, as well as longitudinal images in either the sagittal or coronal plane. Magnetic resonance imaging is the most accurate method of evaluating both the intramedullary extent of a bone tumor and its soft tissue components and relationship to neurovascular structures (Fig. 25–2).

The role of MRI in the work-up of musculoskeletal tumors is becoming better defined. Although many possible pulse sequences can be used for tumor imaging, the most popular has been spin-echo imaging. This sequence is technically easy to implement and provides information about hydrogen density and T1- and T2-weighted images. Another advantage of using MRI is that by varying pulse repetition time (TR) and echo time (TE), the radiologist can drastically change the contrast level between different tissues. This process can be very helpful in trying to distinguish tumor from surrounding normal tissue.[64]

In some instances, MRI is able to determine tumor histology or to determine whether tumors are fluid filled.[28,39] Lipomas have T1, T2, and hydrogen density values that are virtually identical to those of normal subcutaneous fat (Fig. 25–3). However, when spin-echo imaging is used, lipomas reveal a characteristically high intensity that remains high at most spin-echo pulse

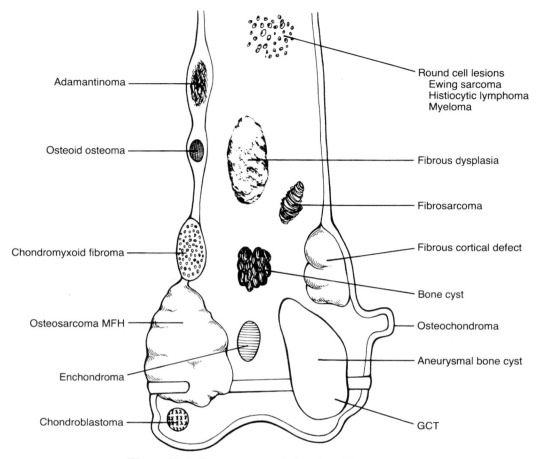

Figure 25–1. Common anatomic location of bone tumors.

Adamantinoma

Osteoid osteoma

Chondromyxoid fibroma

Osteosarcoma MFH

Enchondroma

Chondroblastoma

Round cell lesions
Ewing sarcoma
Histiocytic lymphoma
Myeloma

Fibrous dysplasia

Fibrosarcoma

Fibrous cortical defect

Bone cyst

Osteochondroma

Aneurysmal bone cyst

GCT

sequences. Fluid content may be suspected in a lesion with very long T1 or T2 time. Such lesions, therefore, appear relatively low in intensity on a T1-weighted sequence and become substantially brighter on a more T2-weighted sequence.

The use of intravenous paramagnetic contrast agents in musculoskeletal imaging also helps improve the contrast between tumor and normal tissue.

Biopsy of Bone and Soft Tissue Lesions

The biopsy is an important step in the management of neoplasms of the musculoskeletal system.[48] A principle that permeates orthopedic oncology is the need for a multidisciplinary approach to the diagnosis and management of neoplasms. The accurate prebiopsy staging of the local lesion should be

completed prior to biopsy.[46] Changes induced by the biopsy may alter the local circumstances sufficiently to make it difficult to determine the extent of disease after biopsy or may introduce confusing artifacts on the special studies.

The biopsy procedure must be planned as carefully as the definitive procedure.[46] Details of the biopsy procedure should be the responsibility of the person who will *ultimately* manage the patient. Mankin and coworkers studied a group of 329 patients with malignant primary bone and soft tissue tumors in 1982 and noted both errors in diagnosis and complications of the patients' courses.[32] The biopsy-related problems occurred three to five times more frequently when the biopsy was performed at a referring institution than when performed at the treating center. A large percentage of the patients had to be managed by a less-than-optimal treatment plan, and at least 8 percent had

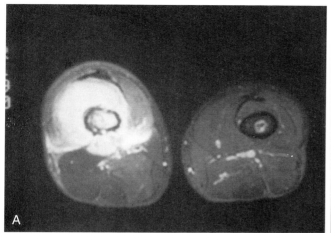

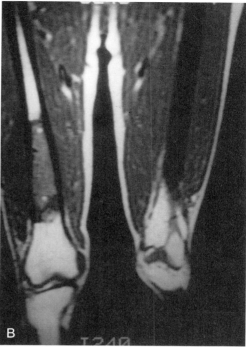

Figure 25–2. MRI scans of a malignant bone tumor (osteosarcoma, malignant fibrous histiocytoma, MFH). *A,* Axial, and *B,* coronal slices of the thigh. The intramedullary extent of the tumor, as well as the soft tissue component, is well visualized. (GCT, giant cell tumor)

a distinctly adverse prognosis because of problems with the biopsy. Almost 5 percent of the patients who might have had a limb-sparing procedure required an amputation as a result of a problem with the biopsy.

SOFT TISSUE TUMORS

All connective tissue can give rise to benign or malignant neoplasms. Confusion may arise when benign lesions become symptom-

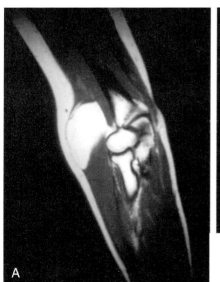

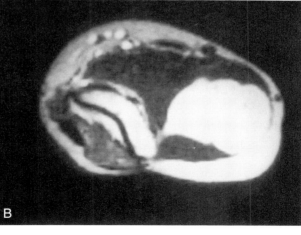

Figure 25–3. *A* and *B,* MRI scans of a lipoma involving the elbow. The tumor has the same signal characteristics as those of the subcutaneous fat.

atic owing to their size, anatomic location, or both. Although benign tumors do not metastasize, local aggressiveness and recurrence can cause significant morbidity.

Patients with a soft tissue sarcoma usually present with a painless, slowly enlarging mass. The length of time from recognition of the mass to presentation varies, but it is often months. This time interval often results from both delayed patient presentation and delayed physician recognition. Many patients are treated for a muscle pull or hematoma. Occasionally the mass may cause symptoms as a result of pressure on adjacent nerves or blood vessels, resulting in paresthesias, weakness, or swelling. About 30 percent of patients will give a history of previous trauma. Patients often associate the development of a soft tissue sarcoma with an injury sustained in the remote past, but direct trauma is not thought to cause soft tissue sarcomas; the injury is only coincidental and may call attention to the presence of a swelling, or there may be intralesional trauma resulting in bleeding and expansion.

Soft tissue sarcomas are usually a disease of adulthood, occurring in persons between 30 and 60 years of age. The sole exception is rhabdomyosarcoma, which occurs in young children.[7] Approximately one half of soft tissue sarcomas are found in the extremities; the remainder arise in the head/neck and trunk.[8] Soft tissue sarcomas may arise from any of the connective tissue elements. The lower extremity is the most common anatomic site; 40 percent of all soft tissue sarcomas occur in this location. The anterior thigh (quadriceps) is the most common compart-

ment, followed by the adductor and hamstrings.

Unlike carcinomas, soft tissue sarcomas disseminate almost exclusively through the blood. Epithelioid, synovial, and alveolar soft part sarcomas may spread through the lymphatic system to regional nodes.[61] Hematogenous spread is manifested by pulmonary involvement. Soft tissue sarcomas usually remain intracompartmental or between compartments where the fascia acts as a good barrier.[18]

SOFT TISSUE TUMOR-LIKE LESIONS

Ganglia

A ganglion is a tumor-like collection of viscous fluid encapsulated by a fibrous sheath. It is most often found on the dorsum of the wrist but can occasionally be found on the dorsum of the foot, the ankle, or knee. It is one of the most commonly encountered tumor-like lesions.[27] These lesions are often associated with tendon sheaths and may communicate with the nearest joint capsule (Fig. 25–4).

Ganglia range in size from 1 mm to 3 cm. Symptoms include pain, discomfort, and cosmetic worries. An occasional patient may have joint instability or paresthesias (from cutaneous nerve compression). Physical examination shows a firm, moveable, cystic-feeling mass that transilluminates. The mass tends to become more tense with age and can obstruct the smooth gliding of

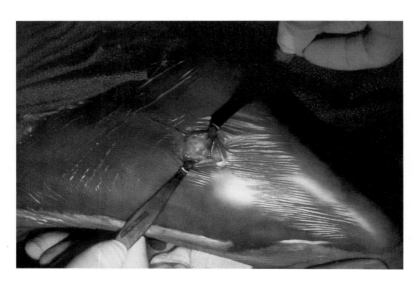

Figure 25–4. Ganglion cyst of the lateral aspect of the foot.

nearby tendons if it is allowed to reach a significant size. Radiographs usually show nothing but a small, soft tissue mass, but they may show extension into adjacent bone.[26,63] The etiology of this lesion has never been elucidated. Theories have included repetitive trauma, connective tissue defects, joint capsule herniation, and articular tissue irritation.[52]

Treatment varies widely. The most common method is marginal excision of the lesion. However, this can yield recurrence rates of up to 20 to 30 percent and leaves a scar that can be cosmetically unacceptable. For these reasons, other clinicians have searched for alternative methods. In the early stages, if the capsule has not excessively matured, the ganglion can be ruptured by manipulation, and the fluid can be massaged into nearby tissue. The fluid will gradually be resorbed. If the ganglion reappears, this process can be repeated until the capsule matures. Aspiration of the ganglion with or without the subsequent injection of steroids and local anesthetics can provide a safe and simple alternative to operative therapy.

Benign Soft Tissue Tumors

Lipoma

Lipomas are the most common benign soft tissue neoplasm. They arise from normal fat and usually appear during adulthood. They may be single or multiple. The location and size of the tumor determine the type of symptoms. Pain is rare, but it may occur secondary to compression of peripheral nerves. The usual complaint is cosmetic (appearance). They are found either subcutaneously or deeply embedded in or between muscle groups. The shoulder girdle and proximal thigh are the two most common sites.[19] Histologically, mature fat cells are present. Surgery is indicated if the mass is painful or enlarging, or there is concern about a malignant degeneration. Simple surgical excision is curative in most cases but is rarely needed as the diagnosis usually can be made clinically. Magnetic resonance imaging and CT scans can be helpful to differentiate these lesions from more malignant processes, for these tumors have signals identical to those of subcutaneous fat.

Neurilemmoma (Schwannoma)

Neurilemmomas originate from the Schwann cell, which is responsible for the supporting structure of the peripheral nerve. These benign growths arise within the nerve and are surrounded by a true capsule composed of the epineurium (Fig. 25–5). They are composed of Atoni A (cellular) and Atoni B (loose myxoid) components. These lesions generally are not associated with von Recklinghausen's disease. They typically present as a painless mass that corresponds to the course of a peripheral nerve. Surgical treatment is indicated for diagnostic purposes or if the lesion is symptomatic. These tumors are usually located eccentrically on the nerve. Resection entails opening the capsule and enucleating the growth from the nerve.

Neurofibroma

Neurofibromas can be divided into two groups: solitary or multiple. Unlike the neurilemmomas, they are not encapsulated, often enlarge the nerves, and may undergo malignant degeneration. Histologically, they consist of varying amounts of cellular, mucinous, and collagenous substances. Multiple neurofibromas are found in patients with von Recklinghausen's disease. These lesions cannot be surgically detached from the underlying nerve. Surgery is indicated only if malignant degeneration is suspected. The central location of their larger nerves

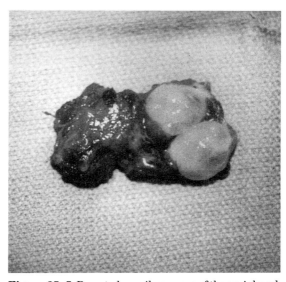

Figure 25–5. Resected neurilemmoma of the peripheral nerve.

and the interdigitation with nerve fascicles make it quite difficult to remove the tumor without producing permanent neurologic damage. Between 20 and 65 percent of patients with neurofibromatosis ultimately develop a sarcoma.

Fibromatosis

The term *fibromatosis* has been used to describe a wide variety of benign or reactive fibroblastic processes. They are divided into superficial or deep forms. The superficial group includes palmar fibromatosis (Dupuytren's contracture), plantar fibromatosis (Ledderhose's disease), and penile fibromatosis (Peyronie's disease) (see Chapter 26). These tumors arise within the superficial fascia, may be familial, and show limited growth potential.

Deep (aggressive) fibromatosis, which appears harmless microscopically, is the most serious of all benign soft tissue tumors. It does not have a capsule and tends to infiltrate far beyond its recognized boundaries (Fig. 25–6). The lesion does not respect fascial borders and thus can attain a large size involving multiple anatomic compartments if left untreated.[19] The most common locations are the neck, shoulder, and pelvic girdle. Death results from intrathoracic or retroperitoneal extension. The clinical history often reveals multiple recurrences despite surgical removal. The appropriate surgical procedure is wide excision. Local recurrence uniformly follows excision with positive margins. Surgical staging studies should be performed prior to resection. Amputation is occasionally required. Radiation and chemotherapy have been utilized as adjuvant treatment for recurrent disease.

Hemangioma

Hemangiomas are benign tumors of the blood vessels. They consist of a variety of types. It is not certain whether these are true neoplasms or vascular malformations. In general, there are two types of hemangioma: generalized and localized. Hemangiomas are classified based upon their pathologic appearance—capillary, cavernous, venous, or arteriovenous. Capillary hemangiomas are the most common type. Most hemangiomas occur during childhood. Venous hemangiomas occur during adulthood, and they are often deeply situated. Intramuscular hemangiomas are rare and are occasionally difficult to differentiate from angiosarcomas. Evaluation may require angiography and venography. Surgery is indicated if symptoms develop. Hemangiomas rarely become malignant.

Giant Cell Tumor of Tendon Sheath

Giant cell tumor of the tendon sheath is a benign lesion involving the tendon sheaths

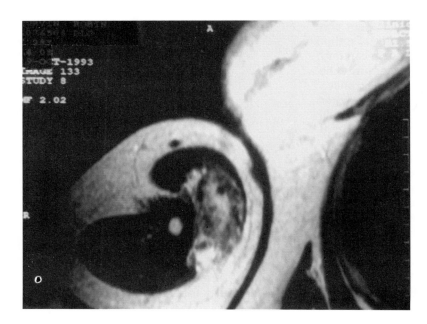

Figure 25–6. Scan of an aggressive fibromatosis of the upper arm.

of the hand and foot. These tumors are small and slow growing; often they can remain the same size for years. The exact etiology is unknown, but previous trauma may be implicated. The typical presentation is a slow growing, painless nodule that is soft but will remain fixed to deep tissue. These tumors range from 0.5 to 4.0 cm in diameter, with lesions of the foot typically being larger than those found in the hand. They are solid and, therefore, not compressible or translucent.

Gross pathologic findings show a small, lobulated mass with an irregular surface. Microscopically, they are moderately cellular, with sheets or whorls of rounded or ovoid synovial cells. Multinucleated giant cells are scattered in a random fashion, and areas of large, foam-filled macrophages or histiocytes are present.

Local excision with a small cuff of tissue is the treatment of choice. These tumors do have the capacity to recur locally in 10 to 20 percent of patients. The recurrences have been shown to take place more commonly from lesions that are hypercellular or have increased mitoses.

Pigmented Villonodular Synovitis

Pigmented villonodular synovitis (synovial xanthoma or villous synovitis) is a benign, tumor-like lesion involving the synovial tissues of joints, tendon sheaths, or bursa. This lesion is characterized by villous overgrowth and pigmentation of the synovial membrane. Pigmented villonodular synovitis usually occurs in the knee but can involve other major joints. The exact pathogenesis is not known. Theories have ranged from neoplastic disorders to localized disturbances of lipid metabolism, post-traumatic reactions, or inflammation. Histologically, pigmented villonodular synovitis is characterized by a 1- to 3-layer pigmented synovial lining. The pigmentation, hemosiderin, is contained in the round synovial fibroblasts or Type B lining cell. This soft tissue lesion can violate bone via a pressure-like phenomenon to cause localized osteoporosis, cystic degeneration, or pathologic fracture (Fig. 25–7).

Treatment consists of wide excision of the soft tissue component with curettage and bone grafting of the intraosseous component.

Malignant Soft Tissue Sarcomas

Malignant Fibrous Histiocytoma

Malignant fibrous histiocytoma (MFH) is the most common soft tissue sarcoma.[62] It usually occurs in adults and is most common in the lower extremity (Fig. 25–8). It may be a secondary sarcoma from radiation. The histologic grade is a good prognosticator of metastatic potential. The lesions may vary significantly in size at the time of diagnosis. Superficial variants may be but a few centimeters in diameter, whereas those arising in the retroperitoneum often obtain a diameter of 15 cm or greater. Approximately 5 percent of MFHs undergo extensive hemorrhagic cystification, often leading to a clinical diagnosis of hematoma. The basic cellular constituents of all fibrohistiocytic tumors include fibroblast, histiocyte-like cells, and mesenchymal cells.

Fibrosarcoma

Fibrosarcomas are malignant spindle cell tumors of bone and soft tissue. Clinical and histologic difficulty usually arises in differentiating low-grade fibrosarcomas from fibromatosis and its variants. This neoplasm usually arises from the fascial and aponeurotic structures of the deep soft tissues. The fundamental cell of this neoplasm is the fibroblast—a spindle cell capable of producing collagen fibers. Treatment consists of wide resection and adjuvant radiation.

Liposarcoma

Liposarcoma is a common soft tissue sarcoma. It has a wide range of malignant potential, depending upon the grade of the individual tumor. Determination of subtype and grade is essential to appropriate management. Grade I liposarcomas rarely metastasize. Unlike other sarcomas, liposarcomas may be multiple and occur in unusual sites within the same individual. Careful evaluation of other masses in a patient with a liposarcoma is mandatory. Occasionally these lesions occur in children. Liposarcomas rarely arise from pre-existing benign lipomas. They can become quite large. The tumors tend to be well-circumscribed and multilobulated (Fig. 25–9). The current histologic classification of liposarcoma recognizes four distinct types. Regardless of the histologic type, the identification of an atypi-

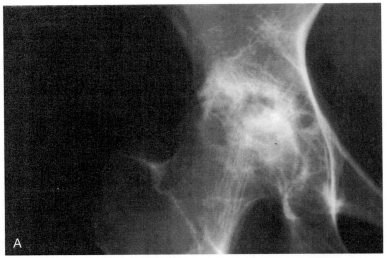

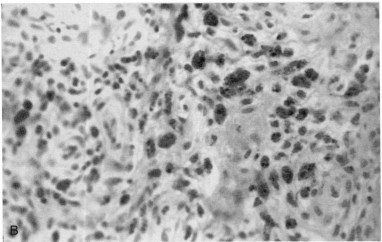

Figure 25–7. *A,* Radiograph of pigmented villonodular synovitis (PVNS) of the hip with erosive cystic degeneration. *B,* Histologic section of PVNS with pigmentation in the synovial fibroblasts.

cal lipoblast is mandatory to establish the diagnosis of liposarcoma.

Synovial Sarcoma

Synovial cell sarcomas are the fourth most common soft tissue sarcoma. They characteristically have a biphasic pattern that gives the impression of glandular formation and suggests a synovial origin. These tumors, however, do not arise from a joint and have a distribution similar to that of other soft tissue sarcomas. Synovial sarcomas occur in a younger age group than other sarcomas. There is a propensity for the distal portions of the extremities; hand, 5 percent; ankle, 9 percent; or foot, 13 percent. The plain radiograph often shows calcifications with a soft tissue mass. Particularly the tumor presents as a deep-seated, well-circumscribed, multi-

nodular firm mass. Actual contiguity with a synovium-lined space is rare. The classic form of the tumor is a biphasic pattern. This implies the presence of two distinct cell populations: spindle cells and epithelioid cells. The plump spindle cells, usually the predominant component, form an interlacing fascicular pattern. The epithelioid cells form either solid nests or glandlike structures.

Epithelioid Sarcoma

Epithelioid sarcoma is an unusually small tumor that is often misdiagnosed as a benign lesion. It occurs in the forearm and wrist one half the time and is the most common sarcoma of the hand. The lesion has a propensity for eventual lymph node involvement. Unlike other sarcomas, it occurs predominantly in adolescents to young adults. When

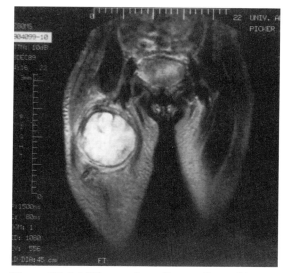

Figure 25–8. MRI scan of a malignant fibrous histiocytoma of the thigh.

it arises in the dermis, it presents as a nodular ulcerative process and often simulates benign cutaneous diseases. The tumor usually arises in the deep soft tissue, particularly in relation to tendons, fascia, and aponeurosis, and presents as a firm, often multinodular, mass. Central nodular hemorrhage or necrosis or both are occasionally encountered. The microscopic characteristics are nodules or granuloma-like collections of epithelioid cells. The characteristic feature is the rather diffuse infiltration of tendinous and fascial structures by small or elongated nests of tumor cells.

Neurofibrosarcoma (Malignant Schwannoma)

Neurofibrosarcomas are malignant tumors that arise from peripheral nerves. They represent about 10 percent of all sarcomas. A large percentage are associated with von Recklinghausen's disease. In general, patients with von Recklinghausen's disease are at high risk for developing sarcomas, and the risk increases with each decade of life. Unlike other sarcomas, a neurofibrosarcoma often presents with neurologic symptoms (pain, paresthesias, and weakness) reflecting its relation to major peripheral nerves. The neoplasm presents as a fusiform or bulbous enlargement of the large nerve, usually within the deep soft tissues. As the nerve enlarges and infiltrates the adjacent soft tissue, its origin from and relation to the nerve structure is frequently obscured. The basic microscopic pattern consists of intersecting spindle cell fascicles, not unlike that observed with fibrosarcoma or liposarcoma. The slender nuclei of the spindle cells tend to be wavy or buckled. A palisading pattern, although not pathognomonic, typifies this entity.

RADIATION/SURGERY AND SYSTEMIC CHEMOTHERAPY

Limb-Sparing Surgery

Limb salvage surgery is a safe operation in select individuals. This technique may be uti-

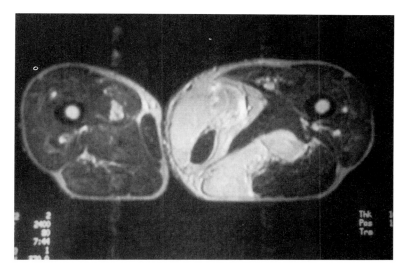

Figure 25–9. MRI scan of a multilobulated liposarcoma of the thigh.

lized for all spindle cell sarcomas, regardless of histogenesis. The successful management of localized sarcomas requires careful coordination and timing of staging studies, biopsy, surgery, and preoperative and postoperative chemotherapy and/or radiation therapy. Preoperative studies allow the surgeon to conceptualize the local anatomy and evaluate the tissue to be resected and reconstructed. The contraindications of limb-sparing surgery are major neurovascular involvement, pathologic fractures, infection, and extensive muscle involvement. The resection of the tumor strictly follows the principles of oncologic surgery. Avoiding local recurrence is the criterion of success and the main determinant of the amount of bone and soft tissue to be removed. It is recommended that a wide margin be achieved with the surgical resection and that at no time should the tumor be entered during surgery.[49] With the advent of neoadjuvant chemotherapy, the resectability of certain tumors has improved, for this allows a less wide margin.[47] Techniques of reconstruction vary, and these include prosthetic replacement, autografting, or allografting (Fig. 25–10). Muscle transfers may be required to restore lost motor power. Adequate skin and muscle coverage is mandatory and may require a free tissue transfer.

Radiation Therapy

Although soft tissue sarcomas were once thought to be radioresistant, it is now recognized that radiation can be useful. When radiation alone is used, effective results are seen only with small lesions (less than 5 cm) and the use of sophisticated techniques designed to deliver 7000 to 8000 cGy over a period of 7 to 8 weeks.[55]

Although radiation alone could not be recommended as the primary treatment for soft tissue sarcomas, many surgeons began to recognize its potential benefit as an adjunct to surgery for local control. The rationale for combining the modalities is to allow a reduction in both the extent of the surgical procedure and the amount of radiation when compared with the extent of either used alone.[16,57]

Radiation can be combined with surgery either preoperatively, postoperatively, or intraoperatively.[13,30,57] Preoperative radiation therapy is administered after the incisional biopsy, with the remaining microscopic tissue left in situ. The total dose administered is approximately 5000 cGy. Between 2 and 3 weeks after the completion of the preoperative radiation, the tumor is resected. The tumor can be removed with a small cuff of normal adjacent tissue; the neurovascular bundle can be dissected from the pseudocapsule, and the lesion stripped from the bone. The wound must be closed carefully to eliminate any residual dead space. The patient's activities should be restricted for 2 to 3 weeks to permit complete healing. Once the wound is healed, additional treatment to

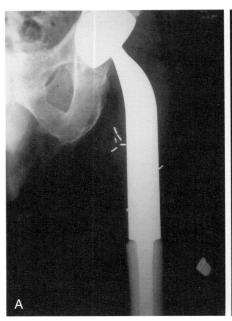
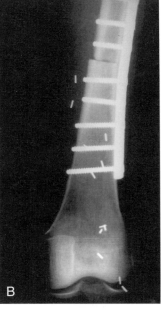

Figure 25–10. Limb-sparing surgery for a high-grade sarcoma reconstructed with *A*, a custommade metallic prosthesis of the proximal femur. *B*, Osteoarticular allograft of the distal femur.

the bed of the tumor is given to bring the total dose to approximately 6500 cGy.[58]

Brachytherapy is an option to postoperative external beam radiation. Brachytherapy is the direct application of radioactive sources at the tumor bed. This administration of radiotherapy to precise depths in the tumor bed permits a higher dose to the tumor sites, sometimes not possible with standard external beam radiation therapy.[2,17] After excision of the tumor, the tumor bed is mapped out to encompass the area of all gross and microscopic tumor plus a margin of at least 1.5 cm. The dimensions of the tumor bed are measured and recorded, and a series of plastic catheters are then inserted percutaneously. Iridium-192 seeds or ribbons are inserted through the catheters to give a temporary implant, which is usually removed after 4 to 5 days.

Brachytherapy offers several theoretic and practical advantages over conventional external radiation therapy in the management of soft tissue sarcomas of the extremities.[44,45] There may be an advantage to applying radiation during the immediate early postoperative period, before the healing process traps the tumor cells in scar tissue that may be less well oxygenated, rendering them more resistant to radiation. The direct application of radiation sources facilitates delivering the dose to the tumor site with maximal sparing of adjacent normal tissue. The disadvantages are that the fall-off of radiation dose can be quite high, and unrecognized areas of tumor-bearing cells may not receive a lethal dose of radiotherapy. In addition, the procedure is cumbersome and often difficult to perform. Brachytherapy can cause wound complications, even though these can be minimized by careful surgical and radiation planning and technique. Brachytherapy is not given to patients who require close medical and nursing support because of the potential exposure to the medical staff.

The value of adjuvant systemic chemotherapy is controversial in the treatment of soft tissue sarcomas. It is given principally in an attempt to eliminate micrometastatic lesions.[25] An early study using the chemotherapeutic agents in vincristine, actinomycin D, and cyclophosphamide were shown to be effective in the treatment of childhood rhabdomyosarcoma.[7] Survival markedly improved using these agents, and this success stimulated an interest in the chemotherapeutic agents in the treatment of adult soft tissue sarcomas. Adriamycin, cisplatinum, methotrexate, and dacarbazine have and are being used in a variety of protocols.[3,6,11,12,14,15,20,35,40,41,51]

There has been no evidence that adjuvant chemotherapy is of benefit in patients with low-grade soft tissue lesions or in patients with soft tissue tumors of the abdomen, retroperitoneum, or viscera. There is conflicting evidence for the benefit of adjuvant chemotherapy in the treatment of high-grade soft tissue sarcomas of the extremity. The reasons for the conflicting evidence are likely due to the lack of a well-controlled prospective study of patients with large (greater than 5 cm), high-grade soft tissue sarcomas, as most of the reported studies have included a variety of histologic grades and all sizes of tumors.[8]

BENIGN BONE TUMORS

Osteoid Osteoma

Osteoid osteoma is the third most common primary benign tumor in bone (11 percent), surpassed only by osteochondroma and nonossifying fibroma. The tumor has a preference for long bones with a predilection for the femur, tibia, humerus, and lumbar spine. All bones, however, may be involved; males are affected more than females at a rate of 2.3 to 1. Pain is the first initial symptom in most cases. Pain is more acute at night and is dramatically relieved with salicylates. The classic radiographic finding is of a well-delineated, smooth, regular, round-to-oval small radiolucency within the cortex that may or may not be calcified and surrounded by dense sclerotic bone (Fig. 25–11). Osteoid osteoma located in the cancellous bone of the metaphyseal region does not usually give the typical sclerotic pattern as seen in cortical bone. Radiographic findings may simulate arthritis or infectious processes. Bone scans are a helpful diagnostic tool and show marked increased uptake. Spontaneous remission has been reported, and conservative treatment has been suggested. Most investigators, however, prefer surgical resection.

Osteochondromas

Osteochondromas are the most common benign bone tumor. They are characteristi-

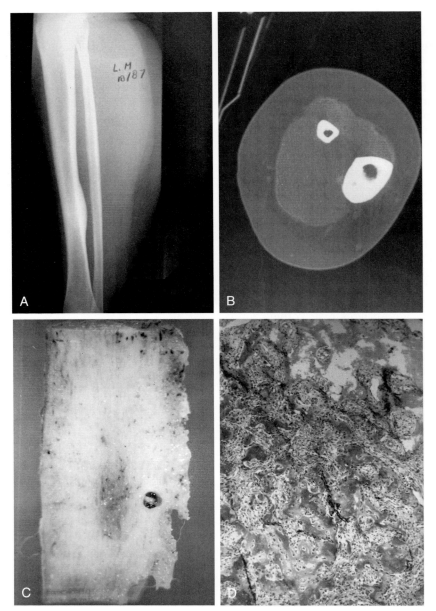

Figure 25–11. Osteoid osteoma of the tibia. *A,* AP radiograph. *B,* CT scan of the tibia delineating the nidus. *C,* Resected specimen—nidus. *D,* Histologic section, demonstrating osteoid osteoma.

cally sessile or pedunculated, arising from the cortex of a long tubular bone adjacent to the epiphyseal plate. Osteochondromas grow with the bone until skeletal maturity is reached. The growth of an osteochondroma during adolescence, therefore, does not necessarily signify malignancy. Pain may be due to local bursitis, mechanical irritation of adjacent muscles, or nerve entrapment. Osteochondromas are usually solitary except in patients with multiple hereditary exostosis. Plain radiographs are usually diagnostic.

Sessile osteochondromas may be difficult to differentiate from periosteal osteosarcomas when they are found in unusual sites, such as the distal posterior femur. Bone scintigraphy and CT may be helpful in distinguishing between these two entities; osteochondromas are contiguous with the marrow space and have little uptake on the scan. Patients with multiple hereditary exostosis are at risk for malignant transformation, usually to a low-grade chondrosarcoma. There is only a very small risk in the solitary osteochondromas. Surgical removal is recommended only for symptomatic osteochondromas or in patients with enlargement of the mass after skeletal maturity.

Chondroblastoma

Chondroblastoma is a lesion of chondroblastic origin occurring predominantly in the epiphysis of the bone in skeletally immature individuals. The typical radiographic feature is a lytic lesion that occupies less than one half of the epiphyseal region with a thin border of sclerosis. Calcification may be present. The tumor is usually surrounded by an intact cortical border. Histologically, the key cell is the polygonal chondroblast, which is encased by reticulum. Frequently, but not always, there is pericellular calcification in a "chicken wire" pattern. The key matrix product is pink-staining chondroid, which may be misinterpreted as osteoid. Also present are osteoclast-like giant cells. Therefore, giant cell tumors must be differentiated. These tumors may be aggressive, with a relatively high rate of recurrence following simple curettage. Local control, though, can be obtained by an augmented intralesional resection or a wide resection.

Enchondromas

Enchondromas are benign cartilage tumors of bone. They are usually painless unless a pathologic fracture occurs. They are quite common in the hands and feet. One of the major problem areas in the field of orthopaedic oncology for both a clinician and pathologist is distinguishing an enchondroma from a low-grade chondrosarcoma. The correlation of symptoms, plain radiographs, and histologic findings is crucial in assessing a cartilage tumor (Fig. 25–12). Radiographic scalloping is a sign of local aggressiveness. Age is also an important indicator of possible malignancy. Enchondromas rarely undergo malignant transformation prior to skeletal maturity. Pain is the other risk factor and is a sign of local aggressiveness and possible malignancy. Currettage with or without bone grafting is usually curative. A pathologic fracture may require internal fixation in addition to curettage.

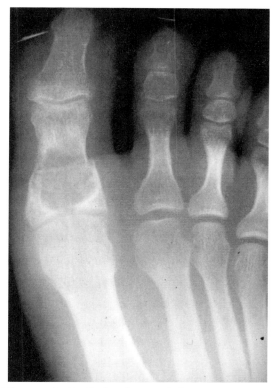

Figure 25–12. Enchondroma of the great toe with pathologic fracture.

Unicameral Bone Cyst

Unicameral bone cysts are benign lesions that occur in the metaphysis or diaphysis of long bones. They represent a reactive process and not a true neoplasm. The most common sites are the proximal humerus and proximal femur. They are usually asymptomatic until a fracture occurs. Radiographically, they are radiolucent and slightly expansile, with well-defined margins. Unicameral bone cysts can be treated by aspiration and injection with methylprednisolone acetate. If this is unsuccessful, then repeat injection followed by curettage and bone grafting is indicated. If a pathologic fracture should occur, it should be allowed to heal before injection is performed.

Aneurysmal Bone Cyst

An aneurysmal bone cyst (ABC) is a solitary, generally eccentric vascular lesion of which the precise nature and histogenesis remain uncertain. Most physicians do not regard it as a true neoplasm. There is the possibility, also, that an ABC might sometimes represent a secondary "blowout" in a pre-existing bone lesion. The lesion most commonly involves long bones or the spine, but any bone may be involved, including flat bones. Nearly 85 percent of patients are under 20 years of age. It is rare under the age of 5 or over 50 years. The radiographic manifestations of an ABC are diverse and may be easily mistaken for a malignant tumor owing to its great rate of growth and tremendous destruction of bone (Fig. 25–13).

Histologically, there are multiloculated cystlike walls filled with blood. There may be exuberant spindle cells, osteoid, and woven bone slivers, as well as osteoclast-like giant cells. The surgical treatment is an intralesional curettage followed by bone grafting. Because of the increased vascularity, angiography followed by embolization may be helpful in very large lesions such as may occur in the pelvis.

Giant Cell Tumor

Giant cell tumors (GCT) of the bone account for 5 percent of all primary bone tumors.[34]

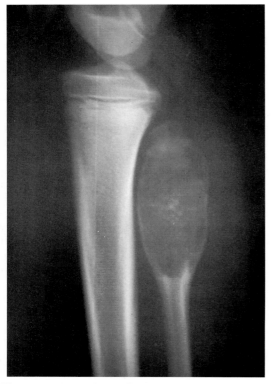

Figure 25–13. Radiograph of an aneurysmal bone cyst of the proximal fibula.

Most GCTs of bone occur in the distal end of the femur, the proximal end of the tibia, the distal end of the radius, and the sacrum.[9,10,21] About 80 percent occur in patients between the ages of 20 and 50 years. Radiographically, the GCT is centered in the epiphysis and has pure lysis with or without a trabeculated appearance (Fig. 25–14).[34] Most lesions are contained within the original bone contours; however, there may be cortical enlargement of the bone's contours. When the tumor gets to a large state and destroys the bone cortex, a pathologic fracture may occur. There may also be an associated soft tissue extension. Other lesions radiographically confused with GCT include aneurysmal bone cyst, chondroblastoma, and the brown tumor of hyperparathyroidism. If a question arises about the possibility of hyperparathyroidism, radiographs of the hands and distal clavicle and a serum parathyroid hormone level should be obtained to exclude this possibility. The typical histologic feature of the GCT is a combination of oval mononuclear cells and benign cells, scattered uniformly throughout the lesion.

The treatment primarily has been aimed at local control of the tumor and preservation of function. Initial attempts to eradicate the tumor with an intralesional curettage resulted in a recurrence rate of approximately 50 percent. This led surgeons to manage these patients with more aggressive treatment, which has ranged from augmented intralesional resection to en bloc resection. The functional results were not as great with such extensive surgery. It is now recommended for Stage I and II GCT to perform an augmented intralesional resection consisting of curettage, high-speed burring to extend the resection, coating the cavity with phenol, and packing the defect with polymethylmethacrylate to provide immediate support. This treatment plan has yielded local control in greater than 85 percent of cases. Alternatives are cryosurgery, which extends the tumor kill but has a significant late fracture rate.

Nonossifying Fibroma (Fibrous Cortical Defect)

Nonossifying fibroma and metaphyseal fibrous defects are benign processes, usually a metaphyseal bone lesion in skeletally immature individuals. Another concept is

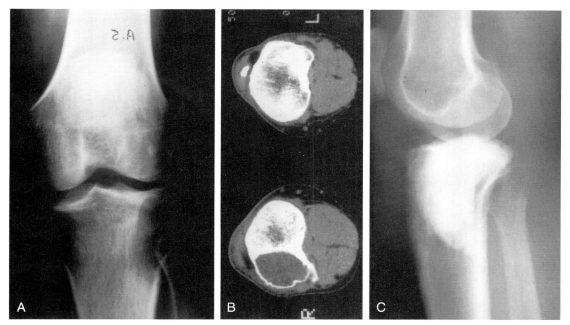

Figure 25–14. *A,* AP radiograph of a giant cell tumor of the proximal tibia. *B,* CT scan delineates a lytic destructive lesion. *C,* Treatment consisted of augmented intralesional resection and the defect packed with polymethylmethacrylate.

that this may represent faulty ossification rather than a true neoplasm. Roentgenographic evidence of cortical defects may be found in approximately one third of growing children, most commonly in the femur and proximal tibia. These lesions may be so large that they predispose to a pathologic fracture. The majority are silent clinically and are discovered incidentally when a region is subjected to roentgenographic study for an unrelated reason. The radiographic appearance is that of an eccentrically located lesion with distinct sclerotic margins (Fig. 25–15). The tumor begins in the metaphysis and appears to migrate toward the center of the bone as the epiphyseal region grows away from it.

Microscopic examination reveals a cellular fibroblastic connective tissue background, with the cells arranged in whorled bundles. Giant cells as well as foam cells are present.

If one is confident of the roentgenographic diagnosis and the structural integrity of the bone is not in question, no treatment need be employed. The progress of the lesion can be followed by serial roentgenograms if the diagnosis is uncertain. If the lesion is large and occupies greater than 50 percent of the diameter of the bone, bone grafting may be desirable. Many of the lesions undergo spontaneous regression-ossification. If a fracture should occur through one of these lesions, it can heal without surgical intervention.

MALIGNANT BONE TUMORS

Osteosarcoma

Osteosarcoma is a malignant spindle cell tumor that produces osteoid, bone, or both. It typically occurs during childhood and adolescence. In patients over the age of 40 years, it is usually associated with a pre-existing disease such as Paget's disease, irradiated bone, multiple hereditary exostosis, or polyostotic fibrous dysplasia.[10] The most common sites of occurrence are the bones of the knee—distal femur, proximal tibia (50 percent), and the proximal humerus (25 percent). Because of its tremendous range of characteristics, osteosarcoma can be misinterpreted as many other benign or malignant entities.

The predominant symptom is pain, which at first may be slight and intermittent. With time, extraosseous extension of the tumor may occur, which causes swelling. Patients may have elevated serum alkaline phosphatase values at the time of presentation. The

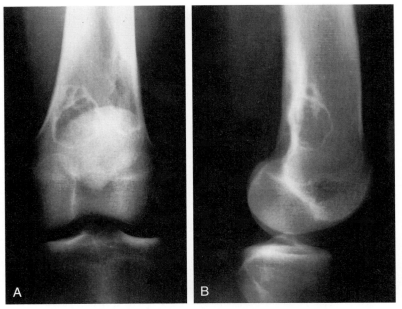

Figure 25–15. *A* and *B,* AP and lateral radiographs of a nonossifying fibroma.

typical radiographic findings are increased intramedullary density and an area of radiolucency. Periosteal elevation and extraosseous extension with soft tissue ossification are also seen (Fig. 25–16). As the neoplasm extends through the cortex, the periosteum may be elevated; this stimulates reactive bone formation and accounts for the radiologic features of the so-called Codman's triangle. Skip areas of metastases may be seen in the same bone.

There are several categories of osteosarcoma. The telangiectatic type contains multiple blood-filled cystic and sinusoidal spaces of variable size. Other categories include surface osteosarcomas—periosteal and parosteal.

Prior to adjuvant chemotherapy, the treatment for osteosarcoma was amputation. Metastasis to the lungs and other bones generally occurred within 24 months. Overall survival ranged from 5 to 20 percent at 2 years. This pattern has been altered by adjuvant chemotherapy. Local control is by surgery; adjuvant chemotherapy is given to control microscopic systemic disease. Several different protocols for chemotherapy currently yield 5-year survival rates as high as 75 percent.[22,23]

The traditional procedure for localized osteosarcoma has been amputation one joint above the tumor, or in some cases transmedullary amputation. Within the past decade it has been shown that limb salvage surgery is as safe as ablative (amputation) surgery in selected sarcomas.

Secondary Osteosarcoma

The term *secondary* applied to osteosarcoma refers to a tumor presenting in association with a pre-existing lesion of the bone. Secondary lesions usually occur in an older population group than primary tumors. Primary lesions in which this may occur are in Paget's disease, sites of previous irradiation, benign bone lesions such as fibrous dysplasia, or in association with orthopaedic implants. Whatever its etiology, the histopathology of secondary osteosarcomas is identical with that of primary osteosarcomas. The prognosis for these tumors is quite poor.

Juxtacortical Osteosarcoma

Juxtacortical osteosarcoma is a distinct, bone-forming, malignant neoplasm that develops in relation to the surface of a bone. This tumor may begin in the periosteum, in the tissue adjacent to the periosteum, or indeed from the cortex itself. These tumors are relatively rare, and the great majority are low grade. Histologically, the periosteal type is observed in patients in the third and

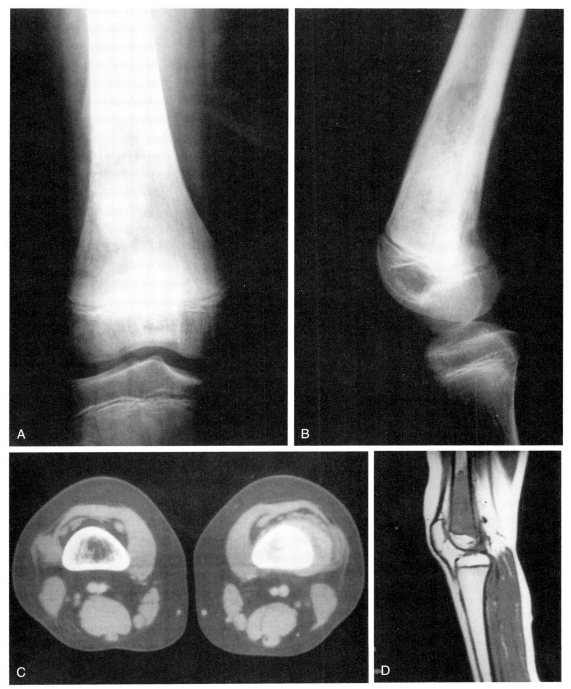

Figure 25–16. *A* and *B*, AP and lateral radiographs showing an osteosarcoma of the distal femur. *C*, CT scan demonstrates the osteoblastic tumor with soft tissue extension. *D*, MRI delineates marrow extension of the tumor.

fourth decades of life and has a characteristic site of predilection for the posterior aspect of the distal femur. Radiographically, the neoplasm presents as a dense oval or spiculated mass attached to the surface of the cortical bone (Fig. 25–17). The radiographic differential includes myositis ossificans, osteochondroma, and juxtacortical chondroma. The histologic diagnosis of a low-grade malignant tumor is usually very difficult to make with-

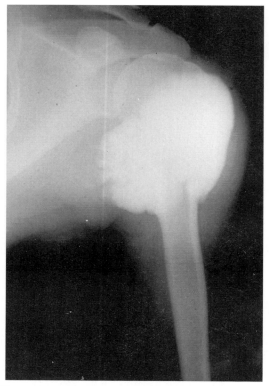

Figure 25–17. Juxtacortical osteosarcoma involving the proximal humerus.

out consideration of the radiographic features. The tumor is slow growing and is usually low grade. Therefore, the prognosis is much better than in other types of osteosarcoma. In principle, the treatment is surgical resection. Adjuvant chemotherapy is not used unless the tumor is of a histologically high grade.

Periosteal osteosarcoma is another type of malignant bone tumor that grows on the surface of bone and is usually located in the midshaft of a bone, occurring most frequently in adolescence. It also may resemble myositis ossificans, and the predominance of cartilage in the lesion may lead to confusion with periosteal chondrosarcoma. The radiographic appearance as well as the histologic identification of osteoid or bone formation by tumor cells helps differentiate this tumor from periosteal chondrosarcoma. The prognosis for periosteal osteosarcoma is somewhat better than for conventional osteosarcoma but worse than that of parosteal osteosarcoma. The small percentage of juxtacortical osteosarcomas that are high-grade tumors carry the same prognosis as that of conventional osteosarcoma.

Chondrosarcoma

Chondrosarcoma is the second most common primary malignant neoplasm of bone. The basic neoplastic tissue is malignant cartilage.[38] There are five types of chondrosarcoma: central, peripheral, myxoma, dedifferentiated, and clear cell. Both central and peripheral chondrosarcomas can arise as a primary tumor or a secondary tumor from a benign cartilage tumor, as in the malignant transformation of multiple hereditary osteochondromas and multiple enchondromas (Ollier's disease).

Half of all chondrosarcomas occur in persons above the age of 40 years. The most common sites are the pelvis, femur, and shoulder girdle.[9] The clinical presentation varies. Peripheral chondrosarcomas may become quite large without causing pain, and local symptoms develop only because of mechanical irritation (Fig. 25–18). Pelvic chondrosarcomas are often large and present with referred pain to the back or thigh, sciatica secondary to sacral plexus irritation, urinary symptoms from bladder neck involvement, unilateral edema due to iliac vein obstruction, or as a painless abdominal mass. Conversely, central chondrosarcomas present with dull pain. A mass is rarely present. Pain, which indicates active growth, is an ominous sign of a central cartilage lesion. An adult with a plain radiograph suggestive of a cartilage tumor but associated with pain has a chondrosarcoma until proved otherwise (Fig. 25–19).

Central chondrosarcomas have two distinct radiologic patterns. One is a small, well-defined lytic lesion with a narrow zone of transition and surrounding sclerosis with faint calcification. This is the most common malignant bone tumor that may appear radiographically benign. In the second type, there is no sclerotic border and it is difficult to localize. The key sign of malignancy is endosteal scalloping. This type is difficult to diagnose on plain radiographs and may go undetected for a long period of time.

In contrast, peripheral chondrosarcoma is recognized easily as a large mass of characteristic calcification protruding from a bone. Its differential diagnosis includes a large benign osteochondroma, periosteal osteosarcoma, and juxtacortical myositis ossificans. Correlation of the clinical, radiographic, and histologic data is essential for accurate diagnosis and evaluation of the aggressiveness of

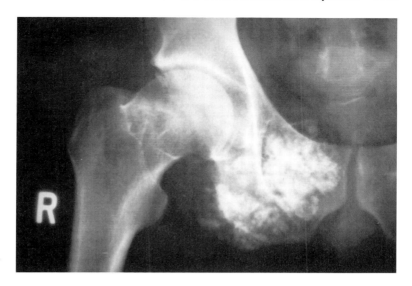

Figure 25–18. Peripheral chondrosarcoma, an exophytic mass involving the pubic bone.

a cartilage tumor. In general, proximal or axial location, skeletal maturity, and pain point toward malignancy even though the cartilage may appear benign.

The treatment of chondrosarcoma is surgical removal. Guidelines for resection of high-grade chondrosarcomas are similar to those of other bone sarcomas. Augmented intralesional resection has been used for central low-grade chondrosarcomas with success. This involves curetting the lesion and extending the margin with cryotherapy. Major advantages are preservation of bone stock and the avoidance of resection. High-grade sarcomas warrant a more aggressive surgical approach.

Malignant Fibrous Histiocytoma

Malignant fibrous histiocytoma of the bone is an aggressive neoplasm that is commonly found in adulthood.[53] Radiographically, it presents as an osteolytic lesion associated with marked cortical disruption, minimal cortical or periosteal reaction, and no evidence of matrix formation. The most common sites are the metaphyseal ends of long bones,

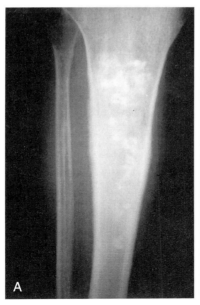
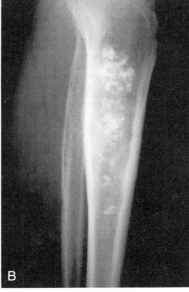

Figure 25–19. *A* and *B*, AP and lateral radiographs: chondrosarcoma involving the proximal tibia.

especially around the knee. Pathologic fracture can be a presentation. The tumor may be multicentric and associated with bone infarcts or other underlying pathologic processes.[53] Microscopically, there is a broad histologic spectrum. Plump, histiocyte-like cells and spindle fibroblastic cells are the main elements. Characteristically, there is the storiform or cartwheel pattern in which the fibroblasts radiate from a central focus. A spindle cell component may resemble fibrosarcoma. Inflammatory cells as well as bizarre tumor cells may also be seen. The treatment for this tumor is similar to that of other high-grade sarcomas. Surgical resection with wide margins and possible adjuvant chemotherapy is indicated. The prognosis for this tumor is poor.

Ewing's Sarcoma

Ewing's sarcoma is a round cell neoplasm that consists of poorly differentiated small cells without matrix production. It tends to occur in young children and is the second most common bone sarcoma of childhood (Fig. 25–20). It may affect the flat and axial bones as well as the long tubular bones.[9,10] When a long tubular bone is involved, it is most often the proximal or diaphyseal portion. Patients may present with systemic signs such as fever, anorexia, weight loss, leukocytosis, and anemia.[37] The most common complaint is pain or mass or both. Localized tenderness is often present with associated erythema and induration. These findings can closely mimic those of osteomyelitis and therefore must be in the differential. Radiographically, the typical pattern consists of a permeative or moth-eaten destruction associated with a multilaminated periosteal elevation or a sunburst appearance. When Ewing's sarcoma occurs in flat bones, these findings may not be present.

The clinical and biologic behavior of Ewing's sarcoma is different from that of

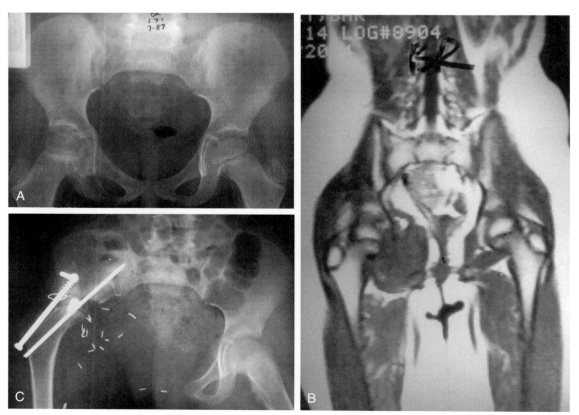

Figure 25–20. *A,* AP radiograph of the pelvis of a 5-year-old girl with Ewing's sarcoma involving the acetabulum and pubic bone. *B,* MRI scan depicting the extensive soft tissue mass. *C,* Radiograph after resection of the tumor with internal partial hemipelvectomy and a reconstruction hip arthrodesis.

other spindle cell sarcomas. It may be associated with visceral and lymphatic involvement. Within the past two decades, the prognosis of patients with Ewing's sarcoma has dramatically improved through the combination of effective adjuvant chemotherapy, improved radiotherapy techniques, and the selected use of limited surgical resection.[37,60]

Chordoma

Chordoma is a rare malignant neoplasm that develops from remnants of the primitive notochord. It constitutes between 1 and 4 percent of primary malignant bone tumors. It ordinarily grows slowly but is locally invasive. Approximately 50 percent originate in the sacrum, 35 percent at the base of the skull, and 15 percent in the true vertebrae.[59] The majority of these tumors are encountered from the fifth through the seventh decades. The symptoms and size of the tumors are usually nonspecific. For sacral tumors, pain, rectal dysfunction, and mass are frequently encountered. Because these symptoms are nonspecific, diagnosis can be delayed for a long period of time.

For sacral tumors, the radiographic findings are characterized by destruction and an expansive ballooning mass. It is often difficult to appreciate the tumor because of overlying gas shadows on the AP x-ray views (Fig. 25–21). Calcification may be present. The tumor is always midline but may have extension laterally. Computed tomography as well as MRI are helpful in delineating the extent of the tumor.

The microscopic appearance is characterized by cells arranged in sheets, cords, or lobules. The physaliferous cell with its vacuolated cytoplasm is the hallmark of the neoplasm. The distinction between chordomas and chondrosarcomas may pose a diagnostic problem.

The major treatment modalities in the management of this tumor are surgery and radiation therapy. Curative surgical resection may be precluded in many patients because of the extent of the tumor. Therefore, adjuvant radiation treatment is used to help achieve local control. The major deficits that may result from extended surgical resection in the sacral region are urinary and rectal dysfunction.[54] A diverting colostomy may be necessary. The overall median survival for all patients with spinal chordomas is 5 years.[59]

Myeloma

Myeloma is a disease of uncontrolled proliferation of plasma cells in the bone marrow. Other names include plasma cystoma and, when present in other forms, multiple myeloma. The clinical manifestations include bone marrow suppression, bone destruction, and hypercalcemia. The diagnosis should be suspected in any patient presenting with bone pain and anemia, particularly if serum chemistry screening reveals an elevated serum globulin level. Serum protein electrophoresis should then be performed to confirm that the increased serum globulin level truly represents a monoclonal

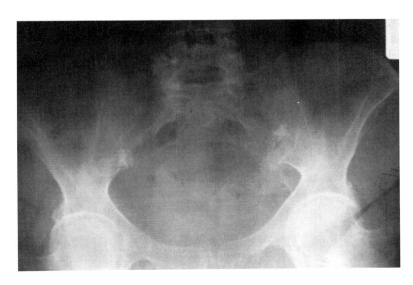

Figure 25–21. Sacral chordoma with destruction seen as loss of the foramen.

gammopathy expressed as a "spike," usually in the gamma globulin region. However, 20 percent of patients show no abnormal serum protein elevation. Bone marrow aspiration or biopsy of the lesion should be performed to establish the diagnosis. The symptoms of local bone lesions are usually effectively palliated by radiation therapy. Pathologic fractures or impending pathologic fractures can be treated by the same methods as in metastatic disease. Systemic chemotherapy consists of an alkaloiding agent plus a corticosteroid.

Metastatic Carcinoma

Metastatic carcinoma to bone is the most common malignant bone tumor and the second most common cause of pathologic fracture. The most common primary tumors that metastasize to bone are thyroid, breast, lung, kidney, and prostate (Fig. 25–22).[29] In the

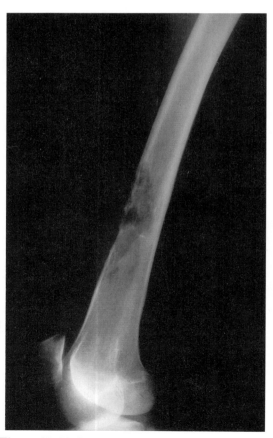

Figure 25–22. Lateral radiograph of the distal femur. Metastatic renal cell carcinoma with impending pathologic fracture.

past decade, the frequency of symptomatic metastatic carcinoma to bone has increased as survival of patients with metastatic carcinoma has increased. Patients presenting with pathologic fractures secondary to metastatic carcinoma but without prior diagnosis should be evaluated so that the primary tumor also may be managed. The screening should include careful physical examination of the thyroid gland, breasts, abdomen, prostate, and rectum. The following tests should be obtained: computed axial tomography of the lung and abdomen, bone scan, serum protein electrophoresis, serum calcium, phosphate, and, in men, acid phosphatase. If the primary tumor is not apparent from these tests, it is probably not necessary to continue to search for the primary carcinoma. It is unlikely that it will be found, and, if found, knowledge of the primary tumor will not lead to a significant difference in the management of the patient.

Management of patients with pathologic fractures secondary to metastatic carcinoma should be directed toward keeping them pain-free and ambulatory. Fractures that can be treated without open reduction and internal fixation while keeping the patient ambulatory and comfortable should be so managed. Fractures that prevent the patient from being comfortable and ambulatory require open reduction and internal fixation. Bedrest is poorly tolerated by patients with metastatic carcinoma and should be kept to a minimum. Polymethylmethacrylate (PMMA) has allowed improved fixation of pathologic fractures associated with metastatic carcinoma, especially when the metastasis has destroyed a large segment of bone or when there are multiple lesions within a single bone.

Lesions within long bones may be treated with either intramedullary fixation or with a sideplate and screws. Lesions within the femoral head or neck may be successfully treated either with replacement arthroplasty or with a plate and side screw.

Blood loss during the stabilization of a metastatic lesion within bone can be a significant threat to the patient's life. Preoperative angiography will identify lesions with a significant blood flow, such as renal cell carcinoma. Preoperative vascular occlusion is the best method of reducing the risk of life-threatening blood loss during the operative procedure for this lesion (Fig. 25–23).

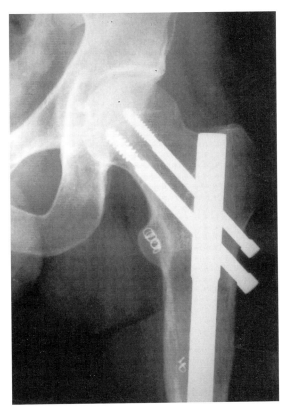

Figure 25–23. Radiograph of a 48-year old man with metastatic tumor. The impending pathologic fracture was treated with embolization and prophylactic intramedullary nailing.

Prophylactic fixation of an impending pathologic fracture is an area of increasing interest. Fixation prior to fracture reduces hospital time and operative risk and permits optimal potential for the preservation of function and activity. The guidelines used as indications for prophylactic internal fixation are (1) persistent pain, (2) 50 percent or more of cortical destruction, (3) primarily a destructive bone lesion, and (4) anatomic location with a particular risk for fracture secondary to high forces. Adjuvant radiation may control the local metastasis but is not curative.

References

1. Alazraki NP, Davis MA, Jones AG, Marty R, NcNeil BJ, Siegel BA: Skeletal system. *In* Kirchner PT (ed): Nuclear Medicine Review Syllabus. New York, New York Society of Nuclear Medicine, 1980, pp 539–586.
2. Anderson LL, Hilaris BS, Wagner LK: A monograph for planar implant planning. Endocurietherapy/hyperthermia. Oncology 1:9, 1985.
3. Antman K, Amato D, Lerner H, et al: Adjuvant doxorubicin for sarcoma: Data from The Eastern Cooperative Oncology Group and Dana-Farber Cancer Institute/Massachusetts General Hospital Studies. Cancer Treat Symp 3:109, 1985.
4. Behr T, Dobozi WR, Badrinath K: The treatment of pathologic and impending pathologic fractures of the proximal femur in the elderly. Clin Orthop 198:173–178, 1985.
5. Belliveau RE, Spencer RP: Incidence and sites of bone lesions detected by ^{99m}Tc-polyphosphate scans in patients with tumors. Cancer 36:359–363, 1975.
6. Bramwell VHC, Rouesse J, Santoro A, et al: European experience of adjuvant chemotherapy for soft tissue sarcoma: Preliminary report of randomized trial of cyclophosphamide, vincristine, doxorubicin and dacarbazine. Cancer Treat Symp 3:99, 1985.
7. Brennan MF, Shiu MH: Multimodality therapy for soft tissue sarcoma. *In* Shiu MH, Brennan MF (eds): Surgical Management of Soft Tissue Sarcoma. Philadelphia, Lea and Febiger, 1989, p 277.
8. Chang AE, Rosenberg SA: Clinical evaluation and treatment of soft tissue tumors. *In* Enzinger FM, Weiss SW (eds): Soft Tissue Tumors. St. Louis, CV Mosby, 1988, pp 19–42.
9. Dahlin DC: Bone Tumors: General Aspects and Data on 6221 Cases, 3rd ed. Springfield, Illinois, Charles C Thomas, 1978.
10. Dahlin DC, Unni KK: Bone Tumors: General Aspects and Data on 8542 Cases, 4th ed. Springfield, Illinois, Charles C Thomas, 1986.
11. Das Gupta TK, Patel MK, Chaudhuri PK, et al: The role of chemotherapy as an adjuvant to surgery in the initial treatment of primary soft tissue sarcomas in adults. J Surg Oncol 19:139, 1982.
12. Dunham WK, Myers JL, Sollaccio RJ, et al: Preoperative intra-arterial doxorubicin and low-dose radiation for high-grade soft-tissue sarcomas of the extremities. AAOS Instr Course Lect 38:419, 1989.
13. Edmondson JH, Fleming TR, Ivins JC, et al: Randomized study of systemic chemotherapy following complete excision of nonosseous sarcomas. J Clin Oncol 2:1390, 1984.
14. Eilber FR, Guiliano AE, Huth J, et al: Limb salvage for high-grade soft tissue sarcomas of the extremity: Experience at the University of California, Los Angeles. Cancer Treat Symp 3:49, 1985.
15. Eilber FR, Morton DL, Eckardt J, et al: Limb salvage for skeletal and soft tissue sarcomas: Multidisciplinary preoperative therapy. Cancer 53:2579, 1984.
16. Eilber FR, Morton DL, Sondak VK, Economou JS: The Soft Tissue Sarcomas. Orlando, Florida, Grune and Stratton, 1987.
17. Ellis F: Tumor-bed implantation at the time of surgery. *In* Hilaris BS (ed): Afterloading: Twenty Years of Experience, 1955–1975. New York, Memorial Sloan-Kettering Cancer Center, 1975, p 263.
18. Enneberg WF, Spanier SS, Malawer MM: The effect of the anatomic setting on the results of surgical procedure for soft part sarcoma of the thigh. Cancer 47:1005–1022, 1981.
19. Enzinger FM, Weiss SW: Soft Tissue Tumors, 2nd ed. St. Louis, CV Mosby, 1985.
20. Gherlinzoni F, Bacci G, Picci P, et al: A randomized trial for the treatment of high grade soft tissue sarcoma of the extremities: Preliminary observations. J Clin Oncol 4:552, 1986.

21. Goldenberg RR, Campbell CJ, Portis RB: Giant cell tumor of bone: An analysis of 218 cases. J Bone Joint Surg 52A:519–664, 1970.

22. Goorin AM, Abelson HT, Frei E III: Osteosarcoma: Fifteen years later. N Engl J Med 313:1637–1643, 1985.

23. Gorrin AM, Frei E III, Abelson HT: Adjuvant chemotherapy for osteosarcoma: A decade of experience. Surg Clin North Am 61:1379–1389, 1981.

24. Heare TC, Enneking WF, Heare MM: Staging techniques and biopsy of bone tumors. Orthop Clin North Am 20:273, 1989.

25. Jaffe KA, Morris SG: Resection and reconstruction for soft tissue sarcomas of the extremity. Orthop Clin North Am 22:161, 1991.

26. Kambolis C, Bullough PG, Jaffe HL: Ganglionic cystic defects of bone. J Bone Joint Surg 55A:496–505, 1973.

27. Kliman ME, Freiberg A: Ganglia of the foot and ankle. Foot Ankle 3:45–46, 1982.

28. Kransdorf MJ, Jelinek JS, Moser RP, et al: Soft tissue masses: Diagnosis using MR imaging. AJR 153:541, 1989.

29. Levy RN: Symposium on metastatic disease of bone. Clin Orthop 169:15–114, 1982.

30. Lindberg RO, Martin RG, Romsdahl MM, et al: Surgery and post-operative radiotherapy in the treatment of soft tissue sarcomas in adults. AJR 123:123, 1975.

31. Lodwick GS, Wilson AJ, Farrell C, et al: Determining growth rates of focal lesions of bone from radiographs. Radiology 134:577, 1980.

32. Mankin HJ, Lange TA, Spanner SS: The hazards of biopsy in patients with malignant primary bone and soft tissue tumors. J Bone Joint Surg 64A:1121–1127, 1982.

33. McNeil BJ: Rationale for the use of bone scans in selected metastatic and primary bone tumors. Semin Nucl Med 8:336–345, 1978.

34. Mirra JM: Bone Tumors: Clinical, Radiographic, and Pathological Correlations. Philadelphia, Lea & Febiger, 1989.

35. Morton DL, Eilber FR, Townsend CM Jr, et al: Limb salvage from a multidisciplinary treatment approach for skeletal and soft tissue sarcomas of the extremity. Ann Surg 184:268, 1976.

36. Orthopaedic Knowledge Update Home Study Syllabus I, II, and III. Chicago, American Academy of Orthopaedic Surgeons, 1984, 1987, 1990.

37. Pritchard DJ, Dahlin D, Dauphine R, et al: Ewing's sarcoma: A clinopathological and statistical analysis of patients surviving five years or longer. J Bone Joint Surg 57A(1):10–16, 1975.

38. Pritchard DJ, Lunke RJ, Taylor WF, Dahlin DC, Medley BE: Chondrosarcoma: A clinicopathologic and statistical analysis. Cancer 45:149–157, 1980.

39. Richardson ML, Kiloyne RF, Gillespy T, et al: Magnetic resonance imaging of musculoskeletal neoplasms. Radiol Clin North Am 24:259–267, 1986.

40. Rosenberg SA, Kent H, Costa J, et al: Prospective randomized evaluation of the role of limb-sparing surgery, radiation therapy, and adjuvant chemotherapy in adult patients with soft tissue sarcomas. Cancer Treat Rep 68:1067, 1984.

41. Rosenberg SA, Tepper J, Glatstein E, et al: The treatment of soft tissue sarcomas of the extremities. Ann Surg 196:305, 1982.

42. Rosenberg SA, Tepper J, Glatstein E, et al: Adjuvant chemotherapy for patients with soft tissue sarcomas. Surg Clin North Am 61:1415–1423, 1981.

43. Schajowicz F: Tumors and Tumor-Like Lesions of Bone and Joints. New York, Springer-Verlag, 1981.

44. Shiu MH, Collins C, Hilaris BS, et al: Limb preservation and tumor control in the treatment of popliteal and antecubital soft tissue sarcomas. Cancer 57:1632, 1986.

45. Shiu MH, Turnbull AD, Nori D, et al: Control of locally advanced extremity soft tissue sarcoma by function-saving resection and brachytherapy. Cancer 53:1385, 1984.

46. Simon MA: Current concepts review: Biopsy of musculoskeletal tumors. J Bone Joint Surg 64A:1253–1257, 1982.

47. Simon MA: Current concepts review: Limb salvage for osteosarcoma. J Bone Joint Surg 70A:307–310, 1988.

48. Simon MA, Bormann JS: Biopsy of bone and soft tissue lesions. J Bone Joint Surg 75A:616–621, 1993.

49. Simon MA, Enneking WF: The management of soft-tissue sarcomas of the extremities. J Bone Joint Surg 58A:317, 1976.

50. Simon MA, Finn HA: Diagnostic strategy for bone and soft-tissue tumors. J Bone Joint Surg 75A(4):622–631, 1993.

51. Sordillo PP, Magill GB, Shiu MH, et al: Adjuvant chemotherapy of soft-part sarcomas with ALO-MAD (S4). J Surg Oncol 18:345, 1981.

52. Soren A: Pathogenesis and treatment of ganglia. Clin Orthop 48:173–179, 1966.

53. Spanier SS, Enneking WF, Enriquez P: Primary malignant fibrous histiocytoma of bone. Cancer 36:2084–2098, 1975.

54. Stener B, Gunterberg B: High amputation of the sacrum for extirpation of tumors. Principles and technique. Spine 3:351, 1978.

55. Suit HD: Sarcoma of soft tissue. CA 28:284, 1978.

56. Suit H, Goitein M, Munzenrider J, Verhey L, Davis KR, Koehler A, et al: Definitive radiation therapy for chordoma and chondrosarcoma of the base of skull and spine. J Neurosurg 56:377, 1982.

57. Suit HD, Mankin HJ, Wood WC, et al: Preoperative, intraoperative, and postoperative radiation in the treatment of primary soft tissue sarcoma. Cancer 55:2659, 1985.

58. Suit HD, Poppe KH, Mankin HJ, et al: Preoperative radiation therapy for sarcoma of soft tissue. Cancer 47:2269, 1981.

59. Sundaresan N: Chordomas. Clin Orthop 204:135–142, 1986.

60. Tepper J, Glaubiger D, Lichter A, Wackenhut J, Glatstein E: Local control of Ewing's sarcoma of bone with radiotherapy and combination chemotherapy. Cancer 46:1969–1973, 1980.

61. Weingard DN, Rosenberg SA: Early lymphatic spread of osteogenic and soft tissue sarcomas. Surgery 84:231–240, 1978.

62. Weiss SW, Enzinger FM: Malignant fibrous histiocytoma. An analysis of 200 cases. Cancer 41:2250, 1978.

63. Willems D, Mulier JC, Martens M, Verhelst M: Ganglion cysts of bone. Acta Orthop Scand 44:655–662, 1973.

64. Zimmer WD, Berquist TH, McLeod RA, Sim FH, Pritchard DJ, Shives TC, et al: Bone tumors: Magnetic resonance imaging versus computed tomography. Radiology 155:709–718, 1985.

CHAPTER 26

Developmental Conditions

- ## PART I

Developmental Conditions in Children

John T. Killian
John Coen

The developmental conditions that are commonly seen in infancy, childhood, and adolescence reflect either normal growth and development of the developing skeleton or an alteration of that process.

BOWLEGS AND KNOCK-KNEES

The natural growth and development of the legs and the effect of legs on the development of normal walking was treated anecdotally until the 1970s. At that time, large-scale surveys of children provided data bases to aid physicians in the diagnosis of developmental bowlegs and knock-knees (genu varum, genu valgum) and to identify pathologic exceptions scientifically.[1]

The newborn infant presents with mild bowlegs. The physiologic varus alignment usually persists from birth to around eighteen months of age and through the initial weight-bearing, cruising, and first steps. Between 18 months and 2 years of age, normal growth and development promote the clinical appearance of knock-knees in the child (Fig. 26–1). This physiologic valgum may be hardly noticeable in some children, whereas in other children it may cause a broad spectrum of concerns in parents and family: child dragging one foot, both feet toeing in, both feet toeing out, no arches in the feet, excessive tripping and falling. The excessive valgus alignment seen at 2 years of age gradually diminishes to normal alignment between 4 and 7 years of age.

Periodic follow-up of these patients and reassurance appear to be all that is necessary once it is determined that a child is well within two standard deviations of normal and appropriate measurements for age.

Children who fall outside this normal growth and development include those with persistent or increasing bowleg deformity after 2.5 years of age, and those who are excessively knock-kneed at 10 years of age with a greater than 3.5-inch gap between the medial malleoli with the knees touching (Fig. 26–2). Such children represent an exception to the usual and customary and should be referred for an orthopaedic evaluation.[2]

METATARSUS ADDUCTUS

Metatarsus adductus is a developmental condition usually associated with intrauterine positioning. The child's foot appears to have an accentuated deviation of the great toe medially, and the lateral four toes may follow

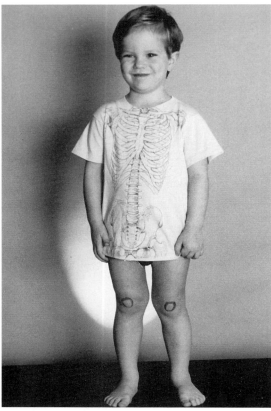

Figure 26–1. This boy, aged 2½, demonstrates the "normal" genu valgum.

as well (Fig. 26–3). The natural history is for metatarsus adductus to resolve spontaneously in most cases by age 3 to 4 months. If it is still present after that time, then treatment in the form of stretching, splinting, taping, or casting may be instituted with generally satisfactory results (Fig. 26–4).

TOEING IN AND TOEING OUT

Internal tibial torsion and femoral anteversion imply that there is an excessive twist in the affected bone more than usual and customary for the child's age. The diagnosis is often determined at age 1 to 3 years in children who walk with a mild in-toeing gait (Fig. 26–5). However, the use of Fillauer or Denis Browne night splints for tibial torsion and twister cables for femoral anteversion have not demonstrated any direct effect on the bone architecture.[3] The rate of improvement with the use of these devices mimics that of the natural history if left untreated.

Occasionally there will be a patient who, at around 7 years of age, has 90 degrees of internal hip rotation and less than 15 degrees of external hip rotation (Figs. 26–3 to 26–9) and may intermittently toe in when tired and with vigorous physical activity. Sitting in the W-position is facilitated when there is excessive internal hip rotation but per se this does not contribute to an in-toeing gait pattern (Fig. 26–10). Such children are usually observed until their adolescent growth spurt to see whether there is any improvement and to determine any functional impairment.

Toeing out is typically seen in the prewalker who has a mild contracture of the external hip rotators or capsule from sleeping prone or from obesity. This resolves spontaneously by 18 months of age and does not usually require night splints or physical therapy.

GROWING PAINS

The physician is frequently asked to evaluate a toddler of approximately 4 years of age who often awakens the parents in the early evening or night complaining of dull aching pains in the lower extremities. The parents will relate that massage, heat, or even anti-inflammatory medications help alleviate the symptoms and allow the child to return to sleep. The child awakens the next morning with no symptoms, but then the symptoms may return again in the evening or night. The physician is often at a loss for a diagnosis based on a history without any evidence of clinical findings, either by laboratory or physical examination. In general there is no limp, no deficits in range of motion, and no warmth, redness, or swelling of the lower extremities. The parents are usually instructed in the use of anti-inflammatory medications to control symptoms and are reassured that this is a time-limited process that, in general, has no long-term sequelae.

SLIPPED CAPITAL FEMORAL EPIPHYSIS

Slipped capital femoral epiphysis is a developmental disorder of puberty that typically affects obese boys. Either acutely or chonically, the capital femoral epiphysis may be displaced from the femoral neck posteriorly and inferiorly. It is felt that excessive body weight, hormones, and an oblique and

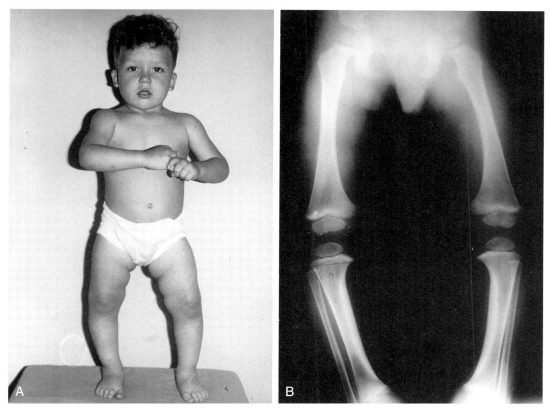

Figure 26–2. *A*, A 3-year-old boy with residual genu varum. *B*, This normal-appearing radiograph was obtained to evaluate for metabolic bone disease or Blount's disease.

altered shape of the growth plate may contribute to the gradual or abrupt displacement of the capital femoral epiphysis.[4] If the displacement occurs acutely and with more than 50 percent displacement of the femoral head, the risk of complications increases (Fig. 26–11). In the adolescent with a chronic slip,

the symptoms may be as subtle as intermittent groin pain and an awkward externally rotated lower extremity. Bilaterality may occur in over 25 percent of the patients, with the other hip often asymptomatic. Treatment of this condition is surgical: screw fixation of the capital femoral epiphysis to the femoral

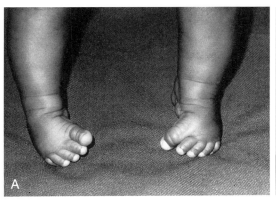
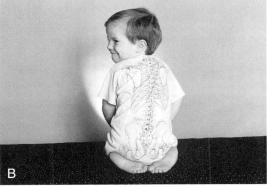

Figure 26–3. *A*, Metatarsus adductus in a 4-month-old that requires treatment. *B*, Sitting position that has anecdotally been criticized for causing metatarsus adductus.

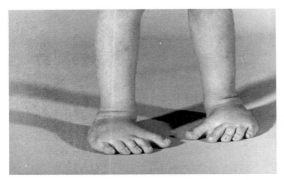

Figure 26–4. A severe residual untreated deformity called "skewfoot."

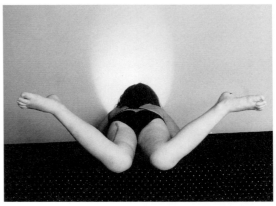

Figure 26–6. Internal hip rotation is measured in the prone position and usually is 45 to 60 degrees.

neck to prevent any additional displacement[5] and to promote physeal closure (Fig. 26–12).

PERONEAL SPASTIC FLATFOOT (TARSAL COALITION)

In contrast to the flexible flatfoot of childhood, the adolescent may present with a painful, stiff foot and some flattening of the longitudinal arch (Figs. 26–13 and 26–14). "Spasm" of the peroneal tendons is noted clinically when the clinician attempts to invert the heel forcibly while checking the range of motion of the foot. This is resisted by involuntary muscle guarding. Radiographs, along with additional imaging modalities such as computed tomography scans, are required to identify the fibrous, cartilaginous, or osseous bar that is limiting motion between the subtalar joint or calcaneal-navicular joint (Fig. 26–15). If nonoperative management, consisting of a reduction in activities, casting, and anti-inflammatory medications, fails to resolve the symptoms, then surgical resection of the bar or arthrodesis of selected joints is indicated and is successful in the majority of cases.[6]

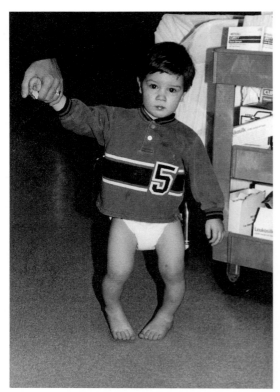

Figure 26–5. A typical 2-year-old toddler who in a 6-month period has experienced a change in his gait pattern, from toeing-out to toeing-in.

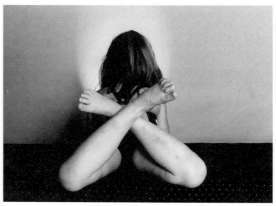

Figure 26–7. External hip rotation in the prone position is usually 30 to 50 degrees.

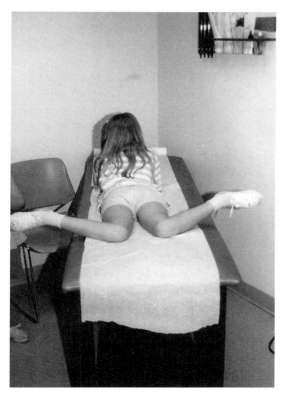

Figure 26–8. A 9-year-old child demonstrating 90 degrees of internal hip rotation.

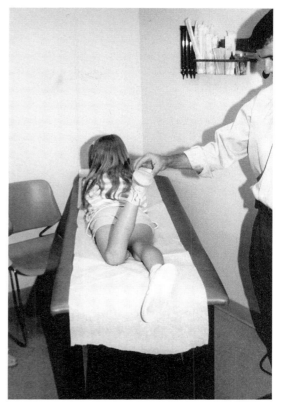

Figure 26–9. There is only 10 degrees of external hip rotation.

OSTEOCHONDROSES

Osteochondroses and osteochondritis are terms that still appear in the medical literature to describe a developmental disturbance of an epiphysis, apophysis, or synchondrosis. Underlying the altered x-ray appearance of the affected area is a reaction of that area to abnormal pressure or compression, tension or traction, or a combination of both. Many of the osteochondroses are still referred to by their eponyms, such as Legg-Calvé-Perthes disease, Kienböck's disease, and Scheuermann's disease. The majority of the osteochondroses represent radiologic curiosities with uneventful clinical outcomes. A few of the significant clinical osteochondroses are presented here.

Legg-Calvé-Perthes Disease

The 3- to 6-year old child (often male, and frequently smaller in size than his peers) presents with a painless but stiff-legged limp. The physical examination reveals a mild-to-moderate hip spasm, involuntary muscle guarding, and limited internal hip rotation. X-ray studies are diagnostic in over 90 percent of the cases, with additional

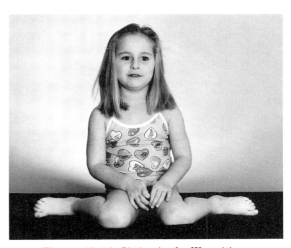

Figure 26–10. Sitting in the W position.

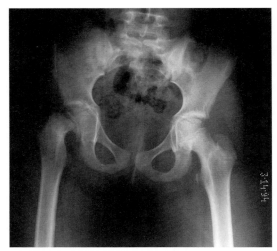

Figure 26–11. Grade II/III slipped capital femoral epiphysis.

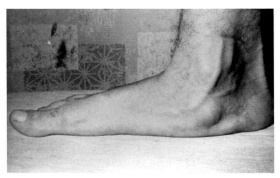

Figure 26–13. A 13-year-old boy with a rigid flat foot.

ing the synovitis in the hip, and promoting healing. Anti-inflammatory medications, crutches, and braces are utilized, and often surgery is required, depending on the amount of hip involvement, age of the patient, and amount of healing incongruity in the hip joint.[7] If the diagnosis of Legg-Calvé-Perthes disease is suspected, referral to an orthopaedist should be made.

modalities, such as bone scan or MRI, being required only rarely. The x-ray changes of fragmentation, resorption, and reossification of the femoral head are usually considered to be diagnostic if only one hip is involved (Fig. 26–16). Symmetric changes in both femoral heads or early acetabular changes are a reason to look for an underlying etiology, such as thyroid disease or bone dysplasia (Fig. 26–17). The treatment is usually aimed at restoring the range of motion, diminish-

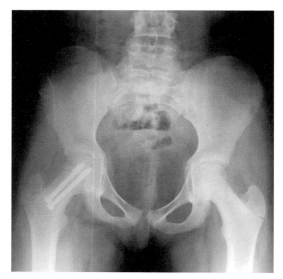

Figure 26–12. Closed reduction and internal fixation of an acute slipped capital femoral epiphysis (SCFE).

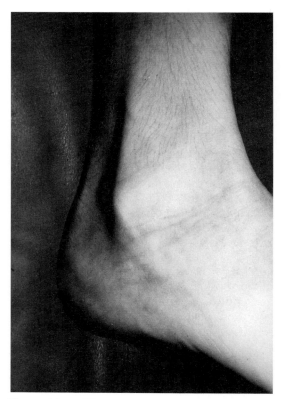

Figure 26–14. The peroneal tendons appear taut over the lateral malleolus.

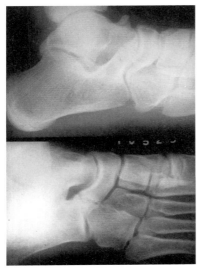

Figure 26–15. Fibro-osseous calcaneal-navicular coalition.

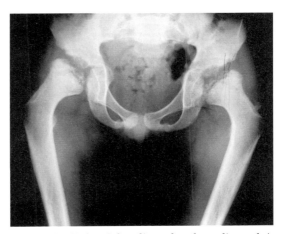

Figure 26–17. A painless limp plus the radiograph in this 8-year-old boy represents a bone dysplasia—multiple epiphyseal dysplasia.

Osteochondritis Dissecans of the Knee

This was originally described in 1887 and is felt to be a result of repetitive microtrauma. Typically the clinician finds this lesion of the knee serendipitously after a radiograph has been obtained for minor trauma to the extremity. The lesion is typically described as a well-circumscribed area on the lateral portion of the medial femoral condyle. Pain or swelling in the knee, effusions, or apparent loosening warrants further evaluation.[8] There is a moderate success rate in obtaining healing of this area with restriction of activities and a brief period of immobilization (Fig. 26–18).

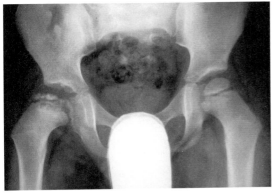

Figure 26–16. A healing whole head involvement in Perthes' disease.

Kienböck's Disease

Originally described in 1910, this disease represents an alteration in the blood supply to the carpal lunate bone. It has a later onset, usually in the patient's twenties, compared with some of the other typical osteochondroses. There is often residual collapse and deformity of the lunate, which contributes to pain and stiffness in the wrist (see Chapter 14).

Sever's Disease

The calcaneal apophysis typically may take on an appearance of markedly increased bone density in children between 5 and 7 years of age. Occasionally the patient will complain of discomfort in the heel with prolonged running and jumping. There is usually no evidence of warmth, redness, or swelling. An intermittent limp may be seen that usually responds to acetaminophen (Tylenol) or nonsteroidal anti-inflammatories. Immobilization is not required; rather, a mild restriction of activities usually allows this to resolve within a matter of weeks.

Freiberg's Disease

Osteochondrosis of the head of the second metatarsal is known as Freiberg's disease, originally described in 1914. The patient

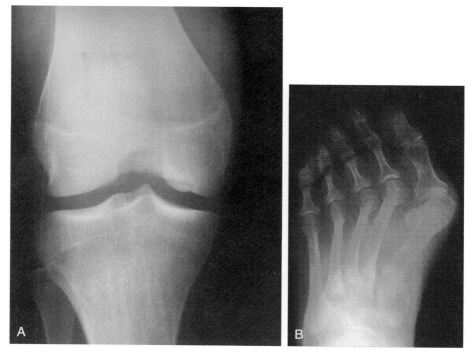

Figure 26–18. *A* and *B,* An osteochondritis dissecans lesion that healed after internal fixation.

may experience pain with prolonged weight-bearing and have some degree of swelling at the metatarsophalangeal joint. Often there is incomplete healing with residual bone deformity of the metatarsophalangeal joint, which may limit dorsiflexion, especially in stair-climbing or running (Fig. 26–19). Weight-relieving metatarsal bars have been used for patients who have prolonged symptoms, and occasionally surgical removal of free-floating joint mice may be warranted.

Panner's Disease

The capitellum of the distal humerus is the site of this osteochondrosis. Typically, between 13 and 18 years of age the capitellum of affected children may develop increased density and fragmentation. In the symptomatic child there may be limitation of elbow flexion and extension, as well as some limitation of pronation and supination. Activities such as gymnastics and baseball may aggravate this condition. Resolution may take as long as 2 to 3 years, and there may be a residual flexion deformity of the elbow.

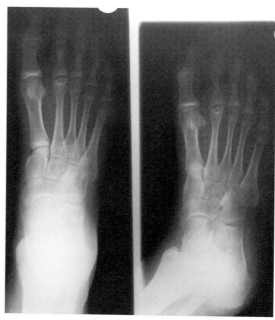

Figure 26–19. Freiberg's infarction of the second metatarsal head with residual flattening and limited range of motion.

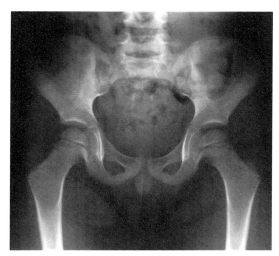

Figure 26–20. AP view of the pelvis demonstrates a bulbous enlargement of the ischiopubic synchondrosis, which should not be misinterpreted as an eosinophilic granuloma or Ewing's sarcoma.

Van Neck's Osteochondrosis

Van Neck's disease is actually the normal appearance of the ischiopubic synchondrosis just prior to fusion. Often there is an irregular, enlarged appearance with occasionally some minor symptoms referable to the hip (Fig. 26–20). In contrast to the other osteochondroses, the x-ray changes should not be interpreted as evidence of ischemic necrosis and should not be confused with a malignancy.

IDIOPATHIC ADOLESCENT SCOLIOSIS

Scoliosis represents a permanent deviation of the spine laterally, combined with spinal rotation. Despite idiopathic adolescent scoliosis being the most prevalent form of spinal deformity, its etiology still remains unknown.[9] As a result of mandatory school screenings in most states, numerous children are referred to their primary care physicians for secondary screenings.[10] A combination of the forward bend test (Fig. 26–21) and the scoliometer is usually effective in eliminating false-positives due to limb length discrepancy, mild paraspinal muscle hypertrophy, and postural roundback. While numerous nonradiographic techniques have been employed to monitor scoliosis and document

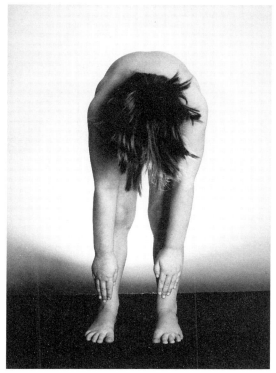

Figure 26–21. The forward bend test is performed with the patient bending forward at the waist and the arms dangling free. Asymmetry in the ribs, scapula, or waist, or deviation of the spine from the midline, can be assessed.

progression, the 36-inch AP scoliosis roentgenogram remains the best. Referral to a pediatric orthopaedist is generally made if the radiograph indicates a scoliotic curve of more than 15 degrees. Many factors are taken into account in trying to predict whether or not the curve will be progres-

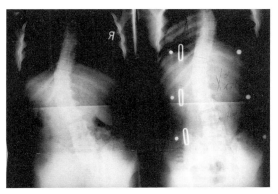

Figure 26–22. A 40-degree thoracolumbar curve is braced in a thoracolumbosacral orthosis (TLSO).

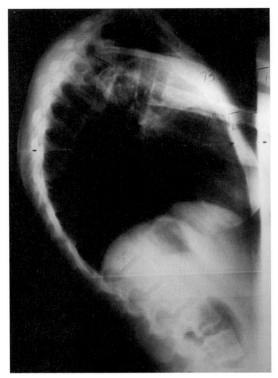

Figure 26–23. Excessive thoracic kyphosis with wedging of adjacent vertebrae.

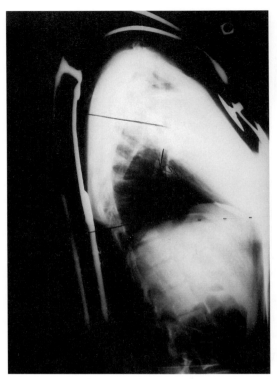

Figure 26–24. The Milwaukee brace provides for gradual correction through continued growth of the spine.

sive.[11] In general, girls have a substantially higher risk of progression than boys. Scoliosis that has an onset prior to 10 years of age is more likely to progress than are minor curves detected at 13 to 14 years of age, and the location of a curve may influence its risk of progression as well.[12] Adolescents who are skeletally advanced and have curves of less than 30 degrees generally are not braced but simply observed until skeletal maturity is reached. Treatment with the use of bracing (Fig. 26–22) is designed to alter the natural history of the progression in those adolescents who are skeletally immature and have a curve that now measures more than 25 degrees.[13]

Curves in the immature child of greater than 40 to 45 degrees or those associated with significant thoracic lordosis (loss of thoracic kyphosis) should be treated surgically. The goal of surgery is to obtain a stable, solid fusion and diminish any decompensation to the left or right.[14]

SCHEUERMANN'S KYPHOSIS

The physician is often consulted for evaluation of an excessive roundness in the back in

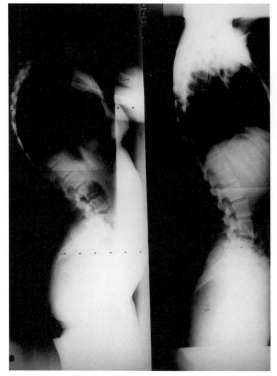

Figure 26–25. A 73-degree kyphosis prebrace, with 2-year follow-up showing a 40-degree kyphosis.

the adolescent boy and girl. Most adolescents have a flexible, postural roundback appearance. There is no associated rigidity in the thoracic spine, and on forward bending the spine has a very smooth contour without a localized "humpback" deformity. Excessive back roundness in general is a benign, self-limited condition that improves as the adolescent completes the growth spurt. Typically, it is not associated with any back pain.

Scheuermann's disease has two presentations. (1) The patient with Scheuermann's disease in the thoracic spine has a localized, increased kyphotic, or "humpback," deformity, which is apparent on a forward bend test (Fig. 26–23). The x-ray views will demonstrate that three adjacent vertebrae are wedge-shaped, and that there is loss of height to the vertebrae.[15] The adolescent may or may not have some discomfort in this area, and, if the wedging and overall kyphosis are significant, may be a candidate for brace wear[16] (Fig. 26–24). Successful brace wear has resulted in permanent reduction of the kyphosis to normal limits (Fig. 26–25).

(2) In the lumbar spine, Scheuermann's disease may manifest as a loss of lumbar lordosis, along with multiple areas of irregularity of the endplate in the lumbar spine. More typically, lumbar Scheuermann's disease is associated with pain and discomfort exacerbated by strenuous physical activity.[17] This is usually a self-limited process that responds to reduction in activities, anti-inflammatory medication, and occasionally outpatient physical therapy modalities. The irregularities that are seen in the lumbar endplate typically are not associated with any long-term degenerative sequelae.

- **PART II**

Developmental Conditions in Adults

John Coen

THE ADULT FOOT

Many conditions of the forefoot can be identified as the source of complaints in patients who present with foot pain. For most of these afflictions, there is an increasing incidence with age, and a female predominance. Footwear is often the reason for the increased problems in women.

Just as a history and physical examination are the starting point in the evaluation of other medical problems, so too are they the first steps in the evaluation of foot pain. The history should include the area of the foot that bothers the patient the most, as well as predisposing and palliative factors. Examination of the foot should include inspection with the patient sitting on an examination table as well as standing. In addition, the gait should be evaluated for the presence of a limp or other abnormalities. Inspection of the footwear is also mandatory, taking note of heel height, toebox size, and patterns of wear on the sole of the shoe.

Deformities of the forefoot are due to a variety of causes: anatomic factors, neuromuscular diseases, connective tissue disorders, congenital anomalies, and trauma.[18] While footwear may not be a cause of forefoot deformities, it is believed to be responsible for the onset of problems in feet that are predisposed to these ailments.

Metatarsalgia

Metatarsalgia is a term for pain in the forefoot related to the metatarsal bones (pain or tenderness over the ball of the foot). The causes of metatarsalgia are divided into three groups.[19] In the first group, pain is due to a localized disease such as a Morton's neuroma (see Chapter 19). The second group is composed of alterations in the biomechanics of the foot due to an overload of the anterior support or an irregular distribution of the metatarsal load. In this instance, a callus is usually located over the prominent and painful metatarsal head. The final group causing metatarsalgia is systemic disease, such as rheumatoid arthritis, in which both fat pad atrophy and increased load on the metatarsal heads occur.

As with other conditions of the forefoot, treatment of metatarsalgia begins with modifications of footwear. Avoidance of high-heeled shoes is the initial step. In addition, shoes with a widened toebox and good support in the sole should be recommended. Inserts that redistribute the load on the metatarsal away from the affected areas are the next measure. If these measures fail or are not realistic for the patient, then surgical options to redistribute weight-bearing more evenly are discussed.

Bunion

A bunion (hallux valgus with a medial metatarsal prominence) is probably the most frequent source of complaints about the forefoot in adults (Fig. 26–26). Bunions are thought to be caused by a variety of factors, both congenital and developmental, involving the first metatarsal bone and soft tissues.[20] Tight footwear may accelerate the formation of a bunion deformity in a foot with these predisposing factors.

The initial treatment of a bunion deformity again centers on footwear. Shoes with a wide toebox to accommodate the medial prominence and a soft pad to cushion the planter surface should be recommended. A variety of commercial appliances are available and can be helpful as well. Surgical correction is considered when these measures fail.

Deformities of the Lesser Toes

A variety of deformities of the lesser toes also can be the source of forefoot complaints. These conditions include mallet toes, hammer toes, and claw toes. These can be distinguished from one another based on the presentation of the involved toe. A mallet toe involves a flexion contracture of the distal interphalangeal joint. A hammer toe involves a flexion contracture of the proximal interphalangeal joint. A claw toe has a flexion contracture of the proximal interphalangeal as well as a hyperextension deformity of the metatarsophalangeal joint (Fig. 26–27). These conditions commonly present with a callus over the involved interphalangeal joint or on the tip of the involved toe. Nail bed deformities also can be seen.

Treatment of these conditions again centers on footwear. Shoes with an adequate toebox or extra-depth shoes should be used. Pads and inserts also can alleviate the areas of pressure but may cause impingement of

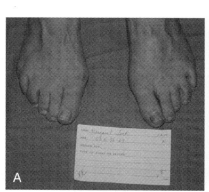
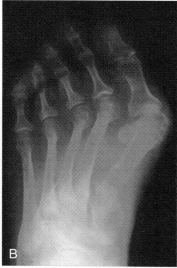
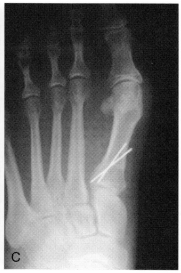

Figure 26–26. *A,* A typical bunion deformity on the right foot with an increased hallux valgus. *B,* AP radiograph demonstrating increased varus of the first metatarsal and increased valgus at the metatarsophalangeal (MP) joint. *C,* Postoperative radiograph following bunionectomy and first metatarsal osteotomy.

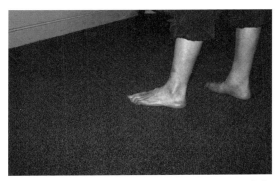

Figure 26–27. Claw toes with hyperextension of the MP and flexion contractures of the interphalangeal (IP) joints.

previously unaffected areas against the shoe. Patients who obtain no relief from these measures can be considered for surgical correction. Modifications of footwear after surgery, specifically the avoidance of shoes with pointed toes, is cruicial to preventing recurrence.

Corns

Corns are keratotic thickenings of the epithelium over a bone prominence.[18] They are called hard corns when they involve the side of a toe coming in contact with the shoe. Soft corns are localized between two toes and are similar to a hard corn but are typically macerated because of moisture. As with other afflictions of the forefoot, inappropriate shoewear is felt to be the etiology of this problem.

Nonoperative treatment of a hard corn consists of shaving the keratotic layers of skin. A "donut" pad may relieve pressure over the involved area. A shoe with a widened toebox is again recommended. Soft corns can be relieved by padding in the web space. Padding is typically lamb's wool, mole skin, felt, or foam. When these measures fail, surgical treatment is recommended. This usually involves excision of the underlying bone prominence.[18, 20] Surgery is usually the preferred treatment for soft corns because attempts at padding are cumbersome.

Ingrown Toe Nails

Ingrown toe nails (onychocryptosis) can affect any of the digits of the foot but are most common in the great toe.[21] Tight shoewear may be the culprit in the formation of the ingrown toe nail. Generally, the nail edges are forced against the nail fold and underlying soft tissue of the nail bed. The normal skin flora of the feet then produce local inflammation, tenderness, and discharge. This eventually becomes a vicious cycle, with a build-up of granulation tissue along the nail fold and chronic drainage (Fig. 26–28).[21]

The initial treatment involves soaking the foot in warm water baths, applying antibiotic ointment, and packing cotton under the nail edge.[21] These measures are frequently unsuccessful, and surgical measures must be considered to provide permanent relief. This typically consists of ablating a wedge of nail matrix, thus narrowing the nail.

DUPUYTREN'S FASCIITIS

Dupuytren's disease causes contractures of the hand and fingers. It is actually a disease of the fascia of the palm and fingers, with the pretendinous bands of the palmar aponeurosis being a common site of the disease. A nodule in this area is pathognomonic of the condition (Fig. 26–29).[22]

Dupuytren's contracture is seen more frequently in people of Northern European, Scandinavian, or Celtic descent. There is also an association with plantar fibromatosis in the instep (Fig. 26–30) and knuckle pads, and involvement of the penis (Peyronie's disease). The age of presentation can vary from the fourth through the seventh decades of life; the condition is more common in men. An associated family history, disease in more than one area, and young age of onset (prior

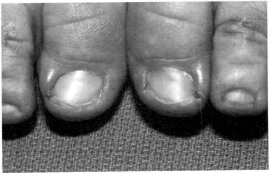

Figure 26–28. Bilateral chronic ingrown toenails with hypertrophy of the lateral paronychial folds.

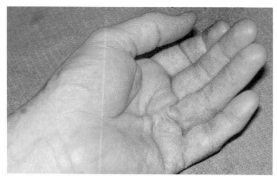

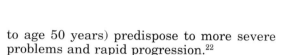

Figure 26–29. Dupuytren's fasciitis with palmar nodules and cords.

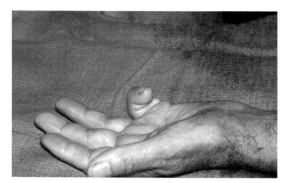

Figure 26–31. Severe contractures of the little finger MP and IP joints secondary to Dupuytren's fasciitis.

to age 50 years) predispose to more severe problems and rapid progression.[22]

There is no reliable nonoperative treatment for Dupuytren's disease. Surgery is the sole means of correcting this condition. When contractures of the metacarpophalangeal joints or the proximal interphalangeal joints develop, prompt referral to a surgeon is indicated (Fig. 26–31). A good rule of thumb for the timing of this referral is when the patient is no longer able to place the palm and fingers flat on a table. Recurrence and progression of the disease after surgical fasciectomy are common, especially in those with factors predisposing to a rapid progression.

OSTEOPOROSIS

Osteoporosis is a term used to describe a diffuse reduction in bone density that usually occurs when the rate of bone absorption exceeds the rate of bone formation (Fig. 26–32).[23] It is commonly associated with aging, or other conditions involving disuse

or immobilization of the body, protein deficiency, and hormonal imbalance.[23,24] This condition is most commonly seen in postmenopausal women. It predisposes to fractures caused by low-energy trauma, especially compression fractures of the spine, hip fractures, and Colles' fractures.

Preventive measures are the best form of therapy in osteoporosis. These include an

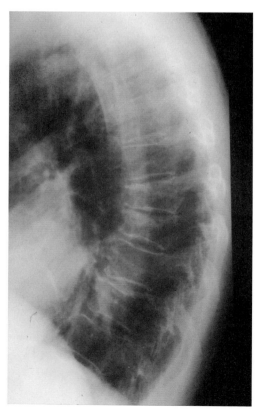

Figure 26–32. Marked osteoporosis of the spine with decreased bone density and multiple compression fractures.

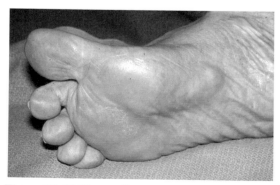

Figure 26–30. Plantar fibromatosis with nodules in the instep.

adequate calcium intake daily (1500 mg per day for postmenopausal and 1000 mg for premenopausal women), increased physical activity, and the use of estrogen or fluoride in women.[23]

References

1. Stahaeli LT, Corbid M, Wyss C, et al.: Lower extremity rotational problems in children. Normal values to guide management. J Bone Joint Surg 67A:39–47, 1985.

2. Kling TF, Jr, Hensinger RN: Angular and torsional deformities of the lower limbs in children. Clin Orthop 176:136–147, 1983.

3. Svennigsen S, Terjesen T, Auflem M, Berg V: Hip rotation and intoeing gait. Clin Orthop 251:177, 1990.

4. Pritchett JW, Perdue KD: Mechanical factors in slipped capital femoral epiphysis. J Pediatr Orthop 8:385–388, 1988.

5. Koval KJ, Lehman WB, Rose D, et al.: Treatment of slipped capital femoral epiphysis with a cannulated screw technique. J Bone Joint Surg 71:1370, 1989.

6. Mosier KM, Asher M: Tarsal coalitions in peroneal spastic flatfoot: A review. J Bone Joint Surg 66-A:976–984, 1984.

7. McAndrew MP, Weinstein SL: A long-term follow-up of Legg Calvé Perthes disease. J Bone Joint Surg 66-A:860–869, 1984.

8. Bradley J Dandy, DJ: Osteochondritis dissecans and other lesions of the femoral condyles. J Bone Joint Surg 71-B:518–522, 1989.

9. Weinstein SL: Idiopathic scoliosis: Natural history. Spine 11:780–783, 1986.

10. Lonstein JE, Bjorklund S, Wanninger MH, et al.: Voluntary school screening for scoliosis in Minnesota. J Bone Joint Surg 64A:481–488, 1982.

11. Lonstein JE, Carlson JM: The prediction of curve progression in untreated idiopathic scoliosis during growth. J Bone Joint Surg 66A:1061–1071, 1984.

12. Weinstein SL, Savala DC, Ponseti IV: Idiopathic scoliosis: Long-term follow-up and prognosis in untreated patients. J Bone Joint Surg 63A:702–712, 1981.

13. Winter RB, Lonstein JE, Drogt J, et al.: The effectiveness of bracing in the nonoperative treatment of idiopathic scoliosis. Spine 11:790–791, 1986.

14. Moskowitz A, Moe JH, Winter RB, et al.: Long-term follow-up of scoliosis fusion. J Bone Joint Surg 62A:364–376, 1980.

15. Ippolito E, Ponseti IV: Juvenile kyphosis: Histological and histochemical studies. J Bone Joint Surg 63A:175–182, 1981.

16. Sachs B, Bradford D, Winter R, et al.: Scheuermann kyphosis: Follow-up of Milwaukee brace treatment. J Bone Joint Surg 69A:50–57, 1987.

17. Blumenthal SL, Roach J, Herring JA: Lumbar Scheuermann's: A clinical series and classification. Spine 12:929–932, 1987.

18. Mann RA, Coughlin MJ: Lesser toe deformities. *In* Jahss, M.H. (ed.): Disorders of the Foot and Ankle, 2nd ed. Philadelphia, WB Saunders, 1991, pp 1205–1228.

19. Viladot A, Sr: The metatarsals. *In* Jahss MH (ed.): Disorders of the Foot and Ankle, 2nd ed. Philadelphia, WB Saunders, 1991, pp 1229–1266.

20. Mann RA, Coughlin MJ: Adult hallux valgus. *In* Surgery of the Foot and Ankle, 6th ed. St. Louis, Mosby–Year Book, 1993, pp 167–296.

21. Lapidus PW: The toenails. *In* Jahss MH (ed): Disorders of the Foot and Ankle, 2nd ed. Philadelphia, WB Saunders, 1991, pp 1573–1594.

22. McFarland RM: Dupuytren's contracture. *In* Green DP (ed.): Operative Hand Surgery, 2nd ed. New York, Churchill Livingstone, 1988, pp 553–589.

23. Turek SL: Orthopaedics, 4th ed. Phildelphia, JB Lippincott, 1984, pp 253–256.

24. Vaswani A, Aloia JF: The osteopenias, rickets, and allied diseases. *In* Dee R, Muuyo E, Hurst LC: Principles of Orthopaedic Practice. New York, McGraw-Hill, 1989, pp 267–271.

CHAPTER 27

Congenital Deformities

Michael Conklin

Strictly speaking, congenital deformities are anomalies that are present at birth. However, many of the skeletal dysplasias and genetic syndromes are not obvious at birth but become manifest during growth and development of the individual. Conditions such as the milder forms of osteogenesis imperfecta and skeletal dysplasia fall into this category. Both congenital anomalies and musculoskeletal disorders that are genetically programmed will be discussed in this chapter.

Etiology

Congenital deformities may be secondary to genetic influences, environmental influences, or a combination of both. Both chromosomal anomalies and single gene mutations may be responsible for musculoskeletal congenital deformities. Many of the chromosomal disorders, with the exception of Down's syndrome (trisomy 21), result in severe congenital defects that are incompatible with life. Single gene disorders are responsible for osteogenesis imperfecta, the skeletal dysplasias, mucopolysaccharidoses, and other congenital deformities.

Environmental influences may be intrauterine or perinatal. Fetal development may be affected by maternal exposure to various chemicals such as thalidomide, irradiation, viruses (e.g., rubella), bacteria (e.g., syphilis), parasites (e.g., toxoplasmosis), dietary deficiencies, hormones, and hypoxia. These teratogens are generally not specific in the anomalies they cause but are dependent on the stage of fetal development at the time of exposure. They may result in multiple anomalies affecting the nervous system, heart, genitourinary system, face and oral cavity, and musculoskeletal system. For this reason, the evaluation of specific musculoskeletal deformities may include imaging of the central nervous system, the heart, and the kidneys.

Many of the musculoskeletal congenital deformities are multifactorial in origin. It is likely that developmental dislocation of the hip and clubfoot fall into this category.

THE SPINE

Congenital deformities of the spine can be classified broadly as failure of segmentation and failure of formation. Failure of segmentation results in congenital fusion of the vertebrae and may lead to spinal deformity. Failure of formation may manifest as failure of formation of a vertebral body with the posterior elements intact, leading to congenital kyphosis or hemivertebrae resulting in congenital scoliosis. Whatever the congenital spine deformity, the evaluation must include imaging of the spinal cord, the heart, and the kidneys, as their development is temporally related to the development of the spine. The suggested work-up includes magnetic resonance imaging (MRI) of the spinal cord, echocardiogram, and renal ultrasound.

Klippel-Feil Syndrome

Klippel-Feil syndrome is a congenital fusion of the cervical spine secondary to failure of segmentation. This may involve two or multiple vertebrae. Associated orthopaedic anomalies include congenital scoliosis and Sprengel's deformity. Other associated congenital abnormalities include cardiac anomalies, renal defects, and deafness.[33]

The degree of deformity is variable and is dependent on the number of vertebrae involved. Patients will have a short, stiff neck with a low posterior hair line and webbing of the neck.[61] Head tilt may or may not be present. Lateral bend is generally more restricted than rotation, flexion, or extension. Radiographs will disclose fusion of a variable number of vertebral bodies and frequently failure of closure of the posterior elements (spina bifida).

When Klippel-Feil syndrome has been diagnosed, orthopaedic consultation should be obtained. Frequently, no treatment is indicated but in those patients with progressive spinal curves, fusion may be required. Later in life the mobile disc spaces between the stiff segments may degenerate, requiring treatment.

Congenital Muscular Torticollis

Torticollis as a general term refers to a rotational deformity of the neck. The specific term *congenital muscular torticollis* refers to a rotational deformity of the neck secondary to a unilateral contracture of the sternocleidomastoid muscle (Fig. 27–1). The etiology of the sternocleidomastoid fibrosis has been debated. It may be secondary to venous congestion and eventual fibrosis, intrauterine malposition, or trauma secondary to a difficult birth.

The differential diagnosis of torticollis includes congenital anomalies of the cervical spine (atlantoaxial anomalies or Klippel-Feil syndrome), neurologic disorders (tumors of

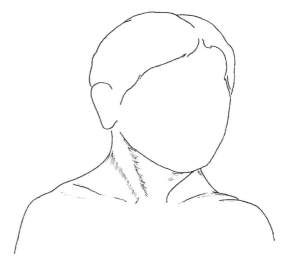

Figure 27–1. Torticollis. Contracture of the right sternocleidomastoid muscle results in chin rotation to the left.

the posterior fossa, cervical cord tumors, or syringomyelia), ocular disorders, rotatory fixation of C1 and C2, and trauma.

Other molding abnormalities may be seen such as plagiocephaly, facial asymmetry, developmental dislocation of the hip (20 percent), and metatarsus adductus.[38] An appropriate prenatal birth and perinatal history should be obtained. Specifically, a history of premature rupture of membranes, oligohydramnios, and breech positioning should be sought. Note any facial asymmetry or plagiocephaly. The sternocleidomastoid muscles should be palpated for fibrosis, masses, or tightness. The position of the head should be noted in regard to head tilt and chin rotation. If the torticollis is secondary to a tight sternocleidomastoid muscle, head tilt will be toward the ipsilateral side, but chin rotation will be away from the pathologic muscle.[19] For instance, in a tight right sternocleidomastoid, the right ear will be tilted toward the right shoulder but the chin will be rotated toward the left. A careful hip examination, including Ortolani's and Barlow's maneuvers, should be done. The feet should be examined for abnormalities.

AP and lateral radiographs of the cervical spine should be obtained to rule out obvious congenital vertebral anomalies.

Treatment should be initiated as soon as the problem is identified. This involves passive stretching of the sternocleidomastoid muscle. Appropriate stretching is demonstrated to the parents. This consists of head tilt away from the tight muscle and chin rotation toward the side of the tight muscle. It is also important to do head tilt and chin rotation with the neck in extension, which further stretches the sternocleidomastoid muscle.

If stretching is begun within the first year of life, the prognosis is good. In the older child with long-established facial asymmetry, it is likely that stretching alone will not resolve the deformity, and surgical release of the sternocleidomastoid muscle is indicated.[13]

Congenital Scoliosis

Scoliosis is defined as a coronal plane curve of the spine. Congenital scoliosis is any scoliosis that results from vertebral anomalies. This may be secondary to failure of formation, failure of segmentation, or a combination of both (Fig. 27–2).

The patient will present with scoliosis or lateral curvature of the spine (Chapter 1). The severity of the deformity will vary with the character of the vertebral anomaly and the age of the patient.[48] The physical examination should include careful inspection of the skin along the back. Cutaneous stigmata such as hairy patches, skin dimpling, or midline lipoma should alert the physician to possible underlying spinal cord anomalies.[49] A careful neurologic examination (Chapter 1) should be carried out. AP and lateral x-ray views of the entire spine should be obtained with the patient standing, when possible (Fig. 27–3). The other imaging studies previously mentioned for congenital spine deformities should be obtained.

Generally, patients with congenital scoliosis and no underlying spinal cord anomalies have a low risk for developing a neurologic deficit. The orthopaedist, however, should be consulted early to monitor the curvature for progression. Progressive curves require fusion.[81]

Congenital Kyphosis

Kyphosis is defined as a sagittal plane curvature of the spine with the apex posterior. Congenital kyphosis can be secondary to failure of formation with an absent or abnormally small vertebral body or can be due to failure of segmentation with congenital fusion of the vertebral bodies and lack of anterior growth. Kyphosis is the most common congenital bone anomaly of the spine leading to neurologic deficits.[44]

Patients will present with a kyphotic deformity that can be anywhere from the cervical to the lower lumbar spine. The deformity will vary in severity depending on the character of the vertebral anomaly. Those with failure of formation tend to have more severe deformities and have a higher risk of developing neurologic deficits than those with failure of segmentation.[80] The kyphosis tends to be sharply angular and rigid.

A careful neurologic examination is strictly indicated. Patients may present with weakness of the lower extremities or upper motor neuron signs such as spasticity and clonus.

Standing AP and lateral x-ray views of the entire spine should be obtained. Tomograms may be helpful to delineate the pathoanatomy. The other imaging studies for congenital spine anomalies should be obtained.

Immediate orthopaedic consultation is indicated. Patients without neurologic deficits may undergo fusion in situ. Those with neurologic deficits require anterior decompression followed by anterior strut grafting and posterior fusion.[11,16]

Myelomeningocele

Myelomeningocele belongs to the family of neural tube defects that encompasses anencephaly, myelomeningocele, meningocele, and lipomeningocele. In myelomeningocele, abnormal neural elements are part of the sac leading to severe peripheral neurologic deficits. Central nervous system abnormalities are also frequently present, including Arnold-Chiari malformations and hydrocephalus.[64]

The etiology of myelomeningocele is unknown. The two main theories include a lack of closure of the neural tube during embryonic development and rupture of a previously closed neural tube. The defect occurs in approximately 1 of 1000 live births in the United States.

Mortality approaches 100 percent in untreated myelomeningocele. Death is generally secondary to infection. During the 1970s, there was an attempt to select patients for treatment by criteria developed by Lorber.[45] Since the 1980s, a large majority of infants with myelomeningocele are aggressively

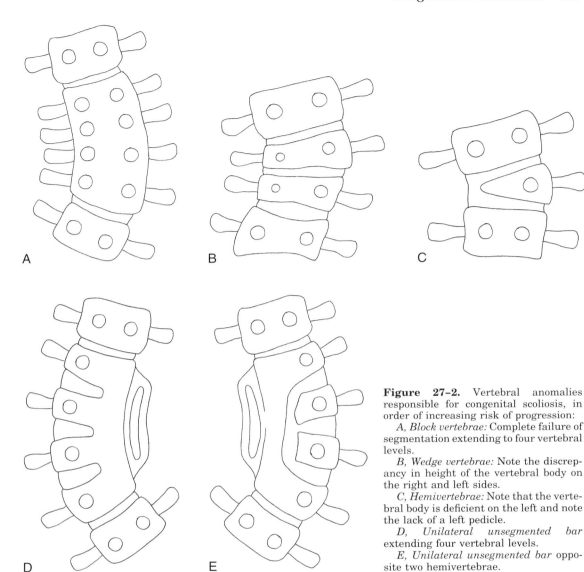

Figure 27–2. Vertebral anomalies responsible for congenital scoliosis, in order of increasing risk of progression:

A, Block vertebrae: Complete failure of segmentation extending to four vertebral levels.

B, Wedge vertebrae: Note the discrepancy in height of the vertebral body on the right and left sides.

C, Hemivertebrae: Note that the vertebral body is deficient on the left and note the lack of a left pedicle.

D, Unilateral unsegmented bar extending four vertebral levels.

E, Unilateral unsegmented bar opposite two hemivertebrae.

treated with initial closure of the defect and shunting of hydrocephalus. For this reason a new natural history is emerging. It has been observed that the neurologic lesion in myelomeningocele is not static but may undergo progressive deterioration because of a number of causes, including hydrocephaly, syringomyelia, Arnold-Chiari malformations, and tethered cord; therefore, careful serial neurologic examination, including upper extremity strength, are indicated during each follow-up visit.

The cause of myelomeningocele is multifactorial. Genetic factors play a role. The incidence in whites is 0.15 percent; in blacks it is 0.04 percent. The incidence rises to 3.2 percent in first-degree relatives. Environmental factors may play a role. Valproic acid has been implicated. Folate deficiency may be a factor.

Prenatal diagnosis can be accomplished through maternal serum alpha-fetoprotein (AFP), amniotic AFP, and ultrasound. The maternal serum AFP test is done at 16 to 18 weeks' gestation and is less invasive than amniocentesis. There is considerable overlap between normal values and those values seen in neural tube defects. If the maternal serum AFP is high, further testing is indicated, such as amniocentesis for AFP or ultrasound. Ultrasound will reliably identify anencephaly, but there is a higher incidence

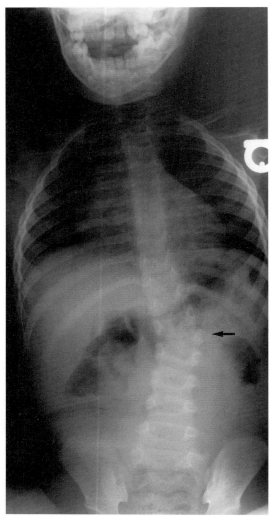

Figure 27–3. Left L2 hemivertebrae *(arrow)* causing left lumbar scoliosis.

of false-negative results in fetuses with myelomeningocele.

With prenatal diagnosis, decision making and treatment begin in the prenatal period. Termination of the pregnancy is an option if the diagnosis is made early. Arrangements should be made to refer the mother and child to a major medical center with a neonatal intensive care unit and pediatric neurosurgery.

From the time of birth the myelodysplasia team involves neurosurgery, urology, orthopaedics, pediatrics, occupational therapy, and physical therapy. Initial neurosurgical treatment generally involves closure of the defect followed by shunting of hydrocephalus, if indicated.[47] It is helpful if both ortho-

paedists and urologists are consulted during the initial hospital stay to establish baseline examinations.

Orthopaedic treatment early in infancy is aimed at establishing a baseline neurologic examination, treatment of hip instability, and assessment of the lower extremities for deformities. The "neurologic level" is defined as the root level corresponding to the most distal muscle with at least four of five (function against resistance) muscle strength; for instance, a patient with quadriceps musculature that will extend the knee against resistance, but with weak or absent foot dorsiflexion and no foot plantar flexion, would be classified as having an L4-level myelomeningocele. Because of the dynamic nature of the lesion, the orthopaedist should repeat the neurologic examination at each visit.

Anteroposterior and lateral radiographs of the spine will disclose the level of the bone lesion (Fig. 27–4). A careful hip examination is carried out, including Ortolani's and Barlow's maneuvers. Initial treatment of hip instability is with conservative measures such as abduction splinting. More aggressive treatment of fixed dislocations or hip subluxation of dislocation later in life is individualized, with the most important factor being the neurologic level.[3,50] Foot deformities, including clubfoot, congenital vertical talus, calcaneal valgus, and valgus feet, are extremely common. Early treatment is with stretching and splinting. Casting of insensate feet may lead to pressure sores. Surgical treatment is indicated in the rigid, deformed foot to provide a stable, plantigrade, and braceable foot. Lower extremity contractures such as hip flexion contractures, hip abduction/external rotation contractures, and knee flexion or extension contractures are treated with stretching and later surgical treatment, if indicated.[24]

Spinal deformities are extremely common in myelomeningocele, including scoliosis, kyphosis, and lordosis. Spine deformities and pelvic obliquity may affect sitting balance and lead to pressure sores. Bracing, surgery, or both may be required to provide a stable spine and a level pelvis.[42,46]

Function and mobility are enhanced through physical therapy, occupational therapy, and bracing. Those with low lumbar or sacral level myelomeningocele may manifest minimal developmental delay in the absence of significant CNS abnormalities. Many children, however, will require an aggressive

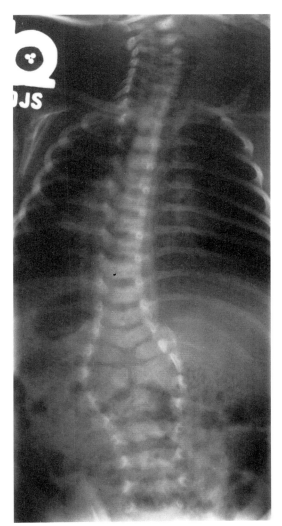

Figure 27–4. Note the wide dysrhaphism seen on the AP spine radiograph in this patient with thoracic level myelomeningocele.

bracing and therapy program to provide upright mobility and control lower extremity deformities and contractures. Complicated and expensive devices, such as the reciprocating gait orthosis, can provide ambulatory ability for even the patient with thoracic level myelomeningocele. However, most patients with high-level myelomeningocele (thoracic and upper lumbar level) will graduate to a wheelchair at adolescence and find this the most efficient means of transportation.[35]

The primary care physician may be the first one to see a myelomeningocele patient with new onset of swelling and redness in an insensate lower extremity. Radiographs of the affected area always should be obtained,

because fractures can frequently simulate infection in these patients.[74] Short periods of casting and early return to braces for ambulation are indicated.

LIMB DEFICIENCIES

Limb deficiencies may be secondary to genetic influences, intrauterine environmental factors, or a combination of both. Tibial longitudinal deficiencies are generally inherited in an autosomal dominant pattern. Many of the other deficiencies are secondary to teratogens.

The classification system of Dundee is simple to understand and apply. According to this system, the deficiency is first classified as transverse or longitudinal. A transverse deficiency involves congenital amputation of all parts distal. A longitudinal deficiency involves a deficiency of the involved bone, with preservation of parts distal or adjacent. Next, the bone or bones involved are stated. Lastly, the deficiency is described as partial or complete in the case of longitudinal deficiencies, or as to level (e.g., midshaft) in the case of transverse deficiencies. For example, radial clubhand is a congenital absence of the radius and would be classified as a "longitudinal deficiency of the radius, complete." Conversely, a congenital amputation of the midforearm with no hand present would be classified as "transverse deficiency of radius and ulna midshaft."

Congenital limb deficiencies may involve any bone or combination of bones. They may involve one or all limbs. They can be associated with spinal anomalies such as scoliosis. For instance, patients with bilateral deficiencies at the proximal humeral level have an almost 100 percent incidence of scoliosis.

Radial Longitudinal Deficiency

Also known as radial clubhand, this is a relatively rare condition characterized by partial or total absence of the radius, with instability of the wrist and radial deviation of the hand. Patients may or may not have hypoplasia or total absence of the thumb or thenar musculature. Other associations may include anomalies of the cardiovascular, gastrointestinal, and genitourinary systems and hematologic abnormalities such as thrombocytopenia and anemia (TAR syndrome) or

Fanconi's anemia.[2] The minimum evaluation, therefore, includes a complete blood count. The condition is frequently bilateral.

The deformity will be obvious at birth. There is shortening of the forearm to a variable degree, with bowing of the ulna, concave radially. The hand will be radially deviated and volarly flexed. The thumb may be normal, hypoplastic, or absent.

Treatment begins in early infancy with stretching or splinting of the hand. Further treatment is individualized. It is important to evaluate the patient's overall function carefully before deciding on operative treatment. Many patients have limitations of elbow flexion and require the volar flexion/radial deviation deformity to get the hand to the mouth. Operative treatment includes centralization of the hand on the distal ulna, frequently combined with an ulnar osteotomy.[8] The thumb hypoplasia or absence may also require surgical treatment.

Fibular Longitudinal Deficiency

Longitudinal deficiency of the fibula is the most common long bone deficiency. Complete absence is more common than partial absence. It is part of a constellation of lower extremity malformations including anomalies of the femur, ball-and-socket ankle joint, tarsal coalition, and longitudinal deficiency of the lateral rays of the foot. The etiology is unknown but likely involves insult to the limb bud before the eighth fetal week.

The affected limb is abnormally short and small, with both the thigh and lower leg affected, the latter to a greater degree. The tibia is shortened and bowed convex anteromedially. There is generally a skin dimple over the apex of the tibial bow. The foot is in equinovalgus with hindfoot stiffness and occasionally absence of the lateral rays of the foot. Upper limb deficiencies may also be seen. Cardiac and renal anomalies are rare.

AP and lateral x-ray views of the femur, lower leg, and foot should be obtained. Leg length films and an AP view of the left wrist for bone age also should be obtained. Radiographs will disclose partial or total absence of the fibula with an anteromedial bow and shortening of the tibia (Fig. 27–5). The femur may show mild hypoplasia or partial absence.

The goal of treatment is to equalize leg lengths and provide a functional foot for

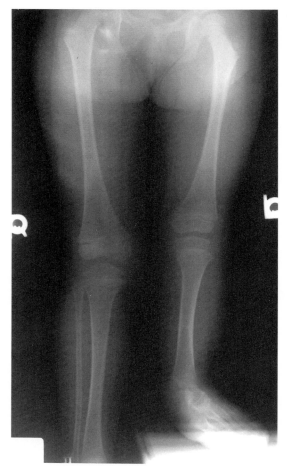

Figure 27–5. Longitudinal deficiency of the left fibula, complete. Note shortening of the femoral and tibial segments and valgus of hindfoot.

ambulation. This may involve forefoot amputation and fitting with a prosthesis or limb lengthening and reconstructive procedures.[15,79] The orthopaedist should be involved early so that the treatment decisions can be made before the child reaches walking age.

Proximal Femoral Focal Deficiency (PFFD)

PFFD is a congenital malformation of the proximal femur and acetabulum resulting from a teratologic insult during limb bud development. Of the various teratogens, only the drug thalidomide has been identified as a definite cause in humans. In PFFD there is no connection between the distal femoral segment and the proximal femoral segment—that is, there is a pseudoarthrosis in the proximal femur. The femoral head may or may not be present. The femur is shortened to a variable degree (Fig. 27–6). Since acetabular development depends on the presence of the femoral head within the joint, the acetabulum will be poorly developed or absent in those patients without a femoral head.[1]

The deformity is obvious at birth. The involved extremity will be shortened, with the foot often at the knee level and the hip flexed, abducted, and externally rotated. Occasionally the deformity is bilateral. Other lower extremity anomalies may be seen, including a fibular longitudinal deficiency. It is important to note that there is also hypoplasia of the gluteal musculature, and even with the best prosthetic fitting or surgical treatment, the patients will walk with a limp.

For those patients with less than 25 percent shortening and a well-developed hip joint, limb lengthening is an option. The family must understand, however, that this will involve multiple procedures and is associated with a high complication rate. The majority of patients will have greater than 25 percent shortening and should undergo early forefoot amputation and knee fusion.[40] It is preferable that the amputation be accomplished before 1 year of age so that the child can be fitted with a prosthesis and begin ambulating at the normal time.

Congenital Pseudoarthrosis of the Clavicle

This is a rare anomaly, the etiology of which is obscure. The deformity is fully present at birth, and the right clavicle is almost always affected. Patients will present with a nontender swelling at the midportion of the clavicle and no history of birth injury. They will not exhibit pseudoparalysis of the arm (lack of voluntary movement), or pain to shoulder range of motion, as would be seen in birth fractures of the clavicle. There will be drooping of the affected shoulder and mild limitation of shoulder abduction.[29]

The pseudoarthrosis is seen just lateral to the midshaft of the clavicle. The bone ends may be enlarged and bulbous, but there will be no fracture callus as would be seen after birth fractures.

The treatment involves excision of the pseudoarthrosis mass, curettage of the bone ends, iliac crest bone graft, and internal fixation. This should be accomplished early, preferably before 4 years of age.[72]

Cleidocranial Dysostosis

This is a rare skeletal dysplasia resulting from a defect in intramembranous ossification. Patients have a partial or complete longitudinal deficiency of the clavicle associated with abnormalities of cranial ossification. On clinical examination, patients will have an increased ability to protract the scapula, occasionally to such a degree as to be able to touch the shoulders together anteriorly. Radiographs will disclose partial or total absence of the clavicles. AP pelvis x-ray views will show a wide pubic symphysis.[27] Generally, there is little disability and no treatment is required.

Sprengel's Deformity

Also known as congenital elevation of the scapula, this rare condition is the result of

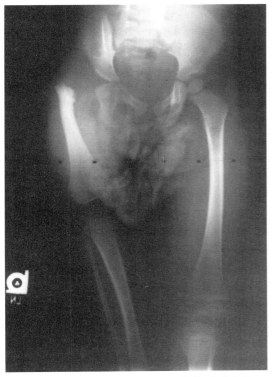

Figure 27–6. Left proximal femoral focal deficiency. Note shortening of the left lower extremity, absence of the proximal femur, and poor development of the acetabulum.

failure of the scapula to descend during fetal development. It is frequently associated with Klippel-Feil syndrome and other congenital spine deformities.[14]

The high scapula presents as a webbing of the neck. Occasionally the condition is bilateral. There is a spectrum of severity from a minimally noticeable asymmetry of shoulder height to a severe high scapula with obvious cosmetic deformity. The shoulder range of motion is restricted to a variable degree, particularly abduction.

Radiographs will disclose the scapula to be high and malformed to a variable degree. It will be rotated in the coronal plane in such a way that the inferior medial corner moves toward the midline. Concomitantly, the glenoid is rotated so that it faces more inferiorly. This, as well as the restricted scapulothoracic motion, is responsible for the decreased shoulder abduction. AP and lateral x-ray views of the cervical spine and thoracolumbar spine should be obtained to rule out congenital spine anomalies. Occasionally, one will see a cervical rib or omovertebral bone.

The goals of treatment are to improve the cosmetic appearance and shoulder motion. In those with a mild deformity, no treatment is indicated. Treatment options for more severe deformities include resection of the superior portion of the scapula, repositioning of the scapula, or a combination of both.[41,82]

Congenital Radioulnar Synostosis

Failure of segmentation of the radius and ulna during fetal development results in a proximal synostosis between the two bones. Clinically, there is a complete lack of rotation of the forearm, with the forearm generally fixed in pronation. Elbow extension may be limited to a mild degree, but otherwise elbow and wrist range of motion are full. Occasionally absence or dislocation of the radial head is seen. The treatment should be individualized, as surgical options are limited. An osteotomy may improve the position of the forearm, but generally it is difficult to reestablish any rotation.[68]

Syndactyly

Syndactyly, or webbing of the digits, results from a lack of differentiation between the digits, occurring somewhere between the sixth and eighth weeks of intrauterine life. This is the most common congenital anomaly of the hand, with an incidence of 1 in every 2250 births. The condition is bilateral 50 percent of the time. It may be familial. Syndactyly can be classified as complete or incomplete. In complete syndactyly, the fusion extends to the most terminal aspect of the digit. Syndactyly can also be classified as simple or complex. In complex syndactyly, there is bone fusion to a variable degree. Syndactyly is commonly associated with other syndromes, such as Apert's syndrome and Poland's syndrome.[6]

The goals of treatment are to improve function and cosmesis. Differential growth of the fingers may result in angular deformity, and therefore separation should proceed in a timely fashion. Thumb-index, ring-little, and index-long finger syndactyly should be separated before 1 year of age. Separation of ring-long finger syndactyly can be delayed until 2 or 3 years of age.

Polydactyly

Polydactyly is the presence of more than five digits on the hand or foot. This is the second most common congenital deformity of the hand, with the incidence being higher in the black population.

Polydactyly on the ulnar side of the hand (postaxial) is the most common form. When it occurs as an isolated anomaly, it is an autosomal dominant trait with variable penetrance. In the black population it commonly occurs as an isolated anomaly, often bilaterally. In whites it may be associated with a variety of syndromes, including acrocephalopolysyndactyly. When a white infant presents with little finger polydactyly, genetic consultation should be considered. Little finger polydactyly may range from a small, pedunculated skin tag with no bone elements to a complete duplication of the finger, including metacarpal. Duplication of the thumb is the most common type of polydactyly in whites. It may be associated with syndactyly of the other digits and is inherited as an autosomal dominant trait.

AP, lateral, and oblique x-ray views of the hand should be obtained to evaluate bone anatomy. The treatment of postaxial polydactyly depends on the degree of duplication. Simple skin tags can be excised and cauterized in the newborn nursery. If bone elements are present, a formal surgical procedure is recommended for excision. This should be accomplished early in life.

The operative treatment of thumb duplication is indicated to improve both cosmesis and function. Improvement in position, stability, configuration, mobility, and adequacy of the web space may be seen. Patients should be referred to the orthopaedist during early infancy for planning of the surgical approach.

Camptodactyly

Camptodactyly is a flexion deformity of the finger, most commonly the proximal interphalangeal joint of the small finger. It usually presents during the first year of life. In two thirds of cases it is bilateral. It is commonly associated with other syndromes. Intermittent splinting, such as a static splint at night, may slow progression. As 80 percent of patients will manifest a progressive deformity, they should be referred to the orthopaedist early in life for consideration of operative treatment.

Cleft Hand

Cleft hand, also known as lobster claw hand, is a rare anomaly, usually bilateral, resulting in congenital absence of the central ray or rays and splitting of the hand into radial and ulnar segments. Associated anomalies include cleft lip and palate, cataracts, deafness, congenital heart disease, and imperforate anus. It is commonly an autosomal dominant trait with incomplete penetrance.

The typical form presents with absence of the entire long finger ray and a V-shaped central defect in the hand.[7] Syndactyly between the thumb and index and small and ring fingers is common. Function is generally good, with grasp and pinch being preserved. Radiographs will disclose absence of the central ray or rays to a variable degree.

Treatment is indicated only if functional deficits are present. Attempts to improve cosmesis are unrewarding. Syndactyly release of the border digits is beneficial. The cleft is then closed at about 18 months of age. Mobilization of the contracted thumb may also help functionally.

DEVELOPMENTAL DISLOCATION OF THE HIP

Developmental dislocation of the hip (DDH) comprises a spectrum of abnormalities ranging from hip instability with capsular laxity to a high dislocation of the hip with severe dysplasia of the acetabulum. To understand DDH, it is imperative to review the embryology of the hip joint. The acetabulum and proximal femur form from a condensation of mesenchyme that progresses to a cartilaginous anlage. Initially, this is a common block of tissue. A cleft forms between the femoral head and acetabulum by 11 weeks. Dislocation can occur at any time after this. Further femoral development and acetabular development are interdependent. For normal acetabular development to occur, a femoral head must be present within the acetabulum. Likewise, for normal formation of the proximal femur, it must be contained within the acetabulum. Therefore, the severity of the pathologic changes seen in DDH is dependent on the timing of the dislocation.[71]

The hip may be dislocated, dislocatable, or subluxable at birth. All three types of typical dislocation of the hip are considered unstable and require immediate orthopaedic consultation and treatment.

Unstable hips are found in 1 of 100 births.[75] Girls are affected five times more frequently than boys. It is more common in children with other abnormalities, such as metatarsus varus and torticollis. Sixty percent of the time it is the left hip only, 20 percent the right, and 20 percent bilateral.

The cause is multifactorial, with both genetic and environmental influences playing a role. Prenatal environmental factors include breech presentation, oligohydramnios, premature rupture of membranes, and tight maternal structures (increased incidence in primiparas). Postnatal factors are apparent in such cultures as the Navajo Indians who wrap their infants in swaddling clothes with the hips adducted and extended. Genetic factors may also play a role. There is a slightly increased incidence in first-degree relatives. Likewise, families with increased ligamentous laxity have a higher incidence of DDH.

Physical findings and treatment options change rapidly in the growing child. Consequently, discussion of physical findings, x-ray findings, and treatment are discussed for three age groups:

Birth to Two Months of Age. A careful hip examination should be performed on all newborn infants. First the child is evaluated both prone and supine for symmetry of the thigh and gluteal folds. The hips and knees are then flexed 90 degrees with the knees together in the midline, and the relative length of each femur is judged by the height of the knees. If one thigh is shorter than the other, this is termed a positive Galeazzi's sign (Fig. 27–7). The hips are abducted fully bilaterally and the amount of abduction is noted. Abduction should be symmetric, and the neonate should have 90 degrees of abduction. Next, Ortolani's and Barlow's maneuvers should be performed with the patient supine on a firm surface. The infant should be relaxed. Ortolani's test is performed as follows: with one hand stabilizing the pelvis, the thigh is grasped with the other hand such that the thumb lies over the medial thigh and the fingers over the greater trochanter. The hip and knee are each flexed 90 degrees. The hip is then gently abducted while upward pressure is placed on the trochanter in an attempt to reduce the femoral head into the acetabulum (Fig. 27–8). A positive test results in a "clunk of entry."[18]

Barlow's maneuver is performed with the hands in the same position and the infant's hip flexed 45 to 60 degrees.[5] Starting with the hip in midabduction, the thigh is brought slowly into adduction while gentle outward pressure is applied to the medial thigh with the thumb (Fig. 27–9). A positive test is felt as a "clunk of exit." Thumb pressure is then released as the hip is again abducted and a "clunk of entry" is noted. Subluxatable hips will not manifest a "clunk of exit" on Barlow's maneuver but instead a sliding feeling or looseness. A teratologic dislocation generally will not show either positive Ortolani's or Barlow's signs but will manifest limited abduction and a positive Galeazzi's sign owing to the fixed nature of the dislocation.

AP pelvis x-ray views should be obtained in all neonates with an abnormal hip examination. Radiographs are generally normal in the child with typical dislocation of the hip in this age group. Those with dislocatable or subluxable hips will be normal. Subtle changes may be found in those children with dislocated hips. The teratologic hip dislocation is identifiable on plain radiograph. Since femoral head ossification does not occur until the ages of 4 to 6 months, interpretation of radiographs centers around the position of the proximal femoral metaphysis. Dislocation will appear as superior migration of the femoral metaphysis in relationship to Hilgenreiner's line (the horizontal line drawn through the triradiate cartilage), and lateral migration of the medial corner of the metaphysis in relationship to the ischium (Fig. 27–10).

Ultrasonography has become popular in the evaluation of the infant hip. Its exact role has yet to be defined, but it is useful in evaluating femoral head position and acetabular morphology before femoral head ossification.[30]

All infants with an abnormal hip examination should be referred for immediate orthopaedic evaluation. Initial treatment in this age group involves abduction bracing. A safe and simple method of abduction bracing is treatment with a Pavlik harness.[53,58,62]

Three to Twelve Months of Age. In the 3- to 12-month age group, positive Ortolani's and Barlow's signs will be lost. As soft tissue structures tighten, those hips that are well reduced will remain so, and those hips that are dislocated will become fixed in their dislocated position, with an inability to feel a "clunk of entry" on Ortolani's maneuver. Instead, in this age group one will see limited abduction (Fig. 27–11), compared with the normal side, and a positive Galeazzi's sign. There will be asymmetry of the skin folds about the thigh and gluteal regions.

An AP pelvis x-ray view will be more useful than in the immediate postnatal period. If the femoral heads have not yet ossified,

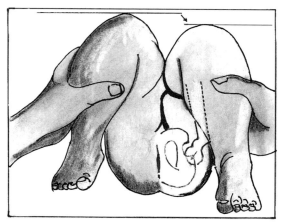

Figure 27–7. Galeazzi's sign. With the hips flexed 90 degrees, the left knee is lower than the right knee due to dislocation of the left hip.

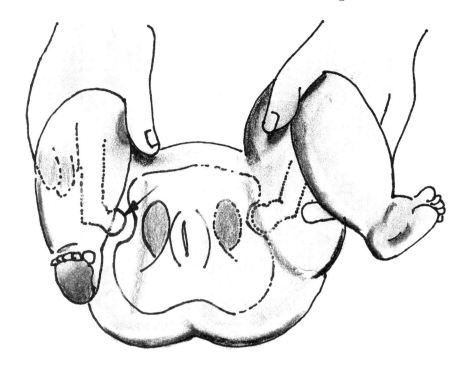

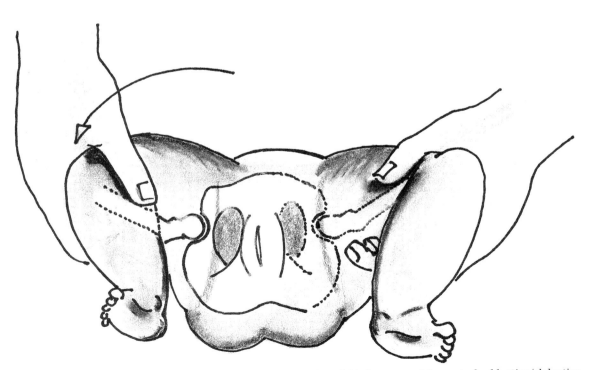

Figure 27–8. Ortolani's maneuver. *A,* Begin with the hip flexed 90 degrees and in neutral adduction/abduction. *B,* Gently abduct the hip while upward-directed pressure is applied over the greater trochanter with the examining fingers.

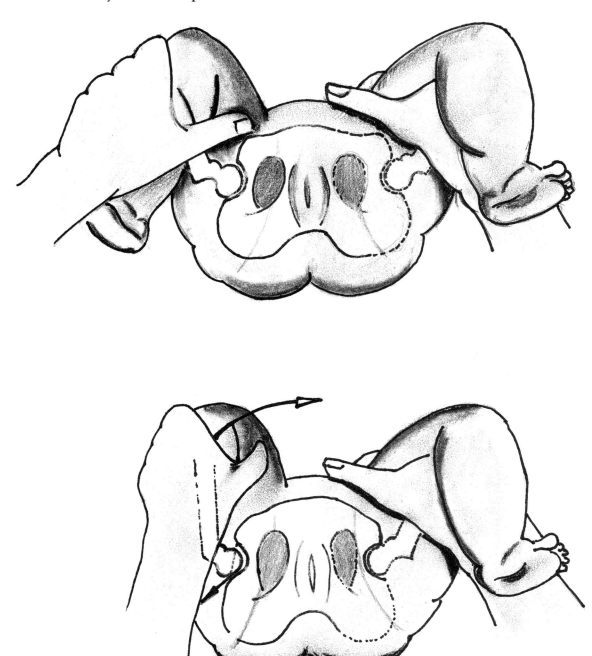

Figure 27–9. Barlow's maneuver. Gently adduct the hip and apply posterior and lateral pressure with the examining hand. Feel for the "clunk" of exit.

one should evaluate the proximal femoral metaphysis for lateral and superior migration as previously described. If the femoral heads have ossified, the ossification center should lie within the inferomedial quadrant formed by Hilgenreiner's and Perkin's lines in the normal hip (Fig. 27–12). Shenton's line, drawn through the superior aspect of the obturator foramen and the medial metaphysis of the proximal femur, should be smooth and unbroken with the leg in a neutral position (adduction of the hip will cause

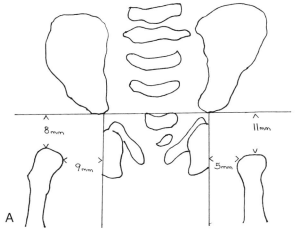

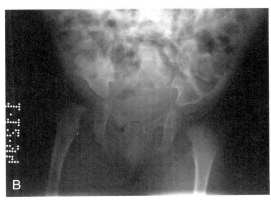

Figure 27–10. Dislocation of the right hip as seen before appearance of the ossific nuclei of the femoral heads. Note superior and lateral migration of the right proximal femoral metaphysis. *A,* Diagrammatic representation. The horizontal line is Hilgenreiner's line. *B,* Radiograph.

Shenton's line to appear broken even in the normal hip). In the dislocated hip, the ossification center of the femoral head will lie outside the inferomedial quadrant (Fig. 27–12), and there will be a break in Shenton's line.

The goal of treatment is a concentric reduction of the femoral head within the acetabulum. Strategies to achieve this involve preliminary traction and closed reduction; closed reduction, arthrogram, and spica casting under general anesthesia; and open reduction and spica cast application.[69,70]

Twelve Months or Greater (After Walking Age). After walking age, patients with DDH will present with an obvious gait abnormality. In unilateral cases, this will appear as a Trendelenburg gait (see Chapter 1). In bilateral cases, patients will have a waddling type of gait, with a trunk shift over the stance phase limb. They will show a positive Tren-

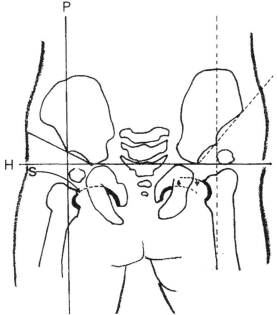

Figure 27–12. Left DDH. Hilgenreiner's line (H) is drawn through the triradiate cartilages. Perkins line (P) is perpendicular to Hilgenreiner's line drawn through the outer margin of the acetabulum. Shenton's line (S) connects the medial metaphysis of the proximal femur with the superior margin of the obturator foreman. In the dislocated left hip, the femoral head lies outside of the inferomedial quadrant formed by Hilgenreiner's and Perkin's line and Shenton's line is broken.

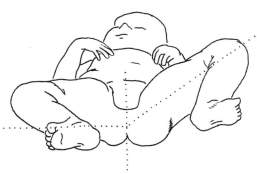

Figure 27–11. Limited abduction of the left hip secondary to developmental dislocation of the hip (DDH).

delenburg sign. Galeazzi's sign will be positive due to superior migration of the proximal femur. Abduction will be limited. Patients will not have a positive Ortolani's or Barlow's sign at this time because the hip will be irreducible.

AP pelvis x-ray views will be diagnostic. By this age the femoral head will be ossified, and there will be obvious lateral and superior migration of the femoral head. The acetabulum will be dysplastic, with an increased acetabular index (Fig. 27–13).

The treatment is aimed at concentric reduction of the femoral head within the acetabulum.[43] Significant acetabular remodeling can occur before 5 years of age. After that period of time acetabular procedures may need to be performed to obtain adequate coverage of the femoral head. Depending on the age of the child, treatment may involve preliminary traction and closed reduction, with adductor tenotomy, open reduction, femoral shortening, varus derotation osteotomy of the proximal femur, acetabular procedures, or any combination thereof.[28,39,59,63,65] As the pathologic changes become more severe and treatment becomes more difficult with time, the child should be referred immediately to the orthopaedist when the diagnosis has been made.

Congenital Abduction Contracture of the Hip

Congenital abduction contracture of the hip results from fetal malposition. It may be associated with an adduction contracture of the opposite hip, torticollis, and positional deformities of the feet. Frequently, children referred to the orthopaedist for DDH prove to have a congenital abduction contracture of the hip, as it is a more common cause of asymmetric abduction than is DDH. Physical findings involve asymmetric abduction, with the affected side held in abduction and external rotation. The opposite side may have a mild adduction contracture. When the hip on the affected side is brought into a neutral position in line with the long axis of the body, pelvic obliquity results, with the iliac crest low on the affected side. In contrast to DDH, Ortolani's and Barlow's signs are negative. AP pelvis x-ray views will show a normal relationship between the proximal femur and acetabulum. The treatment is initiated at birth and involves stretching of the involved hip into adduction.[31]

CONGENITAL DISLOCATION AND SUBLUXATION OF THE KNEE

Congenital dislocation of the knee is much less common than that of the hip. The etiology is multifactorial. Intrauterine positioning has been implicated. It may be associated with Down's syndrome, Larsen's syndrome, and arthrogryposis multiplex congenita. When seeing a child with a congenital dislocation of the knee, one should carefully examine the other joints for abnormalities, particularly the hips and feet.[22,55]

The clinical features will vary in severity from a mild subluxation and hyperextension to a complete anterior dislocation of the tibia on the femur, with severe hyperextension and limitation of flexion. AP and lateral x-ray views of the knee should be obtained. The ossification centers of the distal femur and proximal tibia are frequently not present, but the relationship of the femoral and tibial metaphyses should be noted.

Treatment begins at birth with stretching and serial casting. More severe cases may require traction or open reduction.

Congenital Pseudoarthrosis of the Tibia (Anterolateral Bow)

In spite of the name, true pseudoarthrosis of the tibia is rarely present at birth. Rather, tibial bowing with the apex anterior and lat-

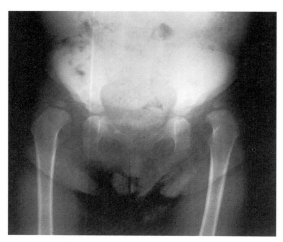

Figure 27–13. Bilateral DDH in a 19-month-old girl. Shenton's line is broken, ossific nuclei lie well outside the inferomedial quandrant, and the acetabulae are dysplastic.

eral is noted. Therefore, the condition is often called anterolateral bowing of the tibia (Fig. 27–14). The condition is extremely rare, being present in approximately 1 per 200,000 live births. Approximately 50 percent of the time it is associated with neurofibromatosis.

Presentation is usually during the first year of life, with anterolateral bowing of the tibia. AP and lateral x-ray views of the leg will show either a cystic lesion or tapering of the tibia, with bone sclerosis at the apex of the bow (Fig. 27–15).[10] Orthopaedic consultation should be obtained. Generally, the child is put in a clamshell orthosis and observed. Fracture frequently occurs through the dysplastic bone when the child begins to walk. Treatment is then aimed at obtaining union. Options include bone grafting and internal fixation, microvascular free fibula transfer, and bone transport using the Ilizarov technique.[26,57,60] The family should understand at the outset that this is a very difficult problem to treat and that amputation is always an option. Many investigators would suggest that after two or three attempts at obtaining union, amputation and fitting with a below-knee prosthesis be carried out.[52]

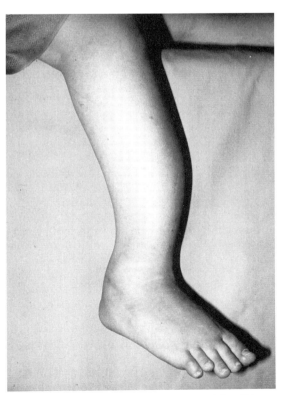

Figure 27–14. Anterolateral bowing of the tibia.

Congenital Posteromedial Bowing of the Tibia

Congenital posteromedial bowing of the tibia and fibula is obvious at birth. The apex of the bow is at the junction of the middle and distal third of the diaphysis, with the apex pointing posterior and medial. The foot is in a marked calcaneovalgus posture, with the dorsum of the foot against the anterolateral surface of the leg.[56] There is, on the average, 10 to 15 percent shortening of the involved tibia.

Radiographs show the obvious bowing, but the cystic or sclerotic changes present in congenital pseudoarthrosis (anterolateral bow) are not seen (Fig. 27–16). The tibial and fibular cortices on the concave side of the bow will be moderately thickened due to stress.

The natural history of posteromedial bow is much more benign than that of anterolateral bow. The bowing spontaneously corrects, with 50 percent of the angulation resolving by 2 years of age. There is no risk of developing a pathologic fracture or pseudoarthrosis. The overall shortening of the tibial segment remains as a constant percentage of the length of the normal side. Serial leg length comparisons should be obtained throughout growth.[37] Generally, the limb length discrepancy can be managed prior to skeletal maturity with epiphysiodesis (growth plate arrest) of the contralateral proximal tibia and fibula.

THE FOOT

Before embarking on a discussion of various foot deformities, the reader is referred to Chapter 10 for a discussion of foot anatomy, and to Chapter 1 for examination techniques. Vanderwilde and coworkers have published standards of the radiographic anatomy of the normal foot.[77]

The radiographic evaluation of children's foot deformities includes AP, lateral, and oblique x-ray views of the foot (standing when possible) and AP and lateral ankle x-ray views. Occasionally it is necessary to obtain forced dorsiflexion and plantar flexion lateral views to evaluate ankle and hindfoot motion.

Calcaneovalgus Foot

Calcaneovalgus is a postural deformity that results in dorsiflexion and eversion of the

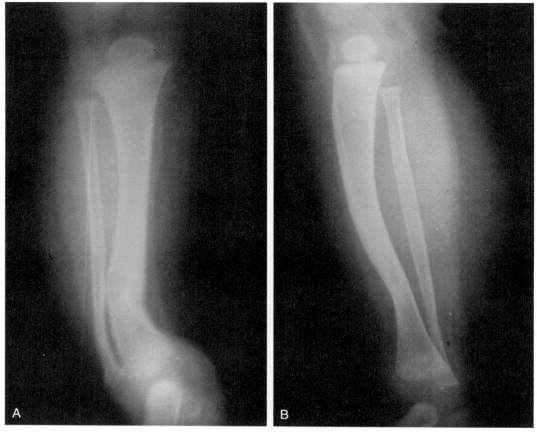

Figure 27–15. Radiographs of a child with anterolateral bowing of the tibia. *A*, AP view; *B*, Lateral view.

foot. In severe cases the dorsum of the foot may be touching the anterolateral surface of the leg. This is the most common foot deformity seen at birth. It may be secondary to intrauterine malpositioning, as there is a higher incidence in firstborn children of young mothers. Clinically, the entire foot, including the hindfoot, is dorsiflexed. This distinguishes calcaneovalgus foot from congenital vertical talus (in which the hindfoot is plantar flexed and the midfoot/forefoot dorsiflexed). If there is doubt about the differential diagnosis, AP and lateral radiographs of the foot can be obtained. These will disclose normal talocalcaneal angles on both AP and lateral views and a normal hindfoot/midfoot relationship.

A careful neurologic examination should be carried out with particular attention taken to demonstrate function of the gastrocsoleus musculature. Occasionally, a calcaneovalgus foot may be seen in neuromuscular conditions such as myelodysplasia. The treatment involves early stretching and occasionally casting or splinting. Generally, the deformity can be corrected within 4 to 6 weeks.

Talipes Equinovarus (Clubfoot)

In clubfoot, the entire foot is in equinus; there is hindfoot varus and forefoot adductus and supination (Fig. 27–17). The deformity may be either positional and respond to stretching and casting, or it may be true clubfoot requiring casting and operative treatment. This relatively common foot deformity is seen in the Caucasian population in a frequency of 1.2 per thousand. It is more common in blacks, orientals and polynesians. It is bilateral in 50 percent of cases.

The etiology is multifactorial. Both genetic and environmental factors play a role. There is a rapid decrease in incidence from first- to second- to third-degree relatives. The deformity is frequently encountered in children with neuromuscular syndromes, such as

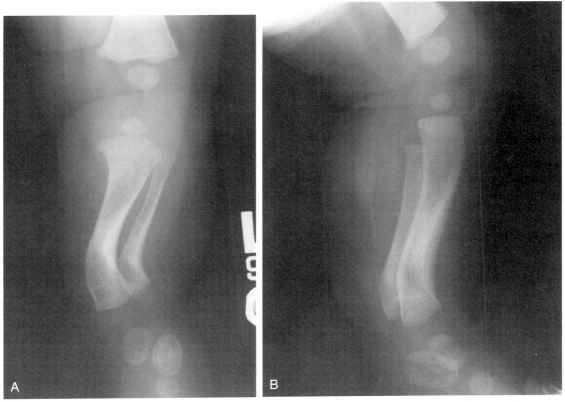

Figure 27–16. Posteromedial bowing of the tibia. Note periosteal new bone formation and thickening of the cortex along the concavity of the bow in response to stress. *A,* AP view; *B,* lateral view.

myelodysplasia and arthrogryposis multiplex congenita.

The deformity is obvious at birth. The severity and rigidity of the deformity are variable. A careful neurologic examination should be performed to rule out neuromuscular causes. The lateral border of the foot is stroked to demonstrate peroneal muscle function (eversion of the foot). Peroneal mus-

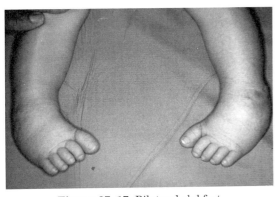

Figure 27–17. Bilateral clubfeet.

cle function may be absent due to neuromuscular causes or due to excessive stretching from the deformity.

In true clubfoot, AP and lateral x-ray views of the foot demonstrate increased parallelism of the talus and calcaneus. The talocalcaneal angle on AP projection will be less than 20 degrees, and on the lateral projection less than 25 degrees (Fig. 27–18). In postural clubfoot, talocalcaneal relationships will be normal. Radiographs are not helpful at birth because the primary ossification centers of the talus and calcaneus are small and round, making it difficult to draw lines through the long axis of the bones.

The orthopaedist should be consulted shortly after birth. This is the best time to initiate serial casting. The foot is casted every 2 weeks into a gradually corrected position. Postural clubfoot will respond to casting alone. True clubfoot will require surgical release within the first year of life.[20,76] Casting is still important in true clubfoot to obtain partial correction of the deformity and to

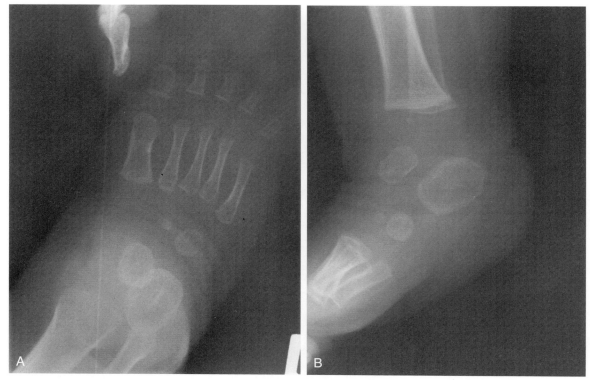

Figure 27–18. Radiographs of a clubfoot in a 4-month-old child. There is a relative parallelism of the talus and calcaneus and hind foot equinus. Note the tibiotalar relationship on the lateral projection. *A,* AP view; *B,* lateral view.

stretch out the soft tissues, facilitating surgery.

Metatarsus Adductus

Metatarsus adductus is a medial deviation of all five metatarsals at the tarsometatarsal joint. The deformity may be present at birth, but when subtle it may go unnoticed for a period of time. There is a variable amount of supination of the forefoot. The lateral border of the foot will demonstrate a convex curve. The medial border of the normal foot is concave, but this will be exaggerated in metatarsus adductus. Grasp the heel firmly in one hand and attempt to correct the deformity to judge its rigidity. Stroke the lateral border of the foot to confirm function of the peroneal musculature. The deformity can be associated with other abnormalities of intrauterine positioning, such as torticollis and DDH.

Plain radiographs will show medial deviation of the metatarsals at the metatarsophalangeal joint. The parallelism of the talus and calcaneus seen in clubfoot is not present.

Treatment for mild, flexible deformities involves stretching exercises by the parents. The heel is grasped firmly and the forefoot corrected by bringing it past the neutral position (the position in which the lateral border of the foot is straight), then holding it for 5 to 10 seconds. The foot is given a 1- to 2-second rest, and the procedure is repeated. This is done in sets of 20. It may be repeated two or three times a day. For a less flexible deformity, serial casting is needed. The casts are changed every 2 weeks. When the deformity has been rendered less severe and flexible by casting, stretching and corrective shoewear are prescribed. Straight-last shoes are used. Use of the Denis Browne bar is discouraged as this may create secondary deformities. For those deformities not responding to nonoperative treatment, surgery may be indicated. This may involve multiple metatarsal osteotomies, osteotomies through the midfoot, or release of tarsometatarsal joints.[9,34]

Congenital Vertical Talus

Congenital vertical talus is also known as congenital convex pes valgus or rocker-bottom foot. It is extremely rare. It may be idiopathic or seen in conjunction with neuromuscular disorders such as myelomeningocele or arthrogryposis.[25]

Clinically, the foot will have a rigid rocker-bottom deformity. The talus is excessively plantar flexed and medially directed in such a way that the talar head is prominent at the apex of the deformity on the plantar medial aspect of the foot. The navicular will be dorsally dislocated, lying on the dorsal neck of the talus, and will carry the rest of the midfoot and forefoot with it. Upon attempts to reduce the midfoot/forefoot by bringing it into plantar flexion, the extensor tendons and peroneal tendons will be tight. A careful neurologic examination should be performed to rule out an underlying cause. Not infrequently, the other foot will have a talipes equinovarus deformity.

The lateral x-ray view is diagnostic (Fig. 27–19). The talus will be excessively plantar flexed in a relatively vertical position. The navicular does not ossify until 3 years of age, but its position can be extrapolated from the position of the metatarsals and cuneiforms. These can be seen to be dorsally dislocated on the talus. On a forced plantar flexion lateral view, the dislocation will be irreducible.

Orthopaedic consultation should be obtained during the neonatal period to begin stretching and serial casting. Open reduction

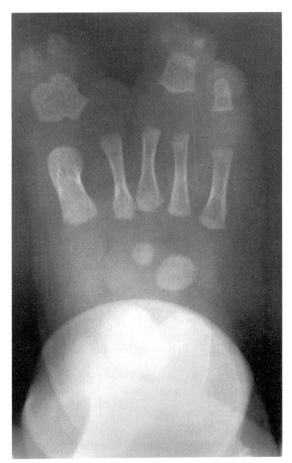

Figure 27–20. Complete, complex syndactyly of the first/second and third/fourth toes.

is indicated in resistant deformities before 1 year of age.[17,23]

Syndactyly

Syndactyly can occur in the foot as well as in the hand (Fig. 27–20). Treatment for syndactyly of the toes is less frequently indicated than in the hand. Cosmetic and functional requirements are not as stringent as with the hand. Release should be performed if syndactyly is associated with progressive angular deformity.

Polydactyly

Polydactyly of the toes is more common in the black population. It is often transmitted as an autosomal dominant trait. It may be

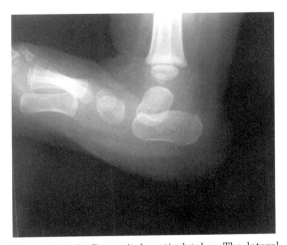

Figure 27–19. Congenital vertical talus. The lateral view shows an increased talocalcaneal angle, excessive plantar flexion of the talus, and dorsal subluxation of the midfoot/forefoot on the head of talus.

associated with polydactyly of the hand and may be seen in a variety of syndromes. Treatment involves excision before 1 year of age for both cosmetic and shoewear considerations.

ARTHROGRYPOSIS MULTIPLEX CONGENITA

Arthrogryposis multiplex congenita (AMC) is characterized by multiple joint contractures or dislocations, muscle fibrosis, and a fusiform appearance to the extremities. In actuality, it is a heterogeneous group of disorders with the classic type being known as amyoplasia. The etiology is a lack of fetal movement due to an abnormality somewhere within the motor unit (anterior horn cell, peripheral nerve, motor endplate, or muscle).

The severity is variable. Patients may manifest multiple joint dislocations and contractures at birth. A teratologic hip dislocation or a hyperextended, dislocated knee or both may be present. Foot deformities such as congenital vertical talus and clubfoot are common.

The extremities are generally fusiform, with a lack of skin creases. Pterygia (skin webbing across the flexor surfaces of the joints) is sometimes seen. Approximately one fifth of patients develop a long thoracolumbar scoliosis. Intelligence is usually normal. In decreasing order of frequency, the patterns of involvement are all four extremities, lower extremities only, and upper extremities only.

A complete discussion of the treatment of AMC is beyond the scope of this text. However, a few basic principles will be mentioned. Physical therapy, bracing, ambulatory aids such as crutches or walkers, and assistive devices for activities of daily living play a major role in the treatment of AMC. Early surgical release of soft tissue contractures is beneficial. This should be followed by aggressive physical therapy and serial casting or splinting. Hip, knee, and foot deformities should be corrected before 1 year of age. The treatment of upper extremity deformities is individualized. Patients can learn to function quite well in spite of what would seem to be devastating deformities.[32,36]

CONGENITAL CONSTRICTION BAND SYNDROME

Constriction band syndrome (CBS), or Streeter's dysplasia, is characterized by ring-like constriction bands about the extremities and occasionally the trunk. The etiology is unclear. Premature rupture of the amniotic sac with the formation of amniotic bands has been implicated. It is nonhereditary.

One or multiple bands may be present. The bands are generally at right angles to the long axis of the digit or limb. The depth of the bands varies from mild skin and subcutaneous involvement to deep bands that cause circulatory compromise. The part distal to the band may swell secondary to lymphatic or venous compromise.

Alternatively, patients may be born with transverse deficiencies of the digits or limbs resulting from in utero amputation. Other congenital anomalies of the hand, such as syndactyly, acrosyndactyly, and brachydactyly, may be seen.[73] Clubfoot and cleft lip and palate are other associated anomalies.

The treatment depends on the severity of the bands. Simple, shallow bands can be observed. Deeper bands, particularly when causing circulatory embarrassment, require immediate orthopaedic referral. The surgical treatment involves excision of the bands and transposition of Z-plasty flaps.[4]

OVERGROWTH SYNDROMES

A variety of syndromes may cause overgrowth of a digit, part of a limb, an entire limb, or true hemihypertrophy. The differential diagnosis of overgrowth syndromes includes neurofibromatosis, hemangiomata, arteriovenous fistula, and Proteus syndrome, to name a few (Fig. 27–21). Treatment is

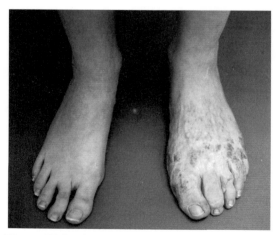

Figure 27–21. Overgrowth of the left foot secondary to hemangiomatosis.

based on the underlying cause and the severity of the overgrowth. Multiple staged debulking procedures may help. Limb length discrepancy may need to be managed with epiphysiodesis. In severe cases of overgrowth, amputation may be necessary.

NEUROFIBROMATOSIS

Neurofibromatosis is a multisystemic hereditary disorder with protean manifestations. It is autosomal dominant with variable penetrance. It is the most common single gene disorder in humans. Neurofibromatosis has been classified by the consensus panel from the National Institute of Health[54] into two types: Neurofibromatosis 1 (NF-1) is the most common and classic form, with multiple café-au-lait spots, neurofibromas, and orthopaedic manifestations. Neurofibromatosis 2 (NF-2) is characterized by bilateral acoustic neuromas and other intracranial and intraspinal tumors but without orthopaedic manifestations.

For the diagnosis of NF-1 to be made, patients must meet two or more of the following criteria:

Six or more café-au-lait spots greater than 5 mm in diameter.
Two or more neurofibromas of any type or one plexiform neurofibroma.
Axillary or inguinal freckling.
Optic glioma or two or more Lisch's nodules.
A first-degree relative with the diagnosis of NF-1.
A typical bone lesion of neurofibromatosis.

Café-au-lait spots are the most common manifestation of neurofibromatosis, being present in greater than 90 percent of patients with the diagnosis. Osseous manifestations of neurofibromatosis may include scoliosis, kyphosis, congenital pseudoarthrosis of the tibia or forearm, overgrowth syndromes, and erosive lesions of bone.

Once the diagnosis of neurofibromatosis has been made, a multidisciplinary approach is appropriate, with the pediatrician, neurologist, orthopaedist, and geneticist being involved. Magnetic resonance imaging of the brain and spinal cord is indicated. AP and lateral x-ray views of the cervical and thoracolumbosacral spine should be obtained. For further discussion of treatment of the orthopaedic manifestations, the reader is referred to the classic article by Crawford and Bagamery.[21]

OSTEOGENESIS IMPERFECTA

Osteogenesis imperfecta (OI) is a heterogeneous group of disorders characterized by bone fragility and other evidence of connective tissue dysfunction, such as dentinogenesis imperfecta and blue sclerae. It is due to a defect in the production or structure of Type I collagen. The phenotype will vary depending on the nature of the mutation.[12]

OI has been classified by Sillence and coworkers[66,67] into four types:

Type I is a mild phenotype with multiple fractures in childhood and decreasing fracture frequency with maturity. There is mild short stature and minimal bowing deformity. It is autosomal dominant.
Type II is the perinatal lethal variety, with 80 percent of children dying before their first year.
Type III is progressive and nonlethal. These patients are generally nonambulators and suffer severe bowing and short stature.
Type IV is of variable severity, falling between Types I and III in regard to deformity, short stature, and fracture frequency.

The presentation depends on the severity of involvement. Those with Types II and III will be born with multiple fractures and severe deformity of the long bones. Patients with Type I may have few fractures during childhood and no obvious bone deformity. Scoliosis may develop and is more common in those with more severe involvement. Although blue sclerae have been considered a hallmark of OI, it should be noted that not all patients with OI will manifest blue sclerae, and that normal infants may have a mild bluish tint to their sclerae. Patients may also have abnormal dentition and conductive hearing loss.

X-ray findings will vary with severity (Fig. 27–22). Patients with Type II OI will be born with crumpled "accordion" femora, bowing of the other long bones, beaded ribs, and poor ossification of the cranium with wormian bones. Fractures may or may not be present. Thin, gracile bones may be seen in patients with Types III and IV OI. Patients with Type III OI frequently will have multiple fractures

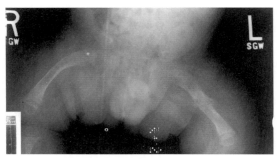

Figure 27–22. Bowing of the right femur and healing fracture of the left femur in a child with osteogenesis imperfecta.

at birth and bowing of the long bones. Patients with Type I OI will present for x-ray evaluation of fracture, and the long bone morphology is frequently normal.

No laboratory test is pathognomonic for OI. Differentiating between child abuse and the milder forms of OI may be important when a child suffers a fracture after minimal trauma or when there is a sketchy history. In Type II (perinatal lethal) OI, the differential diagnosis includes hypophosphatasia and other lethal skeletal dysplasias. Biochemical testing is helpful in the differential diagnosis. This involves skin biopsy under local anesthesia, culturing of dermal fibroblasts, and gel electrophoresis of collagen produced by the fibroblasts. Gel electrophoresis will show abnormalities in greater than 85 percent of patients with a phenotype consistent with OI.[78]

The orthopaedic treatment for perinatal fractures involves early casting and splinting. Those with severe bone fragility will need to have constructed a custom turtle shell type of orthosis so that they can be carried by the parents without suffering fractures. Early osteotomy and intramedullary rodding to correct long bone deformity is frequently indicated and may improve ambulatory function.[51] Scoliosis is difficult to treat with bracing, and early fusion is indicated.

References

1. Aitken GT: Proximal Femoral Focal Deficiency. Washington, DC, National Academy of Sciences, 1969.
2. Alter BP: Arm anomalies and bone marrow failure may go hand in hand. J Hand Surg 17A:566–571, 1992.
3. Asher M, Olson J: Factors affecting the ambulatory status of patients with spina bifida cystica. J Bone Joint Surg 65A:350–356, 1983.
4. Askins G, Ger E: Congenital constriction band syndrome. J Pediatr Orthop 8:461–466, 1988.
5. Barlow TG: Early diagnosis and treatment of congenital dislocation of the hip. J Bone Joint Surg 44B:292–301, 1962.
6. Barot LR, Caplan HS: Early surgical intervention in Apert's syndactyly. Plast Reconstr Surg 77:282–287, 1986.
7. Barsky AJ: Cleft hand: Classification, incidence, and treatment. Review of the literature and report of nineteen cases. J Bone Joint Surg 46A:1707–1720, 1964.
8. Bayne LG, Klug MS: Long-term review of the surgical treatment of radial deficiencies. J Hand Surg 12A:169–179, 1987.
9. Berman A, Gartland JJ: Metatarsal osteotomy for the correction of adduction of forepart of the foot in children. J Bone Joint Surg 53A:498–506, 1971.
10. Boyd HB: Pathology and natural history of congenital pseudarthrosis of the tibia. Clin Orthop 166:5–13, 1982.
11. Bradford DS, Ganjavian S, Antonious D, Winter RB, Lonstein JE, Moe JH: Anterior strut-grafting for the treatment of kyphosis. J Bone Joint Surg 64A:680–690, 1982.
12. Byers PH, Wallis GA, Willing MC: Osteogenesis imperfecta: Translation of mutation to phenotype. J Med Genet 28:433–442, 1991.
13. Canale ST, Griffin DW, Hubbard CN: Congenital muscular torticollis: A long-term follow-up. J Bone Joint Surg 64A:810–816, 1982.
14. Carson WG, Wood WL, Whitesides TE: Congenital elevation of the scapula. J Bone Joint Surg 63A:1199–1207, 1981.
15. Choi H, Kumar SJ, Bowen JR: Amputation or limb-lengthening for partial or total absence of the fibula. J Bone Joint Surg 72A:1391–1399, 1990.
16. Chou SN: The treatment of paralysis associated with kyphosis; Role of anterior decompression. Clin Orthop 128:149–154, 1977.
17. Coleman SS, Stelling FH III, Jarrett J: Pathomechanics and treatment of congenital vertical talus. Clin Orthop 70:62–72, 1970.
18. Coleman SS: Diagnosis of congenital dysplasia of the hip in the newborn infant. Clin Orthop 247:3–12, 1989.
19. Coventry MB, Harris LE: Congenital muscular torticollis in infancy: Some observations regarding treatment. J Bone Joint Surg 41A:815–822, 1959.
20. Crawford AH, Marxen JL, Osterfeld DL: The Cincinnati incision: A comprehensive approach for surgical procedures of the foot and ankle in childhood. J Bone Joint Surg 64A:1355–1358, 1982.
21. Crawford AH, Bagamery N: Osseous manifestations of neurofibromatosis in childhood. J Pediatr Orthop 6:72–88, 1986.
22. Curtis BH, Fisher RL: Congenital hyperextension with anterior subluxation of the knee: Surgical treatment and long-term observations. J Bone Joint Surg 51A:255–269, 1969.
23. DeRosa GP, Ahlfeld SK: Congenital vertical talus: The Riley experience. Foot Ankle 5:118–124, 1984.
24. Dias LS: Surgical management of knee contractures in myelomeningocele. Pediatr Orthop 2:127–131, 1982.
25. Drennan JC, Sharrard WJW: The pathological anatomy of convex pes valgus. J Bone Joint Surg 53B:455–461, 1971.

26. Fabry G, Lammens J, Van Melkebeek J, et al.: Treatment of congenital pseudarthrosis with the Ilizarov technique. J Pediatr Orthop 8:67–70, 1988.

27. Fairbank HAT: Cranio-cleido-dysostosis. J Bone Joint Surg 31B:608–617, 1949.

28. Galpin RD, Roach JW, Wenger DR: One-stage treatment of congenital dislocation of the hip in older children, including femoral shortening. J Bone Joint Surg 71A:734–741, 1989.

29. Gibson DA, Carroll N: Congenital pseudarthrosis of the clavicle. J Bone Joint Surg 2B:644–652, 1970.

30. Graf R: Fundamentals of sonographic diagnosis of infant hip dysplasia. J Pediatr Orthop 4:735–740, 1984.

31. Green NE, Griffin PP: Hip dysplasia associated with abduction contracture of the contralateral hip. J Bone Joint Surg 64A:1273, 1982.

32. Hall JG: An approach to research on congenital contractures. Birth Defects 20:8–30, 1984.

33. Hensinger RN, Lang JE, MacEwen GD: Klippel-Feil syndrome: A constellation of associated anomalies. J Bone Joint Surg 56A:1246–1253, 1974.

34. Heyman CH, Herndon CH, Strong JM: Mobilization of the tarsometatarsal and intermetatarsal joints for the correction of resistant adduction of the forepart of the foot in congenital clubfoot or congenital metatarsus varus. J Bone Joint Surg 40A:299–310, 1958.

35. Hoffer MM, Feiwell E, Perry R, et al.: Functional ambulation in patients with myelomeningocele. J Bone Joint Surg 55A:137–148, 1973.

36. Hoffer MM, Swank S, Eastman F, et al.: Ambulation in severe arthrogryposis. J Pediatr Orthop 3:293–296, 1983.

37. Hofmann A, Wenger DR: Posteromedial bowing of the tibia: Progression of discrepancy in leg lengths. J Bone Joint Surg 63A:384–388, 1981.

38. Hummer CD, Jr., MacEwen GD: The coexistence of torticollis and congenital dysplasia of the hip. J Bone Joint Surg 54A:1255–1256, 1972.

39. Kasser JR, Bowen JR, MacEwen GD: Varus derotation osteotomy in the treatment of persistent dysplasia in congenital dislocation of the hip. J Bone Joint Surg 67A:195–202, 1985.

40. Koman LA, Meyer LC, Warren FH: Proximal femoral focal deficiency. Clin Orthop Rel Res 162:135–143, 1982.

41. Leibovic SJ, Ehrlich MG, Zaleske DJ: Sprengel deformity. J Bone Joint Surg 72:192–197, 1990.

42. Lindseth RE, Stelzer L, Jr: Vertebral excision for kyphosis in children with myelomeningocele. J Bone Joint Surg 61A:699–704, 1979.

43. Lindstrom JR, Ponseti IV, Wenger DR: Acetabular development after reduction in congenital dislocation of the hip. J Bone Joint Surg 61A:112–118, 1979.

44. Lonstein JE, Winter RB, Moe JH, Bradford DS, Chou SN, Pinto WC: Neurologic deficits secondary to spinal deformity: A review of the literature and report of forty-three cases. Spine 5:331–355, 1980.

45. Lorber J: Results of treatment of myelomeningocele: An analysis of 524 unselected cases, with special reference to possible selection for treatment. Dev Med Child Neurol 13:279–303, 1971.

46. Mazur J, Menelaus MB, Dickens DR, et al.: Efficacy of surgical management for scoliosis in myelomeningocele: Correction of deformity and alteration of functional status. J Pediatr Orthop 6:568–575, 1986.

47. McLaughlin JF, Shurtleff DB, Lamers JY, et al.: Influence of prognosis on decisions regarding the care of newborns with myelodysplasia. N Engl J Med 312:1589–1594, 1985.

48. McMaster MJ, Ohtsuka K: The natural history of congenital scoliosis: A study of two hundred and fifty-one patients. J Bone Joint Surg 64A:1128–1147, 1982.

49. McMaster MJ: Occult intraspinal anomalies and congenital scoliosis. J Bone Joint Surg 66A:588–601, 1984.

50. Menelaus MB: The hip in myelomeningocele: Management directed towards a minimum number of operations and a minimum period of immobilisation. J Bone Joint Surg 58B:448–452, 1976.

51. Moorefield WG, Miller GR: Aftermath of osteogenesis imperfecta: The disease in adulthood. J Bone Joint Surg 62A:113–119, 1980.

52. Morrissy RT: Congenital pseudarthrosis of the tibia: Factors that affect results. Clin Orthop 166:21–27, 1982.

53. Mubarak S, Garfin S, Vance R: Pitfalls in the use of the Pavlik harness for treatment of congenital dysplasia, subluxation, and dislocation of the hip. J Bone Joint Surg 63A:1239–1248, 1981.

54. National Institutes of Health: Neurofibromatosis. Consensus Development Conference Statement 6(12):13, 1987.

55. Niebauer JJ, King DE: Congenital dislocation of the knee. J Bone Joint Surg 47A:207, 1960.

56. Pappas AM: Congenital posteromedial bowing of the tibia and fibula. J Pediatr Orthop 4:525–531, 1984.

57. Paterson D: Congenital pseudarthrosis of the tibia. Clin Orthop 247:44–54, 1989.

58. Pavlik A: Stirrups as an aid in the treatment of congenital dysplasias of the hip in children. J Pediatr Orthop 9:157–159, 1989.

59. Pemberton PA: Pericapsular osteotomy of the ilium for treatment of congenital subluxation and dislocation of the hip. J Bone Joint Surg 47A:65–86, 1965.

60. Pho RW, Levack B, Satku K, et al.: Free vascularized fibular graft in the treatment of congenital pseudarthrosis of the tibia. J Bone Joint Surg 67B:64–70, 1985.

61. Pizzutillo PD: Klippel-Feil syndrome. *In* Cervical Spine. Philadelphia, J.B. Lippincott, 1983, pp. 174–188.

62. Ramsey P., Lasser S, MacEwen GD: Congenital dislocation of the hip: Use of the Pavlik harness in the child during the first six months of life. J Bone Joint Surg 58A:1000–1004, 1976.

63. Salter RB, Dubos J: The first fifteen years' personal experience with innominate osteotomy in the treatment of congenital dislocation and subluxation of the hip. Clin Orthop 93:72–103, 1974.

64. Samuelsson L, Bergström K, Thuomas KA, et al.: MR imaging of syringohydromyelia and Chiari malformations in myelomeningocele patients with scoliosis. Am J Neuroradiol 8:539–546, 1987.

65. Schoenecker PL, Strecker WB: Congenital dislocation of the hip in children: Comparison of the effects of femoral shortening and of skeletal traction in treatment. J Bone Joint Surg 66:21–27, 1989.

66. Sillence DO, Senn A, Danks DM: Genetic heterogeneity in osteogenesis imperfecta. J Med Genet 16:101–116, 1979.

67. Sillence DO: Osteogenesis imperfecta: An expanding panorama of variants. Clin Orthop Rel Res 159:11–25, 1981.

68. Simmons BP, Southmayd WW, Riseborough EJ: Congenital radioulnar synostosis. J Hand Surg 8:829–838, 1983.

69. Simons GW: A comparative evaluation of the current methods for open reduction of the congenitally displaced hip. Orthop Clin North Am 11:161–181, 1980.

70. Stromqvist B, Sunden G: CDH diagnosed at 2 to 12 months of age: Treatment and results. J Pediatr Orthop 9:208–212, 1989.

71. Tachdjian MO: Congenital dislocation of the hip. New York, Churchill Livingstone, 1982.

72. Tachdjian MO: Pediatric Orthopaedics, 2nd ed. Philadelphia, WB Saunders, 1990.

73. Tada K, Yonenobu K, Swanson AB: Congenital constriction band syndrome. J Bone Joint Surg 4:726–730, 1984.

74. Townsend PF, Cowell HR, Steg NL: Lower extremity fractures simulating infection in myelomeningocele. Clin Orthop 144:255–259, 1979.

75. Tredwell SJ, Bell HM: Efficacy of neonatal hip examination. J Pediatr Orthop 1:61–65, 1981.

76. Turco VJ: Clubfoot: Current Problems in Orthopaedics. New York, Churchill Livingstone, 1981.

77. Vanderwilde R, Staheli LT, Chew DE, et al.: Measurements on radiographs of the foot in normal infants and children. J Bone Joint Surg 70A:407–415, 1988.

78. Wenstrup RJ, Willian MC, Starman BJ, Byers PH: Distinct biochemical phenotypes predict clinical severity in nonlethal variants of osteogenesis imperfecta. Am J Hum Genet 46:975–982, 1990.

79. Westin GW, Sakai DN, Wood WL: Congenital longitudinal deficiency of the fibula: Follow-up of treatment by Syme amputation. J Bone Joint Surg 58:492–496, 1976.

80. Winter RB, Moe JH, Wang JF: Congenital kyphosis. J Bone Joint Surg 56A:223–256, 1973.

81. Winter RB: Congenital deformities of the spine. New York, Thieme-Stratton, 1983.

82. Woodward JW: Congenital elevation of the scapula. J Bone Joint Surg 43A:219–228, 1961.

Arthritis and Degenerative Conditions

Stuart Stephenson

Virtually all individuals at some time in their life will experience pain in or about one or more areas of their axial or appendicular skeleton. In the majority of cases, these complaints tend to be self-limited and transient and resolve without further sequelae. However, an increasingly large number of patients present to their physician for a more detailed evaluation, diagnosis, and treatment. The most common diagnosis is that of osteoarthritis, but the differential diagnosis is varied (Table 28–1). Osteoarthritis is the most common form of articular disease process and is almost universal in any aging population. In fact, studies have shown that with increasing age, the pathologic process directly correlates with the age of the patient.[3]

OSTEOARTHRITIS

Osteoarthritis is often thought to be either primary, meaning no identifiable etiology, or secondary, inferring that some underlying event or disease process has resulted in specific intra-articular pathologic changes. Primary osteoarthritis, or what is classically also considered wear and tear or age-related

osteoarthritis, presents with very characteristic changes, as well as joint involvement. Universally, this is seen beginning in the fifth decade and increasing throughout the later decades of life. Classic joint involvement includes the distal interphalangeal (DIP) joints of the hands, the thumb (carpometacarpal joint; see Fig. 28–3), the hip joints, the knees, and often the first metatarsophalangeal joints of the feet. Characteristic changes from osteoarthritis are also seen involving the cervical and lumbosacral spine. When an arthropathy presents outside these classic joints or in the younger patient, one should consider the underlying etiology to be other than primary osteoarthritis, and it may have some identifiable initiating event. Despite this somewhat artificial classification, these patients' symptoms may be virtually inseparable and identical.

Pathophysiology of Osteoarthritis

Regardless of the initiating event, the joint destruction seen in osteoarthritis tends to follow a final common pathway. It has been shown that with articular cartilage damage, there is a tremendous metabolic response

TABLE 28–1.
Differential Diagnosis of Arthropathy

Type	Joints Involved	Characteristic Findings
Osteoarthritis	Finger distal interphalangeal, hips, knees, C-spine, lumbar spine, great toe metatarsophalangeal	
Rheumatoid	Spine, wrist, finger metacarpophalangeal and proximal interphalangeal, foot metatarsophalangeal, elbows, shoulders	See Figure 28–1.
Traumatic	Any	
Congenital	Any: especially weight-bearing	Deformity since birth; often short stature; abnormal epiphysis and joint shape on x-ray film
Gout	Knees, great toe metatarsophalangeal joint	Extreme pain and erythema; uric acid elevated; joint crystals on aspiration; response to indomethacin
Charcot arthropathy	Any: especially feet/ankle	History of neurologic disease or diabetes; extreme joint deformity, often with open ulceration; pain minimal despite deformity
Ankylosing spondylitis	Thoracolumbar spine, hips	Male predominance; (+) HLA B-27; limited chest expansion; increasing kyphosis; marked hip flexion contractures
Chondrocalcinosis	Any: especially knees, shoulders	Periarticular and articular joint calcification on x-ray film; CPPD crystals on aspiration; see Figure 28–2
Reiter's syndrome	Any: especially weight-bearing	Urethritis and conjunctivitis; balanitis common; joint involvement asymmetric and acutely inflamed
Psoriatic arthritis	Fingers and toes	Nail bed involvement, classic skin rash; "swollen sausage-like" changes of fingers
Septic arthritis	Any	Febrile, severe pain with joint motion; marked erythema of joint; significant WBC elevation of serum and joint fluid in most cases

at the level of the chondrocyte. Many complex biochemical changes occur, including enzyme release and synthesis, cartilage metaplasia, increasing water content, and an overall change in the morphologic composition of the collagen network itself.[1] It is not known whether this increased metabolic activity is an attempt at repair or the response to continual joint damage.

Not only are physiologic changes occurring at the joint level, but there are mechanical factors as well. This is especially evident in the weight-bearing joints. With changes at the articular level, the joints undergo mechanical changes such that normal joint stress transfer is lost. This probably acts to further joint destruction.

There are also characteristic bone changes in the periarticular area: subchondral sclerosis, bone thickening, and osteophyte formation. These physiologic and mechanical changes occurring simultaneously tend to

perpetuate each other, so that the changes continue in a cyclical fashion and result in progressive joint damage and dysfunction.

RHEUMATOID ARTHRITIS

Rheumatoid arthritis represents the most common form of inflammatory arthritis encountered. In contrast to osteoarthritis, rheumatoid arthritis represents a systemic illness and may involve many different subsystems. Patients presenting with polyarticular complaints, especially with symptoms of fatigue, weight loss, and weakness, should be thoroughly evaluated for the possibility of having rheumatoid arthritis.

Although any joint can be affected, most commonly affected are the small joints of the hands, the wrists, the knees, and the feet. Usually the joint involvement is multiple and often bilateral and symmetric. In the later

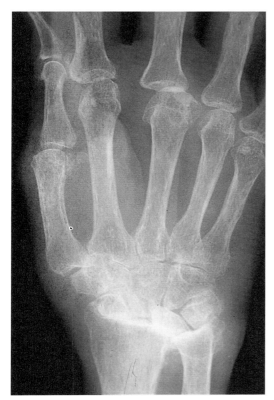

Figure 28–1. Radiograph showing wrist destruction and metacarpal changes characteristic of rheumatoid arthritis.

once the diagnosis has been established, rheumatoid arthritis should be treated medically with the appropriate chemotherapeutic agent. Persistence of symptoms despite adequate medical management can be treated surgically with early synovectomy of the involved joint. Early referral and early surgical synovectomy not only may significantly decrease a patient's symptoms, but also may prolong the time to formation of the characteristic bone and joint changes.[2] Early surgical synovectomy or tenosynovectomy, especially in the hand and knee when appropriate, have been the most useful procedures to date. The remainder of the surgical treatment for rheumatoid arthritis is similar to that of osteoarthritis.

PATIENT PRESENTATION AND EVALUATION

When a patient presents for evaluation of painful joint(s), a careful history and physi-

form of the disease, virtually all joints will be involved.

Hand involvement is almost universal. Early in the disease process, swelling of the proximal interphalangeal joints and the symmetric swelling of the metacarpophalangeal joints is quite common. Classic late deformities are the swan neck deformity, which is hyperextension of the PIP joint with flexion of the DIP joint, and the boutonnière deformity, which is flexion of the PIP joint and extension of the DIP joint. Wrist disease is usually seen with swelling on the dorsal aspect of the wrist and a palpable boggy synovium.

Another joint involved early in the disease process is the knee. Synovial thickening and chronic effusion can be present and can be quite disabling. In the foot, synovitis of the metatarsophalangeal joint is common and will ultimately lead to impressive subluxation of the metatarsal heads.

With a few exceptions, many of the treatments for osteoarthritis are similar to the treatment of rheumatoid arthritis. Initially,

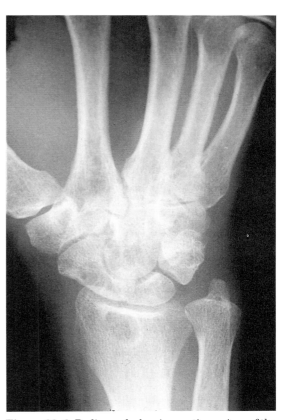

Figure 28–2. Radiograph showing cystic erosions of the distal radius and scaphoid typical of the periarticular changes of calcium pyrophosphate dihydrate (CPPD) crystals.

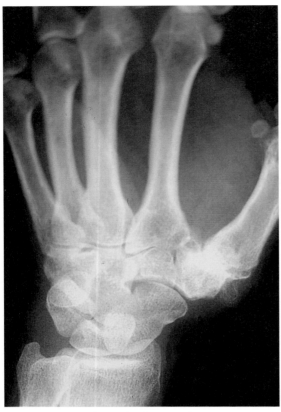

Figure 28–3. Radiograph showing classic carpometacarpal osteoarthritis.

cal examination should always be performed. Specific attention should be directed toward ruling out any of the inflammatory conditions that also result in arthralgic symptoms. The history should review carefully any fevers, rashes, or neurologic changes that would be more indicative of a systemic inflammatory condition. The patient with an osteoarthritic process will more commonly report discomfort and swelling related to activity as well as some component of night pain. Simple overuse symptoms rarely result in night pain and are more commonly the result of some mild periarticular bursitis or tendinitis. In differentiating between primary or secondary osteoarthritis, the patient may relay a past history of trauma, joint injury, occupational activity, and so on, that has resulted in progressive joint symptoms. There may or may not be an enlargement of the joint due either to mechanical changes or intra-articular effusion. Excess warmth is often indicative of an inflammatory process and should be investigated thoroughly to

rule out septic arthritis or crystal-induced change.[2]

Synovial fluid, if analyzed for diagnosis, should have a benign appearance. Usually the fluid is straw colored, clear, or slightly turbid. There should be a very small fibrin clot, with a good mucin clot. If the aspiration is done in an atraumatic manner, the white blood cell count should be in the range of less than 2000 to 3000, with a very low polymorphonuclear count. The glucose level should be approximately that of the serum level. Fluid should also be sent for crystal analysis as well as culture and sensitivity studies. The serum laboratory values should be normal and not indicative of an inflammatory condition. Laboratory values often checked are calcium, phosphorus, alkaline phosphatase, CBC with differential, erythrocytic sedimentation rate, and usually a rheumatoid profile.

Plain x-ray evaluation should, in most cases, be almost pathognomonic. Weight-bearing films are often obtained to show more accurately the mechanical situation. Radiographs should show cartilage space loss, osteophytes, and bone sclerosis limited to the subchondral area. The presence of small cysts in and about the joint is not unusual although they may be seen with other articular disease processes.

TREATMENT

As will be discussed in some detail later, once the diagnosis of primary or secondary osteoarthritis is made, the initial treatment is directed toward controlling symptoms. Depending upon the site of involvement and the activity level of the patient, temporary rest (such as with a removable splint to decrease joint motion) and reassurance often suffice to relieve the patient's symptoms. Often a permanent activity restriction will enable the patient to recover from the acute period of the symptoms, and maintaining this restriction may be all the treatment needed. With involvement of a weight-bearing joint, a cane in the opposite hand significantly lessens joint forces and symptoms.

The use of nonsteroidal anti-inflammatory drugs does appear in a majority of patients to alter the physiologic and biomechanical changes to such a degree that patients report improved symptoms. This alteration, regardless of the mechanism of action, probably serves to decrease the intraosseous and intra-articular pressures to such a degree that patients report symptomatic improvement. However, especially in an increasing number of elderly patients, these drugs do have significant and serious side effects and may not be safely used over a long period of time.

The role of intra-articular steroid injections is likewise controversial, and the mechanism of action is poorly understood. Intra-articular injections do carry the risk of iatrogenic injury, including further cartilage damage as well as the introduction of bacterial contaminants.[4] There is a correlation between long-term intra-articular steroid use and the acceleration of articular or peri-articular degradation.

Weight reduction should be strongly encouraged in obese patients. Forces on the lower extremity are increased three- to four-fold when weight-bearing is applied. Therefore, any mild reduction in overall weight substantially lessens the mechanical forces placed across the joint. Isometric or isotonic exercises may be prescribed in an attempt to strengthen the periarticular structures, with special attention to minimize the amount of transarticular stresses.

SURGICAL ALTERNATIVES

When a patient continues to be symptomatic despite several months of treatment with the foregoing modalities, alternatives for joint reconstruction must be considered. A careful discussion with the patient must be made to determine how much pain is present, how much the lifestyle has been altered by the arthritic joint, and whether or not a surgical procedure and its ensuing rehabilitation are justified. Several general comments can be made about the surgical approach. The patient's age and expectations are key elements. The patient's overall activity level, the number of joints affected, and the degree of deformity all play a role in determining the type and timing of reconstruction.

Depending on the joint involved, several different approaches may be taken. Arthroscopy with joint debridement can be used in certain joints to lessen symptoms and give temporary relief. Osteotomies, a technique in which the alignment of the joint is changed to improve mechanical stress forces, may be

a good alternative in the younger patient. Arthrodesis is a technique in which the joint is fused into a functional alignment but all joint movement is lost. Joint replacement or arthroplasty is continuing to gain widespread acceptance and, despite limitations, tends to offer the best long-term results to the majority of patients.

The key element before a patient is sent for surgical evaluation always should be a careful consideration of that patient's ability to handle a surgical procedure physiologically and emotionally, as well as the ability to participate in postoperative physical rehabilitation.

SURGICAL APPROACHES TO SPECIFIC JOINT INVOLVEMENT

Hand

Characteristic changes seen in the hand include involvement of the distal interphalangeal (DIP) joint characterized by the formation of Heberden's nodes. Mucous cysts over the dorsum of the DIP joint result from the underlying osteophytic spur. These are spur formations with cystic erosion, usually on the dorsolateral aspect of the joint. Lateral deviation of this joint is also common.

Fusion of this joint offers an excellent functional and aesthetic outcome with little interim disability. Similar changes may be seen in the proximal interphalangeal joint, less commonly leading to deformities known as Bouchard's nodes. The treatment is similar to that of the DIP. Osteoarthritis of the trapeziometacarpal joint of the thumb is very common, especially in women over age 45 years. When symptoms interfere with daily activities, an arthrodesis or arthroplasty may be warranted (Fig. 28–3).

Shoulder

Although not usually felt to be a site of primary osteoarthritis involvement, and probably more of a secondary phenomenon, many patients will present with arthritic changes in the acromioclavicular joint (Fig. 28–4).

Care should be taken to differentiate this from simple rotator cuff bursitis or tear (see Chapter 21). With the persistence of symptoms, resection of the acromioclavicular joint, whether by open or arthroscopic

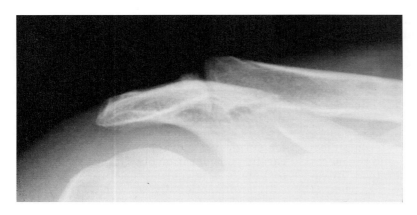

Figure 28–4. Radiograph showing spur formation and narrowing of the acromioclavicular joint.

debridement, often provides dramatic relief from symptoms.

Hip

Patients presenting with hip involvement may report a variety of symptoms. There is a good deal of overlap between the symptoms of lumbosacral osteoarthritis, hip osteoarthritis, and changes involving the knee. A patient may present primarily with knee pain. However, this may be a referred pain from more significant involvement of the hip. Therefore, patients presenting with knee pain should have careful assessment of their hip and knee, including a range of motion examination as well as a screening radiograph (Fig. 28–5).

Hip fusion for the younger patient, although not often done, can provide excel-

lent long-term pain relief with a reasonably good functional return at a very high activity level. Of all the arthroplasty procedures performed, the hip has continued to give one of the best long-term results in patient satisfaction, with good pain relief and little modification of activities.

With recent advances made throughout the 1980s and 1990s, hip replacements can be offered to an increasingly large patient population. Despite continual concerns over prosthetic loosening and ultimate long-term wear, replacement does offer an excellent treatment alternative.

Knee

Patients presenting with osteoarthritis of the knee will also very commonly present with

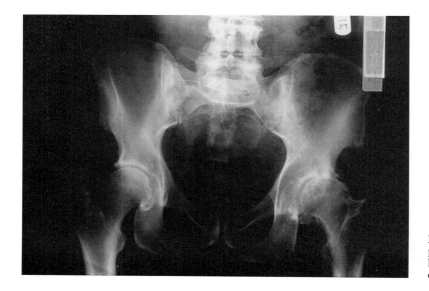

Figure 28–5. Hip film of a patient with the typical acetabular and femoral head changes of osteoarthritis.

a characteristic mechanical deformity. Usually this is a varus or (bow-legged) deformity but can be a valgus (knock-knee) deformity. Standing radiographs are critical in the evaluation of these patients to determine this mechanical alteration (Fig. 28–6).

Depending on the degree of involvement, several different approaches can be taken. Arthroscopic debridement of the joint can provide good temporary relief; however, the patient should have minimal bone changes on radiography. Despite what was initially hoped to be a good solution, the overall results from arthroscopic debridement have not shown substantial long-term improvement in patients and in some cases may even act to accelerate the disease process.

In the young patient, knee fusion can be considered, again allowing good pain relief. However, knee fusion tends to alter gait and sitting comfort or convenience to the point at which acceptance is not widespread.

Prosthetic replacement continues to be the most common procedure performed for osteoarthritis of the knee joint. Despite dramatic improvements in the last 10 years, knee replacement results have not fully duplicated those of the hip. Overall, patient satisfaction is generally good, but postoperative rehabilitation is much more critical, and activity limitations tend to be increased.

Marked mechanical malformation, including the valgus or varus knee, can be treated with alignment osteotomies. These are particularly beneficial in the younger patient with bone changes confined to one side of the knee joint. Restoration of a more normal anatomic alignment allows off-loading of the affected knee compartment and generally provides good results. The major drawback to these procedures is that the patient usually continues to develop further arthritic changes throughout the knee, ultimately requiring prosthetic replacement. As a group, patients who have undergone a realignment osteotomy tend not to do as well as those having a primary arthroplasty.

Foot and Ankle

The ankle is not commonly considered to be a classic joint involved in primary osteoarthritis, but degenerative changes within the ankle joint are becoming more common because of the increasing activity level of the population at large. Often orthotic shoe modification with soft ankle cushioned heel (SACH) heel will suffice, and no surgical procedure is required. If symptoms persist despite orthotic management, nonsteroidal anti-inflammatory agents, and walking aids; an ankle fusion is a functionally acceptable procedure and has minimal effect on the overall gait pattern. Initial attempts at ankle joint replacement have largely subsided owing to the significant difficulty with long-term wear.

Osteoarthritis of the metatarsophalangeal joint of the great toe is quite common. Again, alterations in shoe wear using a more rigid sole can provide long-term and permanent relief. Hallux rigidus presents with pain related to great toe dorsiflexion, usually in men over the age of 40 years. A dorsal bone spur is best seen on the lateral x-ray view. Removal of the bone spur greatly relieves symptoms if done prior to the development of severe arthritic changes in the joint. Although rarely required, fusion of this joint gives the best long-term result. An arthroplasty may be indicated for those patients desiring to maintain joint motion.

Spine

Within the spine, osteoarthritic involvement commonly includes the posterior facet articulations, the vertebral bodies, and the intervertebral discs. Large osteophyte formation may cause neural compromise leading to a

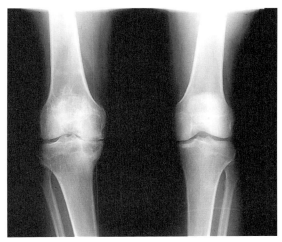

Figure 28–6. Weight-bearing knee film revealing a varus change typical of long-standing osteoarthritis.

variety of radicular and nerve root entrapment symptoms. In the cervical spine, lower segments are usually involved. Patients with cervical spine degenerative arthritis present primarily with shoulder symptoms.

In the lumbar spine, the lower segments again are the most commonly involved and usually result in lumbar canal stenosis. Evaluation by MRI scanning probably gives some of the most sensitive information about the degree of involvement. Surgical decompression with or without the use of spinal fusion continues to be a rapidly evolving area and, with continual development of new techniques, can provide an excellent functional return.

References

1. Adams ME, Grant HOA: Cartilage proteoglycan changes in experimental canine osteoarthritis. J Rheumatol 14:107–109, 1987.
2. Ogilgive-Harris DJ, Basinski A: Arthroscopic synovectomy of the knee for rheumatoid arthritis. Arthroscopy 7:91, 1991.
3. Orthopaedic Knowledge Update. Volume 3, Home Study Syllabus. American Academy of Orthopaedic Surgeons, January 1990.
4. Schumacher HR, et al: Tendon rupture following local steroid injection. Postgrad Med 68:169–175, 1980.

Casting and Splinting Techniques

P. Lauren Savage, Jr.

Victoria R. Masear

Casts and splints are effective ways to immobilize injured extremities in the emergency setting and sometimes for definitive treatment. Splints are usually faster and easier to apply and are frequently utilized in the acute care setting. Casts usually provide more effective immobilization but require more skill and time to apply, and the risk of complications may be higher.

SPLINTING TECHNIQUES

Immediate splinting of injured extremities is an important principle of emergency care. Immediate immobilization can prevent further injury during transport and triage. A number of different types of splints are available. Wire ladder, inflatable splints, preformed metal splints, and plaster splints are some of these options. All have certain shortcomings, but there are three that can be custom-fitted to the extremity: plaster splints, the wire ladder type of splints, and malleable aluminum splints. Inflatable splints are easily used, but they have the disadvantage of being compressive to the

injured extremity, and they may accentuate problems with compartment syndrome. Both malleable aluminum and wire splints may be conformed to the extremity for a custom fit.

Custom-made plaster splints are available in continuous rolls of various sizes, with 10 to 14 layers of plaster and a closed cell foam backing, all encased in stockinette. One has only to cut off the appropriate length and dip the entire splint into water before applying it. This makes for a very rapidly applied customized splint. Custom plaster splints can be made by rolling out strips of plaster and then applying sheet cotton for padding. The sheet cotton may be applied either to the plaster splints themselves or to the extremity. When constructing a custom-made plaster splint, usually about 10 to 14 layers of plaster are used (Fig. 29–1). A few less may be used in an upper extremity, or a few more may be needed in a lower extremity. This can be varied depending on the individual and the size of the splint constructed.

The water into which the plaster is dipped should be room temperature; it should not be warm. Warm dip water will put the patient at

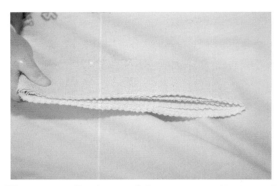

Figure 29-1. Dry layers of plaster prior to dipping and laminating.

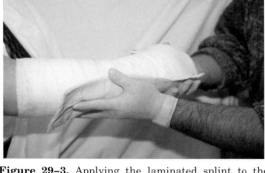

Figure 29-3. Applying the laminated splint to the extremity.

risk for developing a thermal injury since the plaster cures with an exothermic reaction. When the plaster splints are wet, they are laminated together by laying them on a flat surface and pressing them together (Fig. 29-2). The splint is then applied to the extremity, and sheet cotton, an Ace wrap, or both may be used to hold the splint in place (Figs. 29-3 and 29-4).

The advantages of splinting an extremity as opposed to casting are that the splint is a noncircumferential dressing so it is more forgiving with regard to compartment syndrome and swelling. Also, the splint may be removed more easily than a cast in order to check wounds or the condition of the skin. Splints may be used as initial emergency treatment for injuries prior to definitive treatment, and in some cases simple splinting may be appropriate as a definitive treatment. The ulnar gutter splint (see Fig. 29-4) begins at the proximal palmar crease and extends along the ulna to the elbow flexion crease. If the injury being treated is distal to

the wrist, the splint may be extended beyond the metacarpophalangeal (MP) joints to include the fingers.

Long arm posterior splints extend from the axilla across the posterior surface of the elbow and along the ulna to the proximal palmar crease (Fig. 29-5). Coaptation-type splints are U-shaped splints that extend from the axilla down around the elbow and then back proximally around the humerus over the shoulder (Fig. 29-6). The sugartong splint (Fig. 29-7) extends from the MP flexion crease along the volar forearm and wraps around the posterior surface of the elbow, onto the dorsal surface of the forearm, and then distally to the metacarpal heads. This splint will immobilize the entire forearm to supination and pronation, as well as the wrist and the elbow to some degree. Volar and dorsal forearm splints (Fig. 29-8) are applied only to their respective surfaces and may be used to immobilize the wrist as well as the forearm while allowing elbow motion and supination and pronation. Gauntlet-length wrist splints may be used to immobi-

Figure 29-2. Wet plaster layers of splint after they have been laminated together to increase the strength of the splint.

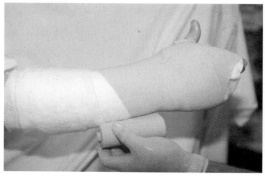

Figure 29-4. Overwrapping with elastic bandage to hold the splint in place.

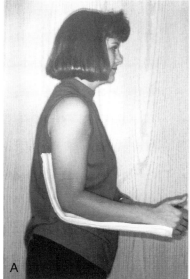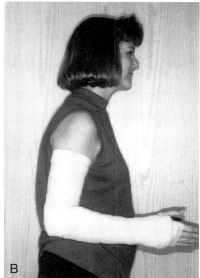

Figure 29–5. Long arm posterior splint extending from the axilla proximally to the palm distally. (From: Lee DH, Nevaiser RJ: Upper extremity fractures and dislocations. *In* Feliciano DV, Moore EE, Mattox KL (eds): *Trauma.* 3rd ed. East Norwalk, CT, Appleton & Lange, 1995.)

lize only the wrist, leaving the forearm free. Hand and digital splints (Fig. 29–9) may be stopped at either the MP joint or over the palm, depending on the level of injury and desired degree of immobilization.

In the lower extremity, splints may be used to immobilize most fractures distal to the middle portion of the femur. Medial and lateral slabs may be applied along the length of the lower extremity on the anteromedial

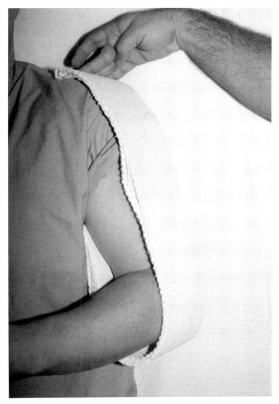

Figure 29–6. Coaptation splint—used for immobilizing middle and proximal third fractures of the humerus.

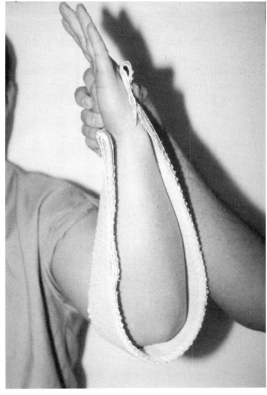

Figure 29–7. Sugartong splint.

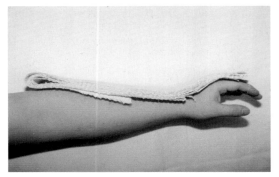

Figure 29–8. Dorsal forearm splint.

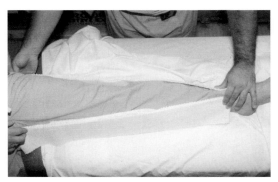

Figure 29–10. Medial and lateral slab splint for the lower extremity.

and anterolateral surfaces of the leg and thigh to immobilize distal femur fractures, fractures about the knee, and proximal tibia fractures (Fig. 29–10). Three-sided splints are used on the lower extremity to immobilize tibia fractures (Fig. 29–11). A posterior splint may be used to immobilize ankle and distal tibia fractures that do not require the heavier and more stable splints (Fig. 29–12). Three-sided splints are made by using a long posterior splint as a foot plate, which extends up the posterior surface of the leg to an appropriate height depending on the level of the fracture. The other two sides of the three-sided splint are applied medially and laterally to add stability and strength to the splint. A U splint and foot plate may be used to immobilize the ankle. This type of splint is constructed by taking a long plaster splint down the lateral side of the leg, under the heel, and then back up the medial side. This splint is kept distal to the knee. A second plaster splint is used as a foot plate to control ankle dorsiflexion and plantar flexion.

CASTING TECHNIQUES

The application of a plaster cast begins with positioning of the patient and the extremity to be casted. The dip water must be room temperature and not warm. Water that is too warm will cause the plaster to set too rapidly and, more importantly, may lead to thermal injury. When applying a cast to the upper extremity, positioning usually involves having the patient lie supine. The shoulder is abducted to 90 degrees, the elbow is flexed 90 degrees, and the digits are held up toward the ceiling. Finger traps or an assistant may be used to hold the digits and keep the arm positioned appropriately. Lower extremity casts are best applied with the patient sitting for the short leg cast and with the patient supine for either a long leg cast or a cylinder cast. For the application of the short leg and for some long leg casts, a footrest with a thin metal plate is helpful to keep the ankle at neutral position while applying the cast.

After positioning the extremity, the next step is to pad it adequately. The stockinette

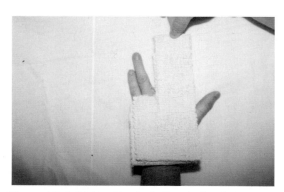

Figure 29–9. Digit splint, including the hand, for immobilizing the long and index rays.

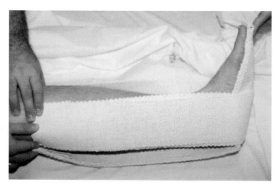

Figure 29–11. Three-sided leg splint for immobilizing an unstable ankle and distal tibia fractures.

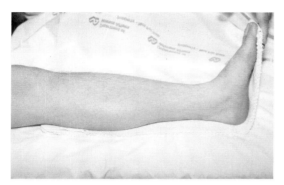

Figure 29–12. Posterior splint.

used as the first layer frequently will make the cast more comfortable and make the edges more durable. It will also help protect the patient from sharp edges of the cast. The stockinette may be applied only at the upper and lower ends, or it may be applied over the entire length of the extremity (Fig. 29–13). Three- or four-inch stockinette is preferable in the upper extremity; four- or six-inch stockinette usually works well in the lower extremity. The stockinette will expand its

circumference but will not stretch much in length.

An appropriate wadding or padding should then be chosen. There are several different varieties, but a cotton padding that stretches is more forgiving. Some padding or wadding has no stretch built into it and is more difficult to use. An appropriate width (4, 5, or 6 inch for the lower extremity and usually 2, 3, or 4 inch for the upper extremity) is chosen. The padding is rolled distally to proximally. The padding is rolled on with as few wrinkles as possible, using tears to go around joints and to advance up or down the extremity as necessary. Padding is applied with approximately 50 percent overlap (Fig. 29–14). An extra layer of padding over the heel or elbow and over the malleoli and other bone prominences will lessen problems with pressure points. Too much padding will cause the cast to fit rather loosely, will decrease the control over fracture immobilization, and increase the amount of movement possible within the cast.

An appropriate-sized plaster roll is then chosen. Usually three or four inches in the upper extremity and two inches if the thumb

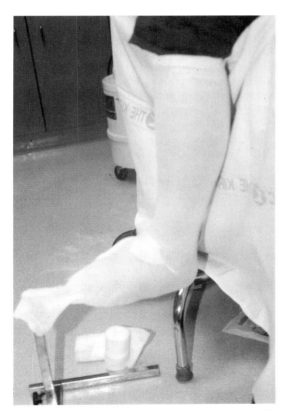

Figure 29–13. Application of a short leg cast, stockinette application.

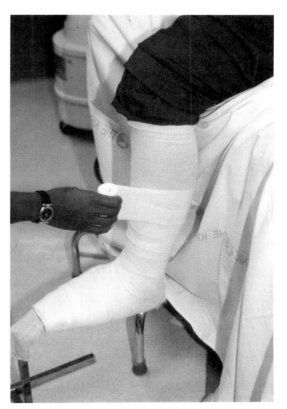

Figure 29–14. Application of sheet cotton.

is included in the cast are needed. The plaster roll is dipped into the bucket, then the center of the plaster is creased or compressed into the middle at the ends. This will keep the plaster roll from slipping out through the center. The plaster is then rolled on smoothly, beginning distally and proceeding proximally. It is not pulled tight. The roll should always be kept near the extremity to guard against stretching the plaster tightly. Tucks are taken in the plaster to turn corners or advance up the extremity. Each roll of plaster is smoothed over as it is applied, so that a strong laminate is formed between the layers. The plaster roll is advanced such that 50 percent overlap of the width of the plaster roll occurs as one advances along the extremity (Fig. 29–15). There is a tendency to place more plaster on the flexion surface of the ankle, knee, and elbow and the cast will become excessively thick in these regions. This puts the extremity at risk for thermal injury in these areas, as well as making it more difficult to remove the cast. If the extensor surface of the elbow or ankle appears to

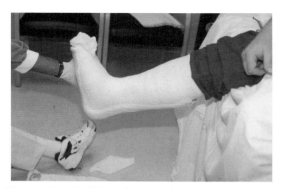

Figure 29–16. Using plaster splints to reinforce the heel of the cast.

be too thin, then several splints may be used to thicken these regions (Fig. 29–16), instead of going repeatedly about the extremity with a plaster roll, which will create excessive layers of thickness on the flexion surface. At the proximal and distal ends of the cast usually two or three layers are applied successively, because these areas tend to be some of the thinner and weaker areas of the cast. The stockinette and cast padding are then pulled back over these initial layers, and subsequent layers are applied to make a neat cast edge (Fig. 29–17). Attention should be paid to edges of the cast so that sharp points are not left protruding to cause discomfort or injury. Once application of plaster is complete, trimming of the cast around the toes or digits is frequently necessary (Fig. 29–18).

Upper Extremity Casts

The thumb spica cast is a short arm gauntlet, which extends from the proximal forearm to

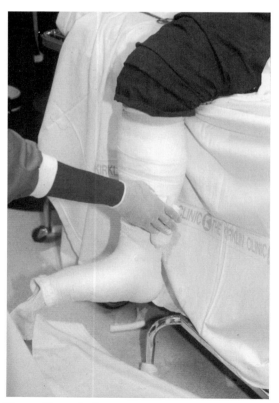

Figure 29–15. Rolling on the cast—rolling paster with 50 percent overlap.

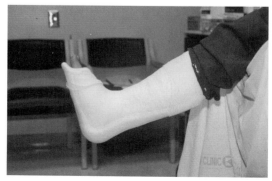

Figure 29–17. Finishing the cast edges.

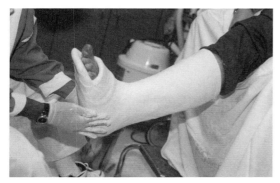

Figure 29–18. A completed short leg cast.

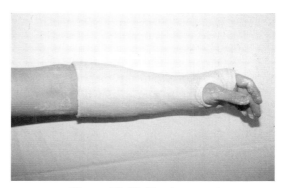

Figure 29–20. Short arm cast.

the proximal palmar crease but includes the thumb (Fig. 29–19). This cast is used for the immobilization of scaphoid or thumb fractures, or other instances in which immobilization of the thumb is desired.

The short arm cast extends from the proximal forearm to the proximal palmar flexion crease volarly and to the metacarpal heads dorsally (Fig. 29–20). Careful attention should be paid to the thumb hole and to the palm. Sharp edges should be avoided around the thumb. The cast should allow full flexion of the MP joints, as these will be at great risk for stiffening if they are immobilized. Extending the cast to the MP joints dorsally will not inhibit motion of these joints but will help control swelling.

The long arm cast (Fig. 29–21) is extended proximally to the axilla. One must be careful that too much plaster is not placed into the elbow flexion crease. If the cast is thin over the extensor surface of the elbow, a few plaster splints may be used locally in this area and incorporated into the cast. The short arm cast is used for immobilization of fractures of the distal radius or ulnar styloid fractures

or wrist injuries. Long arm casts are more appropriate for injuries to the middle third of the radius or ulna or injuries about the elbow.

Lower Extremity Casts

Short leg casts are applied with the patient in the sitting position, with the foot resting

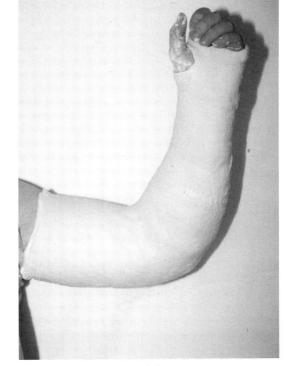

Figure 29–21. Long arm cast.

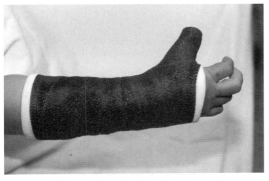

Figure 29–19. Thumb spica cast.

on a thin narrow metal foot plate. The ankle is positioned in neutral. Stockinette is applied to the leg and foot, and excess stockinette on the anterior surface of the ankle is removed. Stockinette is left long over the toes so there will be plenty to turn back. Cast padding is then applied over the toes. If one wishes to have a foot plate under the toes, the cast padding will need to extend distal to the tip of the great toe. If a foot plate is not desired, then cast padding can be stopped at the great toe MP joint.

Proximally the cast should be carried to or above the level of the tibial tubercle anteriorly and should be short enough posteriorly to be comfortable when the knee is flexed to 90 degrees. This will mean that the cast will have to be higher anteriorly than posteriorly. When rolling the plaster, one should begin distal to the toes if a foot plate is desired. Extra splints are used to reinforce the bottom of the cast in the area over the heel that will tend to be thin. After the cast has been applied, the toe section should be trimmed so that the fifth toe is visible. If a foot plate is not desired, stockinette and padding are then turned back to the level of the web spaces and another roll of plaster applied to hold the padding back. If a toe plate is desired, only the top portion of plaster is trimmed so that all toes are visible dorsally and the plaster on the sole is left intact beneath the toes (see Fig. 29–18). This area usually needs to be reinforced with more plaster to make the toe plate strong. Cast material at the proximal edge of the cast is then turned back and a roll or a splint applied about the cast circumferentially to hold back this material.

Application of the long leg cast begins with the same technique as the short leg cast. The details regarding finishing the foot of the cast are the same for the long and short casts. Once a short leg cast is begun, the plaster layers are left thin proximally so that the thigh section may be incorporated into the short leg cast. The patient may then be turned to the supine position and a leg holder placed under the short leg cast such that the knee is flexed to approximately 30 or 35 degrees. At this point, the layers of the cast are carried proximally. Layers of plaster are begun below the knee over the short leg cast and rolled proximally to incorporate the two sections. Failure to apply appropriate over-

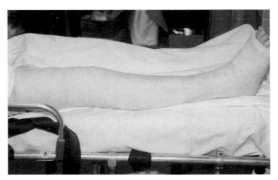

Figure 29–22. Long leg cast.

lap layers of plaster between the leg and thigh sections of the cast will result in the cast being very weak about the knee, and it will eventually break at this point. Extra padding over the distal femoral condyles and patella may be necessary to avoid pressure points in these areas. Application of the long leg cast should be proximal to the greater trochanter on the lateral surface and to within about 2 fingerbreadths of the groin medially (Fig. 29–22). Frequently, additional cast material in the form of splints will be incorporated across the knee to strengthen the cast in this region. This also helps avoid the accumulation of excess plaster over the knee flexion crease.

The cylinder cast extends from just proximal to the malleoli up to the greater trochanter (Fig. 29–23). This cast leaves the foot and ankle free but immobilizes the knee. Application of the cylinder cast begins distally with the rolling of six or more layers of sheet cotton padding. This should be above the level of the malleoli. The application of plaster begins several centimeters proximal to the

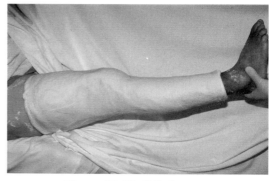

Figure 29–23. Cylinder cast.

edge of the sheet cotton at the distal end of the cast. When the sheet cotton at the distal end of the cast is turned back, an area of approximately three cm should be left between the malleoli and the lower end of the cast. If this much space is not left the cast invariably will irritate the malleoli.

The cast is then rolled proximally and the knee is kept in 5 to 10 degrees of flexion. The cast is continued proximally, and plaster is taken up to the greater trochanter on the lateral surface and as high as possible medially. The proximal edges of sheet cotton and stockinette are then turned distally and another layer applied to smooth these edges. While the cast is still malleable, it is important to apply a supracondylar mold and a suprapatellar mold. This mold keeps the cast from simply sliding down the leg. Once cast application is complete, the area over the Achilles tendon may be trimmed 1 or 2 cm and the sheet cotton in this area folded proximally. Irritation about the Achilles tendon and malleoli will be the primary problem, so adequate padding in this area, keeping the cast well proximal to the malleoli, is important.

COMPLICATIONS OF CASTING

Some of the minor complications of casting have already been mentioned: irritation to the skin caused by rough edges about the plaster and impingement of the cast on flexion surfaces of the extremity. More serious complications of casting include skin necrosis secondary to pressure, compartment syndromes, significant thermal injuries, and severe maceration of the skin secondary to immersion injury if the cast becomes wet.

An injured, swollen extremity treated with a circumferential dressing or cast is at increased risk for compartment syndrome, which, if overlooked early in its clinical course, may have a catastrophic outcome. Frequent neurovascular checks of the casted extremity are essential. These include checking capillary refill and also looking at the color of the digits to make sure they are not dusky or cyanotic. Pin-prick and light touch sensation also should be checked. Pain with passive range of motion is a classic sign. Active motion is also important, and if the patient can actively move the digits or toes, this is a good sign of normal compartment pressures. If the patient complains of severe,

unrelenting pain or that the cast simply feels too tight, then it should be split. Taking a quarter-inch strip of plaster out of the cast, spreading it slightly, and cutting the sheet cotton usually relieves the feeling of tightness. Thermal injuries are more likely with thick casts or splints, warm water dips, and fast-setting plaster. If the patient states that the cast or splint is burning the skin, it should be removed immediately and the skin checked.

Maceration can be a significant problem. If a cast has gotten wet and is made of plaster, there will probably be no way of drying it. The cast needs to be removed and reapplied after the skin has been checked. Even fiberglass casts can lead to serious problems with maceration of the skin. Casts made of fiberglass and Gore-Tex padding on top of a Gore-Tex lining can lead to problems with skin maceration even though the cast itself is not harmed by the moisture. If the cast is not thoroughly dried with warm air following exposure to or immersion in water, then significant skin problems may occur.

Pressure points inside of casts also occur. If the patient complains of pain, it is usually best to check the skin over the area. Occasionally, patients will complain of pain for some time, which then subsides. If the pain was in response to an area of pressure, this pain will be relieved only when the skin has necrosed in that area. This problem tends to occur more frequently in individuals who are immobilized in hip spica or long leg casts and who keep the leg elevated for long periods of time with pressure on the heel.

SUMMARY

1. Injured extremities are usually best splinted to prevent further trauma during transport or triage.

2. Splints tend to be more forgiving for swelling since the plaster is not circumferential.

3. The neurovascular status of extremities with circumferential bandages, whether splints or casts, should be checked frequently. A compartment syndrome is a catastrophic complication if it is not appreciated early in its course. Neurovascular checks should include tests of light touch and pinprick sensation, capillary refill, pain with

passive motion, and the ability to move toes and fingers actively.

4. The important technical aspects of splinting and casting include leaving the MP joints free in upper extremity splints and casts so they will not get stiff; flexing the ankle to 90 degrees whenever possible as long as it does not displace a fracture or is not otherwise contraindicated; adequately padding the ends and openings of all casts, including the thumb hole on upper extremity casts; avoiding placing too much plaster in flexion creases and instead using splints on the extensor surfaces opposite the flexion creases; using adequate padding applied so that it is smooth and will not indent the skin; making sure all toes are visible when casts or splints are applied to the lower extremity; being cognizant of the threat of thermal injury secondary to the exothermic reaction of gypsum-impregnated bandages when using them to make splints or casts.

Suggested Reading

1. Charnley J: The Closed Treatment of Common Fractures. Edinburgh, Churchill Livingstone, 1961, pp 1–67.
2. Colton CL: The history of fracture treatment. *In* Browner BD, Jupiter JB, Levine AM, et al. (eds): Skeletal Trauma. Philadelphia, WB Saunders, 1992, pp 3–31.
3. Harkess JW, Ramsey WC, Harkess JW: Principles of fractures and dislocations. *In* Rockwood CA, Green DP, Bucholz RW (eds): Fractures in Adults, 3rd ed. Philadelphia, JB Lippincott, 1991, pp 23–56.

Index

Page numbers in *italics* indicate illustrations.
Page numbers followed by t indicate tables.

ABC (aneurysmal bone cyst), 277–278, *278*
Abduction, defined, 1
  of fingers, 19
  of foot, 123
  of hip, 21
  of shoulder, 12, *13*
Abduction contracture, of hip, congenital, 318
Abductor digiti minimi, palpation of, 20
Abductor pollicis brevis, palpation of, 20
Abductor pollicis longus, in thumb metacarpal
    fractures, 191, *192*
  tendinitis of, 246–247, *247, 248*
Abductor pollicis longus tendon, in Bennett's fracture,
    191–192, *192*
Abscess(es), in osteomyelitis, 48
  pulp (felon), 251, *252*
  web space, 253
Acetabulum, computed tomographic scanning of,
    69, *70*
  fractures of, *66,* 68–71
    and posterior hip dislocation, *73,* 73–74
    classification of, 69–70, *70, 71*
    management of, 70–71
    radiographic evaluation of, 69, *69–70*
Achilles tendon, 228, *228*
  and cylinder cast, 345
  continuity of, Thompson test for, 31
  reflex of, 30
  retrocalcaneal bursitis and, 240
  tendinitis of, 239
Acromial fracture, 143
Acromioclavicular joint, dislocations of, 147–148, *148, 149*
  in clavicle fracture, 145
  osteoarthritis of, 333, *334*
  separation of, 243
Acromioclavicular ligament, in clavicle dislocation,
    147, 148
Adduction, defined, 1
  of fingers, 20

Adduction *(Continued)*
  of foot, 123
  of hip, 21–22
Adductor pollicis, in thumb metacarpal fractures, 191,
    192
Adolescent(s), apophyses of, 239
  clavicle fracture in, 145
  epithelioid sarcoma in, 272–273
  femoral fracture in, 86
  gonorrheal septic arthritis in, 255–256
  idiopathic scoliosis in, *297,* 297–298
  osteosarcoma in, 279
  patellar fractures in, *103,* 104
  peroneal spastic flatfoot in, 291–292, *294, 295*
  Scheuermann's kyphosis in, *298,* 298–299
  slipped capital femoral epiphysis in, 242, 290–291,
    294
  spondylolisthesis in, 61
  tibial fractures in, *104,* 105, *105,* 106
  traction apophysitis in, 239, 241, 242–243
Adson's maneuver, in thoracic outlet syndrome, 225, *225*
Advanced Trauma Life Support protocols (American
    College of Surgeons), 206
Aerobic dancers, sesamoiditis of, 137
Allen's test, 143, 224
  in ulnar artery thrombosis, 224
Allis's reduction maneuver, 74, *74*
Ambulation, aids for, in gait examination, 6
  delay in, evaluation of, 3
AMC (arthrogryposis multiplex congenita), 324
American College of Surgeons, 206
American Spinal Injury Association (ASIA), 206
Amputation(s), fingertip, *197,* 197–198
  of osteosarcoma, 280
  replantation of, 44, *44,* 198
Anaerobic cellulitis, *vs.* gas gangrene, 43
Anaerobic myonecrosis, 43

Anal wink, 207
Anatomic snuffbox, 17, 176
Aneurysm(s), *222,* 222–223, *223*
Aneurysmal bone cyst (ABC), 277–278, *278*
Animal bites, 254
Ankle(s), anatomy of, 117, *118,* 122–123
    arthritis of, surgery and, 335
    dorsiflexion of, 30, *30*
    extension of, neurologic examination of, 25
    fracture-dislocation of, 124
    fractures of, 117–127, *123–127*
        classification of, 124–125
        evaluation of, 123–124
        in children, 127
        open, 122
        radiographic imaging of, *123–124,* 124
        treatment of, 125–127, *127*
    ligamentous injuries of, 117–127
    neurologic examination of, 30–31
    orthopaedic evaluation of, 27–31
    osteoarthritis of, 335
    palpation of, 28–29
    plantar flexion of, neurologic examination of, 26
    range of motion of, 30, *30*
    splits for, 340, *340, 341*
    sprains of, 117–121, *119–121*
        diagnosis of, 117, 119t
        eversion, 117, *119*
        grading of, 118
        injuries simulating, 117, 119t
        inversion, 117, 118, *119*
            anterolateral ankle pain and, 121
        radiographic evaluation of, 117, 119–120,
            120–121
        recalcitrant, pathology associated with, 119,
            120t
        treatment of, 118–119
    stability of, 123
Ankylosing spondylitis, joints involved in, 330t
Anterior cord syndrome, 42, 207
Anterior drawer test, 117, 119, *120*
    for anterior cruciate ligament injury, 95, *95*
Anterior hip. See *Hip, anterior.*
Antibiotic therapy, for bite injuries, 254
    for felon, 251
    for hand infections, 250
    for infection of diabetic foot, 256
    for nail bed injury, 188
    in acute hematogenous osteomyelitis, 48
    in open fracture, 41, 114
    intravenous, 251
Antishock trousers, in pelvic fracture, 66
Apophysis(es), calcaneal, 295
    of adolescent, 239
    pain at, 239
Apprehension sign, positive, in patellofemoral joint
    dislocation, 99
Arch, medial, exaggeration of. See *Pes cavus.*
    flattening of. See *Pes planus.*
Arcuate complex, 89
    and lateral collateral ligament injury, 94
Arcuate ligament, 64, *64*
Arm. See also *Forearm.*
    casts for, 343, *343*
    hyperabduction of, 225
    motor innervation of, 201, *202, 203*
    muscles of, 159
    neurologic examination of, 16–17
    orthopaedic evaluation of, 15–17

Arm *(Continued)*
    physical examination of, in brachial plexus injury,
        209
    range of motion of, 16, *16*
    reflexes of, 16–17
    sensory examination of, 16
    splints for, 338–339, *339–340*
    vascular status of, in brachial plexus injury, 209
Arterial injuries, 221–222
    associated with clavicle fracture, 146
    diagnosis of, 221
    early management of, 222, *222*
    injection and, 225
    physical examination of, 221–222
Arterial lacerations, 222, *222*
Arterial thrombosis, in upper extremity, 223–226
Arteriovenous fistulas, 223
Arthralgia, evaluation of, 331–332
Arthritis, 329–336, 330t. See also specific condition,
        e.g., *Osteoarthritis.*
    evaluation for, 331–332
    pyogenic, 253–254
    rheumatoid, 330t, 330–331, *331*
    septic, 46–47
    treatment of, 332–333
        surgical alternatives in, 333
Arthrodesis, 333
Arthrogryposis multiplex congenita (AMC), 324
Arthropathy, differential diagnosis of, 330t
Arthroplasty, 333
    of hip, 334
    of knee, 92
Arthroscopy, 333
    of knee, 91
    of meniscus, 93
Articular cartilage, of knee, 88
        injuries to, 90–92, *92*
Articular fractures, of hand, 191–196. See also
        specific joint.
Artificial turf, and turf toe, 137
Athletes, and ulnar collateral ligament injuries, 194
    metatarsal fracture in, 134–135
Athletic injuries. See specific activity, e.g., *Baseball;*
        specific area injured, e.g., *Cruciate ligament.*
Automobile accident, total hip arthroplasty with,
        36, *37*
Automobile grease, and high-pressure injection
        injuries, 35
Axillary artery, and proximal humerus, 150, 151
    and scapula, 143
    injury to, 221
Axillary nerve, 208, *209*
    and proximal humerus, 150, 151
    sensory distribution of, 14, *14*
Axon, 199, *200*
Axonotmesis (grade II injury), 199, *201*

Babinski reflex, 30–31
Baby. See *Infant.*
Back, physical examination of, in spinal injury, 51
Back board, in spinal column injury, 50
Back pain, in children, 61
    in spinal column injuries, with radicular pain,
        60–61
    low, in spinal column injuries, 59–60
        with spondylolisthesis, 61–62
        with spondylolysis, 61
Bacterial arthritis, 46

Ballet dancers, and rupture of flexor hallucis longus
    (FHL), 235
    metatarsophalangeal joint injury and, 137–139, *139*
    tendinitis in, *240*
Barlow's maneuver, 314, *316*
Barton's fracture, 172, *173*
Baseball, and hamate fracture, 183
    and little league elbow, 244
    and little league shoulder, 243–244
    and stress fractures, 243
Basketball, and Jones' fracture, 134–136, *135*
    and jumper's knee syndrome, 241
Bennett's fracture, 191–193, *192*
    fixation of, 192
    reverse, 193
Biceps, 159
    reflexes of, 16–17
Biceps tendon, rupture of, 231
Bigelow's reduction maneuver, 74, *74*
Billroth, Theodor, 113
Bimalleolar fractures, 125, *126*
Biopsy, of neoplasms, management of, 266–267
Birth history, 3
Birth (obstetric) palsies, 210
Birth trauma, and clavicle fracture, 145, 146
    and humeral shaft fracture, 156
Bite injuries, 250–251, 254
    animal, 254
    human, 254, *255*
    spider, 256
Bladder, in pelvic fracture, 38
Block vertebrae, 307
Blood loss, from arterial injury, 221
    from metastatic carcinoma lesion, 286
    in brachial plexus injury, 210–211
    in clavicle fracture, 146
    in femoral shaft fracture, 81
    in pelvic fracture, 38, 65–66
Blood pressure, in femoral shaft fracture, 81
Blood supply, to proximal humerus, 149–150
    to scaphoid, 180
Blood vessels, benign tumors of, 270, 324, *324*
    entrapment of, by fracture fragments, 45, *45*
Böhler's angle, 129–130, *130*
Bone(s), demineralization of, 258–259
    infection of, 47–48
    of hand, fractures of, 185
        injuries to, 185–198. See also under specific
            injury or part of hand.
        evaluation of, 186
        management of, 186–187, *187, 188*
    stress fracture of, 237
    tumors of, 263–267, 264t, 275–287. See also specific
        tumor, e.g., *Enchondromas.*
        benign, 275–279
        biopsy of, 266–267
        history and physical examination of, 263–264
        laboratory evaluation of, 264
        malignant, 279–287
        radiographic staging of, 265–266
Bone cyst, aneurysmal, 277–278, *278*
    unicameral, 277
Bone dysplasia, 293, *295*
Bone marrow, infection of, 47–48
Bone scan, in reflex sympathetic dystrophy, 259, *259*
    in tumor staging, 265
    of metatarsal stress fracture, 136, *137*
    three-phase, in acute hematogenous
        osteomyelitis, 47
Boutonnière deformity, *234,* 234–235

Bowleg(s), 289, *291*
    of lateral collateral ligament injury, 89, 93, 94, *94*
Boxer's fracture, 190, *190*
    and human bite injury, 254, *255*
Brachial artery, and humeral shaft, 156, 157
    injury to, 221
Brachial plexus, anatomy of, 208, *209*
    and proximal humerus, 150, 151
    and scapula, 143
    in shoulder injury, 143
    injuries to, 208–211, *209–211*
        causes of, 208, *210*
        open, 210–211
        physical examination for, 209–210
        prognosis in, 211
        symptoms of, 208–209
        traction, 203–204
Brachioradialis, reflex of, 17
Bracing, in idiopathic adolescent scoliosis, *297, 298*
    of collateral ligament injury, 94, *94*
    of infant hip dislocation, 314
    vs. immobilization, of injured knee, 90
Brown recluse spider, bite of, 256
Brown-Séquard lesion, 42
Brown-Séquard syndrome, 207
Bruit, of aneurysm, 223
Buerger's disease, 223
Bulbocavernosus reflex, 52, 207
Bunion(s), 300, *300*
Burst fracture, lumbar, 59, *60*
Burst (comminuted) fracture, vertebral, 58, *58*

Café-au-lait spots, 325
Calcaneal apophysis, 295
Calcaneal stress fractures, 238, *238*
Calcaneal-navicular coalition, fibro-osseous, 295
Calcaneocuboid joint, injury to, 132–133
Calcaneofibular ligament, 117
    in ankle sprains, 118, *118*
Calcaneovalgus foot, 319–320
Calcaneus, defined, 27, *27*
    fractures of, 128–130, *129–130*
    traction apophysitis of, 239
Calcaneus fractures, intra-articular *vs.* extra-
        articular, 130
    treatment of, 130
Calcium, for osteoporosis, 302–303
Calf, Achilles tendon rupture and, 228, *228*
    gastrocnemius muscle rupture and, 229
    plantaris tendon rupture and, 228, *228*
    strength of, 6
Callus, of metatarsal stress fracture, 136, *137*
    plantar, of metatarsal fracture, 133, *135*
Camptodactyly, 313
Cannulation, as injection trauma, 225
Capital femoral epiphysis, slipped, 290–291, *294*
Capitate, and lunate, radiographic evaluation of,
        174–175, *176*
    fractures of, 182–183
Carcinoma, metastasis of, to bone, *286,* 286–287, *287*
Carpal bones, dislocations of, 174–175, *176–179,*
        178–179, *181*
    and scapholunate dissociation, 175–176, *179*
    fracture-dislocations of, 178–179, *181*
    fractures of, 179–184, *182–184*
        scaphoid, 179–180, *182*
    instabilities of, 174–175, *176–179*
Carpal bossing, 193

Carpal height index, 175
Carpal lunate, Kienböck's disease and, 295
Carpal tunnel syndrome (CTS), 215–216, *216*
 tests for, 213, *213*
 vs. pronator syndrome, 215
Carpometacarpal (CMC) joint(s), of finger, injuries of, 193
 of thumb, 191
 fractures of, 191–193, *192*
 osteoarthritis of, *332*
Carrying angle, of elbow fracture, 15, *15*
Cartilage, of femoral head, in acetabular fracture, 69–70
 of knee, articular, 88
 injuries to, 90–92, *92*
 meniscal, 88, *89*
 tumors of, 264t
Casting, complications of, 345
 of ankle fracture, 126
 of ruptured Achilles tendon, 228
 techniques for, 340–345, *341–343, 346*
Casts, lower extremity, 343–345, *344*
 upper extremity, 342–343, *343*
Cat bites, 254
Cauda equina syndrome, 207
Causalgia, 261
CBS (constriction band syndrome), 324
Central cord syndrome, 42–43, 207
Cervical collar, in spinal column injury, 50
Cervical lordosis, 4, *6*
Cervical spine, congenital fusion of, 305
 flexion/extension of, 7, *9*
 fractures of, 55–56, *56–58*, 58
 fracture-subluxation of, 55–56, *56*
 inspection of, 6
 lateral bend of, 7, *9*
 lower, injuries to, *57*, 57–59, *58*
 neurologic examination of, 7
 orthopaedic evaluation of, 6–7
 osteoarthritis of, 336
 palpation of, 6–7
 range of motion of, 7, *9*
 roentgenographic evaluation of, 52–53, *54*
 rotation of, 7, *9*
 subluxation of, 54
 upper, injuries to, 54–57, *54–57*
Charcot arthropathy, joints involved in, 330t
Chauffeur's fracture, 172, *174*
Child (children), bowlegs in, 289, *291*
 congenital deformities in, 304–326. See also specific
  deformity, e.g., *Talipes equinovarus (clubfoot).*
 developmental dislocation of hip in, 317–318, *318*
 distal phalanx of, epiphyseal plate injury to, 187
 Ewing's sarcoma in, 284–285, *284*
 fingertip amputation replacement in, 197, 198
 fracture(s) of, ankle, 127
  clavicle, 145
  elbow, 161–162
  femur, 83–86
  forearm, 165
  hand, 185
  humeral shaft, 156
  knee, classification of, 101–103, *102*
   distal femoral and metaphyseal, 101–104, *102*
  scapula, 144
  tibia, 114–115
  tibial, *103, 104*, 104–106, *105*
 Freiberg's disease in, 295–296, *296*
 genu valgum in, "normal," 289, *290*

Child (children) *(Continued)*
 genu varum in, 289, *291*
 glenohumeral joint dislocation in, 152
 growing pains in, 290
 herpetic whitlow in, 253, *253*
 hip dislocation in, 75
 knee of, 101–106
  anatomy of, 101
 knock-knees in, 289, *290*
 Legg-Calvé-Perthes disease in, 293–294, *295*
 metatarsus adductus in, 289, *291, 292*
 osteochondritis dissecans in, 91–92, *92*, 294–295, *296*
 osteochondroses in, 292–297
 osteosarcoma in, 279
 Panner's disease in, 296
 proximal metacarpal epiphyses of, injury to, 193
 puncture wounds of foot in, 256
 radial head dislocation in, 163
  reduction of, 164
 rhabdomyosarcoma in, 268
 Sever's disease in, 295
 toeing in/out in, 290, *292–293*
 torticollis in, 305–306, *306*
 van Neck's osteochondrosis in, 296–297, *297*
Child abuse, and femoral neck fracture, 75, 77
 and humeral shaft fracture, 156
 and pediatric knee fracture, 103
 vs. mild osteogenesis imperfecta, 326
Children, ankle fractures in, 127
 back pain in, 61
Chondroblastoma, 277
 vs. enchondroma, 277
Chondrocalcinosis, joints involved in, 330t
Chondromalacia, 91
 of first metatarsophalangeal joint, 239
Chondrosarcoma, 282–283, *283*
 periosteal, *vs.* periosteal osteosarcoma, 282
 vs. chordoma, 285
Chordoma, 285, *285*
Chromosomal anomalies, 304
Chronic pain syndromes, 258–262
 factitious, 261–262
Circulation, in compartment syndrome, 38
 in pelvic fracture, 65
Circumferential casting, 112
Clavicle, cleidocranial dysostosis and, 311
 congenital pseudoarthrosis of, 311
 dislocations of, 147–149, *148*
 distal, osteolysis of, 243
 fractures of, 145–147, *146, 147, 148*
  at birth, 145, 146
  classification of, 145, *146*
  injuries associated with, 146
  radiographic evaluation of, *146*, 146–147
 orthopaedic evaluation of, 11–14
Claw toe, 300, *301*
Claw toes, 240, 241
"Clayshoveler's fracture," 58
Cleft hand, 313
Cleidocranial dysostosis, 311
Clonus test, 30
Clostridium perfringens, 43
 and hand infection, 255
Clostridium tetani, and hand infection, 255
Clot dissolvers, in arterial injection injury, 225
Clubfoot (talipes equinovarus), 320–322, *321, 322*
Clubhand, radial, 309–310
CMC joint. See *Carpometacarpal (CMC) joint(s).*

Coaptation splint(s), 157, *157,* 338, *339*
Cold injury, 226
Cold sensitivity, in ulnar artery thrombosis, 224
Collateral ligament, lateral, 89, 93, 94
    medial, 89, 93–94, *94*
    radial, of proximal interphalangeal joint, 195
        of thumb metacarpophalangeal joint, 194
    ulnar, baseball pitchers and, 244
        of thumb metacarpophalangeal joint, 194, *194*
Colles' fracture, 170–171, *171*
Comminuted (burst) fracture, vertebral, 58, *58*
Common digital nerve, in Morton's neuroma, 219–220
Compartment syndrome, 38–41, *41*
    and casting, 345
    and elbow fractures, 161–162
    classic signs of, 39
    common areas for, 38
    in metatarsal fractures, 133
    in tibial fracture, 111
    of leg muscles, 241
    of shoulder injury, 143
    treatment of, 40–41
Compartmental pressures, measurement of, in
        shoulder injury, 143
Compound fracture, 41. See also *Fracture(s), open.*
Computed tomography, in tumor staging, 265
    of acetabulum, 69, *70*
    of ankle, 123
Congenital abduction contracture, of hip, 318
Congenital arthritis, joints involved in, 330t
Congenital constriction band syndrome (CBS), 324
Congenital deformities, 304–326. See also specific
        deformity or part of body affected.
    causes of, 304
    of foot, 319–324
    of hand, 323, *323*
    of hip (congenital dislocation), 313–318, *314–318*
    of knee (congenital dislocation), 313–318, *314–318*
    of spine, 304–309
Congenital dislocation/subluxation of knee, 318
Congenital kyphosis, 306
Congenital muscular torticollis, *305,* 305–306
Congenital posteromedial bowing, of tibia, 319, *321*
Congenital pseudoarthritis, of clavicle, 311
    of tibia (anterolateral bow), 318–319, *319, 320*
Congenital radioulnar synostosis, 312
Congenital scoliosis, 306, *307, 308*
Congenital vertical talus, 323, *323*
Constriction band syndrome (CBS), congenital, 324
Conus medullaris syndrome, 207
Coracoclavicular ligaments, in clavicle dislocation,
        147
    in clavicle fracture, 145
Coracoid fracture, 143
Corns, 301
Coronal, defined, 1
Coronal plane, deformity of. See *Scoliosis.*
Cortical defect, fibrous (nonossifying fibroma),
        278–279, *280*
"Cortical ring" sign, *177*
Corticosteroids, local injections of, 237, 241, 244
Costoclavicular ligament, 147
    in clavicle fracture, 145
Counterforce brace, 245
Cruciate ligament, *95,* 95–98, *96, 97*
    anterior, 89, *95,* 95–97, *96, 97*
    posterior, 89, *97,* 97–98
Crush injuries, of metatarsals, 133
Crystalloid, in hypotension of spinal injury, 42
CTS (carpal tunnel syndrome), 213, 215–216, *216*

Cubitus valgus, 15, *15*
Cubitus varus, 15, *15*
Cylinder cast, *344,* 344–345
Cyst, bone, 277–278

Dancers, ballet, and rupture of flexor hallucis longus
        (FHL), 235
    metatarsophalangeal joint injury and, 137–139,
        139
    tendinitis in, *240*
    Morton's neuroma in, 219–220
Dapsone, for spider bite, 256
Debridement, arthroscopic, 335
    in gas gangrene, 44
    of injection injuries, 36
Deep palmar arch, anatomy of, 223, *224*
Deep venous thromboses, 38
Deformity, evaluation of, 2–3
Degenerative arthritis, post-traumatic, in hip
        dislocation, 75
Deltoid ligaments, *118*
    and malleolar fracture, *125*
Dental personnel, herpetic whitlow in, 253, *253*
DeQuervain's tendinitis, 246–247, *247, 248*
Dermatomal distribution, 4, *5*
Dermatomes, cervical, 52, 54t
    lumbar and sacral, 52, 54t
    sensory, 52, *53*
    thoracic, 52, 54t
Developmental conditions, 289–303
    in adults, 299–303. See also specific condition, e.g.,
        Bunion(s).
    in children, 289–299. See also specific condition,
        e.g., *Bowleg(s).*
Developmental history, 3
Diabetic foot, infections in, 256–257
    prevention of, 256–257
Die-punch (lunate load) fracture, 172–174, *175*
Diesel oil, and high-pressure injection injuries, 35
Digit splint, 339, *340*
Digital arteries, anatomy of, 223
Digits. See also *Finger(s); Thumb.*
    amputation of, 44, *44*
    fractures of, malrotation of, 189
    pallor of, 225–226
DIP joints. See *Interphalangeal joint(s), distal.*
Dislocation(s), 34
    classification of, *31,* 33–34, *34*
    defined, 34
    facet, 57, *57*
    occipital-C1, 54
    of acromioclavicular joint, 147–148, *148,* 149
    of carpal bones, 174–175, *176–179,* 178–179, *181*
    of clavicle, 147–149, *148*
    of elbow, 162–164, *164*
    of finger carpometacarpal joints, 193
    of finger distal interphalangeal joints, 196
        proximal interphalangeal joints, 195, 196, *196*
    of glenohumeral joint, 151–154, *152, 153, 154*
    of hip, 72–79, *73, 74*
        developmental, 313–318, *314–318*
    of interphalangeal joint(s), 196
    of knee, 45–46, *46,* 318
        types of, 45, 46
    of metacarpophalangeal joints, 193–194
    of metatarsophalangeal joints, 137–139, *139*
    of patellofemoral joints, 98, 99
    of radioulnar joints, distal, 177–178, *180*

Dislocation(s) *(Continued)*
  of scapula, 143–145, *144, 145*
  of sesamoids, 138
  of shoulder, 142–154. See also specific joint, e.g.,
    Glenohumeral joint.
  of sternoclavicular joint, 147, 148, 149
  of thumb interphalangeal joints, 196
  of ulna, 163, *164*
  subtalar, 131–132
  vascular trauma from, 44–45
Dislocation/subluxation, of knee, congenital, 318
Dog bites, 254
Dorsal block splint, 195
Dorsal intercalary segment instability (DISI), *178*
Drop foot, 6, *8*, 27
Drug use, and thrombosis of ulnar artery, 223
Dundee limb deficiency classification system, 309
Dupuytren's fasciitis, 301–302, *302*
Dysostosis, cleidocranial, 311
Dysplasia, Streeter's, 324

Edema, of hand, self-inflicted, 241
Effusion, knee, following trauma, 106–107
Eikenella corrodens, and hand infection, 250
Elbow, dislocations of, 162–164, *164*
    causes of, 163
    imaging of, 164
    injuries associated with, 163
    physical examination of, 163
    radiographic evaluation of, 163
  extension of, 16
  flexion of, 16, *16*
  fractures about, 157–162, *159–162*
    causes of, 160
    classification of, 159, *160*
    treatment of, 162, *162*
    valgus and, 15, *15*
  lateral condyle fracture of, valgus and, 15, *15*
  muscles of, 159
  neurologic examination of, 16–17
  orthopaedic evaluation of, 15–17
  overuse syndromes of, 244–245
  palpation of, 16
  physical examination of, 160
  radiographic evaluation of, 162
  range of motion of, 16, *16*
  supracondylar humerus fracture of, varus and,
    15, *15*
Elderly, distal radius fractures of, 169
  knee of, 109
  proximal humerus fractures of, 150
  tendon ruptures in, 227
  tibial plateau fracture of, 107, *108*
Electromyography (EMG), 203, 213
Emboli, and ulnar artery thrombosis, 224–225
Embolism, fat, 36–37, *37*
  pulmonary, 37–38, *39*
Embolization, angiographic, in pelvic fracture, 38
Emergency care, 35–48
  of acute hematogenous osteomyelitis, 47–48
  of arterial injury, 222
  of compartment syndrome, 38–41, *41*
  of dislocation of knee, 45–46, *46*
  of fat embolism, 36–37, *37*
  of gas gangrene, 43–44
  of injection injuries, 35–36, *36*
  of open fractures, 41, *42*
  of pelvic fracture, 38, *40,* 65–66

Emergency care *(Continued)*
  of pulmonary embolism, 37–38, *39*
  of septic arthritis, 46–47
  of spinal injury, 41–43, 50, 206
  of tibial fracture, 111, 114
  of traumatic amputation, 44, *44*
  of vascular injuries associated with fractures and
    dislocations, 44–45, *45*
Enchondroma, 277, *277*
Epicondyle, femoral, lateral, iliotibial band syndrome
    and, 241–242
  humeral, medial, stress injury to, 244–245
  of humerus, lateral, palpation of, 15
  medial, palpation of, 15
Epiphysis(ses), and pediatric knee fractures, 101–104,
    102
  femoral, capital, slipped, 290–291, *294*
  of hand, 185
  of long bones, infection of, 47
  tibial, proximal, displacement of, *103,* 104–105
Eponychial fold, and paronychia, 252
Eponychium, 197, *197*
Equinus, defined, 27, *27*
Erythema, in hand infection, 251
Erythrocyte sedimentation rate, in osteomyelitis, 48
Essex-Lopresti fracture-dislocation, 159
Eversion test, of ankle, 117
Ewing's sarcoma, *284,* 284–285
Excessive lateral compression syndrome (lateral
    patellofemoral compression syndrome), 99–100
Extensor carpi ulnaris tendinitis, 248
Extensor digiti quinti (EDQ), 233
Extensor digitorum communis (EDC), 233
Extensor indicis proprius (EIP), 233
Extensor lag, in mallet finger, 233–234, *234*
Extensor pollicis brevis, tendinitis of, 246–247, *247,*
    248
Extensor pollicis longus (EPL), 233
Extensor pollicis longus tendinitis, 248
Extensor tendon (distal phalanx), terminal, rupture
    of, 196, *196*
Extensor tendons, of hand, injuries to, 233
    rupture of (mallet finger), 233–234, *234*
  palpation of, 18
Extremity(ies), lower. See *Lower extremity(ies).*
  upper. See *Upper extremity(ies).*
Eyelid, drooped, in brachial plexus injury, 209, *210*
Eyes, in brachial plexus injury, 209, *210*

Facet dislocations, 57, *57*
False aneurysm, 222, *223*
Family history, 3
Farm injuries, antibiotic therapy for, 251, 254
Fascia, fatigue failure of, 237
Fascicles, 199, *200*
Fasciitis, Dupuytren's, 301–302, *302*
Fasciotomy, for vascular trauma, 45
  in compartment syndrome, 40–41
Fat embolism, 36–37, *37*
  treatment of, 37
Fatty tissue, tumors of, 264t
Felon (pulp abscess), 251, *252*
Femoral. See also at *Femur.*
Femoral artery, in fractures of distal femur, 107
  superficial, injury to, 221
Femoral condyle, in knee dislocation, 45, *46*
Femoral cutaneous nerve, lateral, entrapment of, 219

Femoral epiphysis(ses), capital, slipped, 290–291, *294*
distal, 101
Femoral head, fractures of, 72, *73*
transcondylar or indentation, in anterior hip
dislocation, 72–73
in Legg-Calvé-Perthes disease, 293–294, *295*
osteonecrosis of, in hip dislocation, 75
reduction of, in developmental dislocation of hip,
318
Femoral neck, fractures of, 75, *76–78*
displacement of, 75, *76*
stress fracture of, 242
Femoral nerve supply, 203, *204*
Femoral shaft, 81–83
fractures of, 81–83
classification of, 81–82
in children, 83–86
anatomy of, 83–84, *84, 85*
causes of, 84
history in, 84
physical examination of, 84–85
radiographic evaluation of, 85–86
treatment of, by age, 85–86
isolated, 82
prognosis for, 82–83
radiographic assessment of, 81
treatment of, 82, *82*
Femoral triangle, palpation of, 21
Femur. See also *Femoral* entries.
chronic osteomyelitis of, *48*
distal, fractures of, 107, *107, 108*
epiphyses of, 101–104, *102*
fractures of, 81–86. See also *Femoral shaft,
fractures of.*
classification of, 81–82
in children, 83–86
anatomy of, 83–84, *84, 85*
diagnosis of, 84–86
physical examination in, 84–85
radiologic evaluation of, 85–86
treatment of, 86
mechanism of injury in, 84
long-term prognosis for, 82–83
radiographic assessment of, 81
treatment of, 82, *82*
vascular trauma and, 45, *45*
growth plate injuries of, 101–104, *102*
metaphysis of, 103
proximal, migration of, 314, *317*
physeal plate of, 101
radiographic evaluation of, 81
sulcus of, flattening of, in patellofemoral instability,
98, *98*
Fibroma, nonossifying (fibrous cortical defect),
278–279, *280*
Fibromatosis, 270, *270*
Fibrosarcoma, 271
Fibrous cortical defect (nonossifying fibroma),
278–279, *280*
Fibrous histiocytoma, malignant, 283–284
Fibrous tissue, tumors of, 264t
Fibula, fracture of, 110, 123
palpation of, 25
Fibular longitudinal deficiency, 310, *310*
Fibular tunnel syndrome, *218,* 218–219
Figure-of-eight immobilizer, for clavicle fractures,
147, *147*
Finger(s), acute suppurative tenosynovitis of, 253
carpometacarpal joints of, injuries to, 193
congenital flexion deformity of, 313

Finger(s) *(Continued)*
contractures of, 301–302, *302*
psychologic origin of, 261
extension of, 16
extensor tendons of, injury to, 233
flexion of, 16
flexor tendons of, rupture of, 232
mallet, 233–234, *234*
metacarpophalangeal joints of, injuries to, 193–194
range of motion of, 19–20
syndactyly of, 312
Fingernail, and paronychia, *252,* 252–253
infection of, *252,* 252–253
Fingertip, amputation of, *197,* 197–198
anatomy of, 197, *197*
felon of, 251, *252*
fracture of, 187–188, *188*
herpetic whitlow of, 253, *253*
injuries of, 196–198, *197*
replantation of, 198
Finkelstein's test, 247, *247*
First dorsal interosseous muscle, palpation of, 20
Fish-mouth incision, contraindicated for felon, 251,
252
Fistulas, arteriovenous, 223
Fixation, external, in pelvic fracture, 38, *40,* 66
internal, for femoral neck fracture, 75, *76, 78*
for intertrochanteric fractures, 77, *79*
for metatarsal fracture, 134–135
of pelvic fracture, 66–68, *67–68*
intramedullary, 82, *82*
Flatfoot, spastic, peroneal (tarsal coalition), 291–292,
294, 295
Flatfoot (pes planus), 27, *28*
Flexor carpi ulnaris tendinitis, 248
Flexor digitorum profundus, avulsion of, 232–233
Flexor digitorum profundus tendons, 231, 232
Flexor digitorum superficialis tendons, 231–232
Flexor hallucis longus (FHL), 235
Flexor hallucis tendinitis, *240*
Flexor tendons, palpation of, 18
Flexor tenosynovitis, 232
vs. septic arthritis, 254
Foot (feet), alignment of, 27–28, *28*
anatomy of, 128, *129*
arthritis of, surgery and, 335
articular cartilage of, 239
calcaneovalgus, 319–320
congenital deformities of, 319–324. See also specific
deformity, e.g., *Talipes equinovarus (clubfoot).*
developmental conditions of, 299–301
diabetic, infections in, 256–257
prevention of, 256–257
dislocations of, 128–140
subtalar, 131–132
fifth metatarsal of, 238, *238*
flat, 27, *28*
fracture-dislocations of, tarsometatarsal, 133, *134*
fractures of, 128–140
calcaneal, 128–130, *129–130*
metatarsal, 133–136, *135, 136*
stress, 136, *137,* 238, *238*
midtarsal, 132–133
sesamoid, 136–137, *138, 139*
talar, 130–131, *131, 132*
in myelomeningocele, 308
malalignment of, ligament sprain from, 239
medial arch of, posterior tibial tendon rupture and,
230, *230*
nerve entrapment in, *218,* 218–219

Foot (feet) *(Continued)*
  neurologic examination of, 30–31
  orthopaedic evaluation of, 27–31
  osteoarthritis of, 335
  overuse syndromes of, 237–240, *238, 240*
  palpation of, 28–29
  plantar-flexed (in equinus). See *Drop foot.*
  position of, in ankle injury, 123
  puncture wounds to, 256
  range of motion of, 30, *30*
  rheumatoid arthritis of, 331
  sensory examination of, *26,* 27, 30
  susceptibility of, to injury, 128
  syndactyly of, 323, *323*
Foot drop, in fibular tunnel syndrome, *218,* 218–219
Foot eversion, neurologic examination of, 26
Foot inversion, neurologic examination of, 26
Football, and turf toe, 137
Football players, and rupture of flexor hallucis longus
  (FHL), 235
  Jones' fracture in, 238, *238*
Forearm, acute suppurative tenosynovitis of, 253
  anatomy of, 165
  and biceps tendon rupture, 231
  fractures of, 165–168, *166, 167*
    causes of, 165
    injuries associated with, 165
    physical examination of, 165
    radiographic evaluation of, 165–166, *166*
    reduction of, anesthesia for, 166–167
    treatment of, 166–168
  intersection syndrome of, 247–248
  motor innervation of, 201, *202*
  neurologic examination of, 16–17
  orthopaedic evaluation of, 15–17
  pronation and supination of, 16, *17*
  range of motion of, 16, *17*
  sensory examination of, 16
Forearm splint, 338, *340*
Forefoot, alignment of, 27–28, *28*
  anatomy of, 128
  deformities of, 299
  developmental conditions of, 299–301
Forward bend test, 297, *297*
Fracture(s). See also *Fracture-dislocation(s); Fracture-
  subluxation(s).*
  and fat embolism, 36–37, *37*
  Bennett's, 191–193, *192*
  bimalleolar, 125, *126*
  buckle, 34
  C1, 55
  cervical, 55–56, *56–58*
  classification of, *31,* 33–34, *34*
    by displacement, *32,* 34
    Salter-Harris, *32*
  closed, 111, *112,* 112t
    definition of, 111
  comminuted, *31,* 34, 111, *113*
    definition of, 111
  complete, definition of, 111
  compound, 41
  definition of, 110–111
  description of, to orthopaedic surgeon, 110–111,
    114
  diagnosis and disposition of, commandments for,
    110
  elbow, 157–162, *159–162*
  femoral, distal, 107, *107*
  greenstick, 34

Fracture(s) *(Continued)*
  incomplete, 111, *111*
    definition of, 110–111
  Jones,' 134–136, *135*
  metacarpal, 190–191, *190–192*
  metatarsal, 133–136, *135, 136*
  midtarsal, 132–133
  oblique, *31,* 34
  odontoid, 55–56, *56*
  of acetabulum, 68–71, *73,* 73–74
  of ankle, in children, 127
  of base of thumb metacarpal (Bennett's, Rolando's),
    191–193, *192*
  of carpal bones, 179–184, *182–184*
  of clavicle, 145–147, *146, 147,* 148
  of distal radius, 169–174, *170–174*
  of elbow, carrying angle of, 15, *15*
  of femoral head, 72, *73*
  of femoral neck, 75, *76–78*
  of femur, in adults, 81–83
    in children, 83–86
  of finger carpometacarpal joints, 191–193, *192*
  of finger distal and thumb interphalangeal joints,
    196
  of forearm, 165–168, *166, 167*
  of hand joints, 191–196. See also specific joint.
  of hip, 72–79
    femoral head, 72, *73*
    femoral neck, 75, *76–78*
    intertrochanteric, 75–78, *79*
    subtrochanteric, 78–79
  of humeral shaft, 156–157, *157, 158*
  of humerus, proximal, 149–151, *150*
  of pelvis, 63–68
  of phalanx, distal, 187–188, *188*
    middle, 188–190, *189*
    proximal, 188–190, *189*
  of proximal interphalangeal (PIP) joints, 194–195,
    195
  of scapula, 143–145, *144, 145*
  of sesamoids, 136–137, *138, 139*
  of shoulder, 142–154
  of talus, 130–131, *131, 132*
  of tibia, 110–115
    consequences of, 114
    in children, 114–115
  of tibial plateau, 107–108, *108*
  of toes, 139–140, *140*
  of wrist, 169–184
  open, 41, *42,* 86, 111, *112,* 112t
    classification of, 41, 112t
    definition of, 111
    Gustillo-Anderson classification of, 112t
    of ankle, 125
  patellar, in children, *103,* 104
  pathologic, prophylactic fixation of, 287
  patterns of, 111, *111*
  pelvic, 38, *40*
    associated (complex), 69, *71*
    elemental, 69, *70*
    intra-articular, 69–70
  Rolando's, 191–193, *192*
  shortening of, 34
  spiral, *31,* 34, 111, *113*
    definition of, 111
  stress, metatarsal, 136, *137*
    sesamoid, 137, *137*
  tibial, eminence, in children, *104,* 105
    proximal, in children, *103,* 104–105
  tibial tuberosity, in children, *105,* 106

Fracture(s) (Continued)
  transverse, 31, 34, 111, 113
    definition of, 111
    vascular trauma from, 44–45, 45
Fracture fragments, entrapment of blood vessels
  by, 45
Fracture-dislocation(s). See also Fracture(s); Fracture-
  subluxation(s).
  and arterial injury, 221
  Essex-Lopresti, 159
  Galeazzi's, 168
  Lisfranc, 133, 134
  midtarsal, 132–133
  Monteggia's, 163, 164
  of ankle, 124
  of carpal bones, 178–179, 181
  of fifth metacarpal/hamate, 193
  of lumbar spine, 59
  of metatarsals, 133, 134
  tarsometatarsal, 133, 134
Fracture-subluxation(s). See also Fracture(s);
  Fracture-dislocation(s).
  C2, 55–56, 56
  of cervical spine, 55–56, 56
  of lumbar spine, 59
Fragments, osteochondral, 91, 92, 92
Freiberg's disease, 295–296, 296
Frostbite, 226
Fungal infections, of hand, 250
"Funny bone," 205, 216
Furuncle, 253

Gait, "antalgic," 5
  disturbance of, 3
  evaluation of, 4–6, 8
  of toddler with developmental dislocation of hip,
    317–318
  phases of, 5, 8
Galeazzi's fracture, 165, 166
Galeazzi's fracture-dislocation, 168
Galeazzi's sign, 314, 314
Ganglion (ganglia), 268–269, 269
Gas gangrene, 43–44
  treatment of, 44
  vascular, 43
Gastrocnemius, in lateral patellofemoral compression
  syndrome rehabilitation, 99
  medial, rupture of, vs. plantaris tendon rupture,
    229
Genu valgum, 4, 7
  "normal," in children, 289, 290
Genu varum, 4, 7
  in children, 289, 291
Giant cell tumor, 278, 279
  of tendon sheath, 270–271
  vs. chondroblastoma, 277
Glenohumeral joint, and proximal humerus, 149
  dislocations of, 151–154, 152, 153, 154
    causes of, 151–152
    injuries associated with, 152
    neurologic examination of, 153
    radiographic evaluation of, 152, 153
    reduction of, 152, 153
    treatment of, 153–154
  immobilization of, 153, 153–154
  radiographic evaluation of, 144, 144
  subluxations of, 151

Glenoid fracture, 143
Gluteus medius, strength of, 23. See also
  Trendelenburg test.
Godfrey, posterior sag sign of, 97, 97
Golf, and hamate fracture, 183
Golfer's elbow, 245
Gonorrhea, joint manifestations of, 255–256
  septic arthritis of, 255–256
Gout, joints involved in, 330t
Gower's test, 6
Gram-negative infections, 255
Grease, and high-pressure injection injuries, 35
Great toe, 128, 129. See also Lesser toes; Toe(s).
  extension of, neurologic examination of, 25
  flexion of, neurologic examination of, 26
  fracture of, displaced, 140, 140
  metatarsophalangeal joint of, injury to, 137–139,
    139
    osteoarthritis of, 335
    sprains and strains of, 137–138
  sesamoids of, 136–137, 138, 139
    fracture of, 136–137, 138, 139
Greater trochanter, tendinitis at, 242
Grip strength, 170
Gripping, and intersection syndrome, 248
Growing pains, 290
Growth disturbances, from physeal fracture, 104
Growth plate, fractures of, 32
  and pediatric knee fractures, 101–104, 102
Gunshot wounds, and arterial injury, 221
  and brachial plexus injury, 210, 211
  as nerve injury, 205
  to hand, 186–187
  vascular trauma from, 45
Gustillo-Anderson classification, of open fractures,
  111, 112t
Guyon's syndrome, 217

Haemophilus influenzae, and hand infection,
  250
  in osteomyelitis, 47
Hallux rigidus, 239, 335
Hallux valgus, 300, 300
Hamate, fractures of, 183
Hammer toe, 300
Hamstring, in anterior cruciate ligament injury, 97
  in collateral ligament injury, 94, 94
  in femoral shaft fracture, 81
  in lateral patellofemoral compression syndrome
    rehabilitation, 99
Hamulus process, fractures of, 183
Hand. See also Finger(s); specific joint, e.g.,
  Carpometacarpal (CMC) joint(s); Thumb.
  anatomy of, 223, 224
  and wrist, overuse syndromes of, 246–249, 247,
    248
    tendinitis of, 246–249
  arterial thrombosis of, 223, 224
  arthritis of, surgery and, 332, 333
  "attitude" of, 17, 18
  bones of, fractures of, 185
  cleft, 313
  contractures of, 301–302, 302
  evaluation of, 17–20
  flexor tendons of, 231
    avulsion injury to (Jersey finger), 232–233
    enlargement of (trigger finger), 231–232
    rupture of, 232

Hand (*Continued*)
fractures of, articular, 191–196. See specific joint or fracture.
multiple, 187
open, 186–187
furuncle of, 253
injection injuries to, 35–36, *36*
injuries to, 185–198. See also under specific injury or part of hand.
evaluation of, 186
management of, 186–187, *187, 188*
intrinsic positive (intrinsic plus) position of, 186, *187*
neurologic examination of, 20
normal, alignment of, 189, *189*
osteoarthritis of, *332,* 333
palpation of, 18
polydactyly of, 312–313
position of function of, 251, *251*
rheumatoid arthritis of, 331
rotational alignment of, 190
sensory examination of, 20, *21*
sensory innervation of, 201, *202*
syndactyly of, 312, 313
tendons of, extensor, injuries to, 233
rupture of (mallet finger), 233–234, *234*
flexor, avulsion injury to (Jersey finger), 232–233
enlargement of (trigger finger), 231–232
rupture of, 232
"Hangman's fracture," 57, *57*
Hawkins' sign, 131
Head, physical examination of, in spinal injury, 51
Heavy lifting, and biceps tendon rupture, 231
Heel. See also *Hindfoot.*
in calcaneus fractures, 128, *129*
"Heel spur" syndrome, 239
Hemangioma, 270, 324, *324*
Hemarthrosis, and anterior cruciate ligament injury, 95
in tibial eminence fracture, 105
in tibial plateau fracture, 107, *108*
intra-articular, in fractures of distal femur, 107
Hematoma, 45, 221, *222*
subungual, drainage of, 188
of toe, 139
Hemivertebrae, 307, *308*
Hemorrhage, control of, in arterial injury, 222
Hemosiderin, 271
Herpes simplex, and hand infection, 250
Herpetic whitlow (herpes simplex), 253, *253*
Heterotopic bone, formation of, 227
High-pressure injection injuries, 35–36, *36*
Hilgenreiner's line, 314, *317*
Hindfoot. See also *Heel.*
anatomy of, 128
dorsiflexion of, 320
Hip, abduction contracture of, congenital, 318
abduction of, test for, 21–22, *22*
adductors of, neurologic examination of, 22
anterior, dislocations of, 72–73, *74*
reduction of, 72, 74, *74*
arthritis of, surgery and, 334, *334*
dislocation of, 72–79
and femoral head fractures, 72, *73*
complications of, 75
developmental, 313–318, *314–318*
in children, 75
in myelomeningocele, 308
embryology of, 313
extensors of, neurologic examination of, 23

Hip (*Continued*)
flexion contracture of, Thomas test for, 21, *22*
flexors of, neurologic examination of, 22
fractures of, femoral head, 72, *73*
femoral neck, 75, *76–78*
intertrochanteric, 75–78, *79*
subtrochanteric, 78–79
fusion of, 334
neurologic examination of, 22–23
orthopaedic evaluation of, 20–24
osteoarthritis of, 334, *334*
overuse syndromes of, 242
painful, gait in, *9*
palpation of, 20–21
posterior, dislocation of, 73–75, *74*
CT scan of, 74
reduction of, 73–74, *74*
range of motion of, 21–22
rotation of, 290, *292, 293*
evaluation of, 22, *23*
sensory examination of, 23
Hippocrates, on ankle fractures, 122
Histiocytoma, fibrous, malignant, 271, *273,* 283–284
History, orthopaedic, 1–3
Hook of hamate, fractures of, 183
Horner's syndrome, in brachial plexus injury, 209, *210*
Human bite injuries, 191, 254, *255*
Humerus, distal, 157–158
condylar fracture of, 159, *160*
supracondylar fracture of, 15, *159*
fracture of, braces for, 157, *158*
palpation of, 15
proximal, epiphysiolysis of, 243
fractures of, 149–151, 150, *150*
classification of, 150, *150*
displaced, 151
radiographic evaluation of, 150, *150*
shaft of, fractures of, 156–157, *157, 158*
"Humpback," *298, 299*
Hyperabduction maneuver, 225, *225*
Hypotension, acute, in spinal cord injury, 42
"Hypothenar hammer syndrome," 224
Hypovolemic shock, in pelvic fracture, 65–66

Idiopathic adolescent scoliosis, *297,* 297–298
Iliac crest, palpation of, 20
Iliac spines, superior, anterior, palpation of, 20
posterior, palpation of, 20–21
Iliac wing fracture, *66*
Iliolumbar ligament, 64
Iliopatellar ligament, 90
Iliotibial band, 89
Iliotibial band syndrome, 241–242
Ilium, 64, *64*
Immobilization, casting techniques for, 340–345, *341–343,* 346
in intertrochanteric fractures, 75–76
in spinal column injury, 50
of ankle fracture, 126
of clavicle, 147, *147–148*
of Colles' fracture, 170
of dislocated elbow, 164
of distal radioulnar joint dislocations, 177, *180*
of forearm fractures, 167, *167*
of hand fractures, 187
of scaphoid, 179–180
of shoulder, 145, *145,* 151, *153,* 153–154

Immobilization *(Continued)*
    splinting techniques for, 337–340, *338–340,* 346
    vs. bracing, of injured knee, 90
Impingement injection, 244
Impingement syndrome, of shoulder, 243–244
Incision, fish-mouth, contraindicated for felon, 251,
    252
Infant, birth (obstetric) palsies of, 210
    developmental dislocation of hip in, 313–318,
        314–318
    femoral fracture in, 86
    hip dislocation in, 75, 313–318, *314–318*
    hips of, orthopaedic evaluation of, 20
    radial head dislocation in, 163
    with myelomeningocele, 308
Infection(s), gram-negative, 255
    mycobacterial, 254–255
    of foot, 250–251, 256–257. See also specific
        infection or organism.
    of hand, 250–251, *251.* See also specific infection or
        organism.
    of joint, 46
    streptococcal, anaerobic, 43
    tetanus, 255
    wound, and gas gangrene, 43, 255
Infrapatellar tendinitis, and jumper's knee syndrome,
    241
Injection injuries, 35–36, *36,* 225
Innervation, segmental, of muscle groups, 51–52, 52t
Innominate bones, 64, *64*
Interosseous nerve, posterior, entrapment of, *217,*
    217–218
Interphalangeal joint(s), distal, 197, *197*
    and boutonnière deformity, *234,* 234–235
    and swan neck deformity, 234, *234*
    Heberden's nodes in, 333
    of thumb and fingers, dislocations of, 196
    proximal, and Boutonnière deformity, *234,* 234–235
    and swan neck deformity, 234, *234*
    Bouchard's nodes in, 333
    condylar fractures of, 195
    dislocations of, 195–196, *196*
    fractures of, 194–195, *195*
Intersection syndrome, 247–248
Intertrochanteric fractures, 75–78, *79*
    treatment of, 76–78, *79*
    nonoperative, 77
    operative, 77–78
Intracompartmental tissue pressures, measurement
    of, 40, *41*
Intramedullary fixation, 82, *82*
Intraperiosteal aspiration, 47
Intrinsic positive (intrinsic plus) position, of hand,
    186, *187*
Inversion test, of ankle, 117
Ischemia, of compartment syndrome, 39–40
Ischiopubic synchondrosis, normal, 296–297, *297*
Ischium, 64, *64*

Jogging, and gastrocnemius muscle rupture, 229
Joint(s). See also specific joint, e.g., *Patellofemoral
    joint.*
    arthritic, surgery for, 333–336
    arthroscopic debridement of, 335
    aspiration of, in acute hematogenous
        osteomyelitis, 47
    in septic arthritis, 47
    congenital contractures of, 324

Joint(s) *(Continued)*
    decompression of, in septic arthritis, 47
    infection of, 46
    in hand, 251
    malalignment of, 237
    of hand, fractures of, 191–196. See also specific
        joint.
    painful, evaluation of, 331–332
    pyogenic arthritis of, 253–254
Jones' fracture, 134–136, *135*
    delayed union of, 238, *238*
    stress form of, 135, *135*
Judet-Letournel radiographic views, 69, *69,* 70
Jumper's knee syndrome, 241
Juncturae tendinum, 233

Kienböck's disease, 295
    fracture of lunate, 180–181, *183*
Klippel-Feil syndrome, 305
Knee. See also *Patella.*
    anatomy of, 88–90, *89, 90*
    arthritis of, surgery and, 334–335, *335*
    bracing of, 88, 90
    dislocation of, 45–46, *46*
        and popliteal artery, 221
        popliteal angiography in, 46
        types of, 45, 46
    dislocation/subluxation of, congenital, 318
    extension of, 25, *26*
        neurologic examination of, 25
    extensor tendons of, rupture of, 230
    flexion of, 25, *26*
        neurologic examination of, 25
    fractures about, 88–115, *106–109*
        classification of, 108
        treatment of, 108–109
        vascular trauma from, 45, *45*
    fusion of, 335
    ligamentous injuries of, 88–115. See also specific
        ligament, e.g., *Collateral ligament.*
    locking of, 92, 93
    muscle and tendon injury to, 229
    neurologic examination of, 25–27
    orthopaedic evaluation of, 24–27
    osteoarthritis of, 334–335, *335*
    osteochondritis dissecans of, 294–295, *296*
    overuse syndromes of, 241–242
    palpation of, 25
    pediatric, 101–106
        anatomy of, 101
        fractures about, classification of, 101–103, *102*
            distal femoral and metaphyseal, 101–104,
            102
    range of motion of, 25, *26*
    rehabilitation of, 90
    replacement of, 335
    rheumatoid arthritis of, 331
    sports injuries to, 88–100. See also specific
        structure involved, e.g., *Meniscus (menisci),
        injuries to.*
    valgus deformity of, 24–25
    varus deformity of, 24
Knee jerk (patellar tendon) reflex, 27
Knee pain, and osteoarthritic hip, 334
Knock-knees, 289, *290*
Knuckle, depressed, 190
Kyphosis, congenital, 306
    Scheuermann's, *298,* 298–299
    thoracic, 4, *6, 7, 10*

Laceration(s), and extensor tendons of hands, 233
  and flexor tendons of hands, 232
  arterial, 222, *222*
  nerve deficit with, 204–205
  of flexor hallucis longus, 235
  of muscles and tendons, 228
  vascular trauma from, 45
Lachman's test, for anterior cruciate ligament injury,
    95, *95*
Lateral, defined, 1
Lateral buttress knee sleeve, 90
Lateral buttress patellofemoral knee sleeve, 99
Lateral patellofemoral compression syndrome
    (excessive lateral compression syndrome), 99–100
Leg, casts for, 343–344, *343–344*
  lateral, and peroneal tendon rupture, 229–230
  length of, 20, 242
  neurologic examination of, 25–27
  orthopaedic evaluation of, 24–27
  overuse syndromes of, 240–241
  palpation of, 25
  range of motion of, 25
  splints for, 339–340, *340–341*
Legg-Calvé-Perthes disease, 293–294, *295*
Lesser toes, 128, *129*. See also *Great toe; Toe(s).*
  deformities of, 300–301, *301*
  metatarsophalangeal joint dislocation of, 138–139
  neurologic examination of, 26
Ligament(s). See also specific ligament, e.g.,
    Collateral ligament, medial.
  fatigue failure of, 237
  of ankle, 117, *118*
  of knee, 88–90
    cruciate, injuries to, anterior, 95–97, *95–97*
        posterior, *97*, 97–98
    medial and lateral, injuries to, 93–94
  of pediatric knee, 101
  of pelvis, 64, *64*
    CT scan for, 66
  of wrist, injuries to, 169–184
Limb deficiencies, 309–313. See also specific
    condition, e.g., *Syndactyly.*
  classification of, 309
Limb lengthening, 311
Limb-sparing surgery, 273–274, *274*
Lipoma, *267*, 269
  magnetic resonance imaging for, 265–266, *267*
Liposarcoma, 271–272, *273*
Lisfranc's fracture-dislocations, 133, *134*
Lister's tubercle, 18, 248
Little League elbow, 243
Little League shoulder, 243
Little toe, 128, *129*
Lobster claw hand, 313
Log-rolling, in spinal column injury, 50, 51
Long arm posterior splint, 338, *339*
Long leg cast, 344, *344*
Long leg splint, for closed tibial fracture, 111–112
Lordosis, cervical, 4, 6
  lumbar, 4, 6
Low back pain, chronic, 61
Lower cervical spine, *57*, 57–59, *58*
Lower extremity(ies), casts for, 340–342, *340–344*,
    343–345
  contractures of, in myelomeningocele, 308
  innervation of, 203, *204*
  overuse syndromes of, 237–243. See also specific
      site, e.g., *Foot (feet).*
  splints for, 339–340, *340–341*

Lubricating oils, and high-pressure injection
    injuries, 35
Lumbar compression fracture, 59, *59*
Lumbar lordosis, 4, *6*
Lumbar radiculopathy, 61
Lumbar spine, in Scheuermann's kyphosis, *298,*
    299
  injuries to, 59, *59, 60*
  osteoarthritis of, 336
Lunate, fractures of, 180–181, *183*
  Kienböck's disease and, 180–181, *183*
Lunate load (die-punch) fracture, 172–174, *175*
Lunotriquetral ligament injury, in triquetrolunate
    dissociation, 177, *178*
Lunotriquetral tear, 175, *178*

Maceration, in casting, 345
MacMurray's test, 92, *93*
Magnetic resonance imaging (MRI), and anterior
    cruciate ligament tear, 95, *97*
  and osteochondral lesions of talus, 120–121
  and radicular pain, 61
  in tumor staging, 265–266, *267*
  of meniscus injury, 93
Maisonneuve's fracture, 123, *125*
Malleolus, fibular, lateral, 123
  fracture of, 125, *125*
  posterior, of tibia, 123
  tibial, medial, 123
Mallet finger, 196, *196*
Mallet splint, 196
Mallet toe, 300
Manual labor, repetitive, and carpal tunnel syndrome,
    249
March fracture, 237–238
Mass, evaluation of, 3
Maternal serum alpha-fetoprotein (AFP), 307
McConnell taping, in lateral patellofemoral
    compression syndrome rehabilitation, 99
Mechanism of failure, in overuse syndromes, 237
Medial, defined, 1
Median nerve, 20, *21, 208, 209*
  and humeral shaft, 156
  and pronator syndrome, *214,* 214–215
  and supracondylar process, 159
  compression of, in distal radius fracture, 173
  entrapment of, *214,* 214–215
  function of, assessment of, 161
  in carpal tunnel syndrome, 215, *216*
Median nerve supply, 201, *202*
Meniscectomy, partial, 93
Meniscus (menisci), 88, *89*
  injuries to, 92–93, *93*
  tears of, with tears of anterior cruciate ligament, 93
Meralgia paresthetica, 219
Metacarpal(s), fractures of, 187
    complications of, 191
    immobilization of, 190–191
    palpation of, 18
    thumb, base of, fracture of, 191–193, *192*
Metacarpal neck fractures, 190, *190*
  following human bite injury, 254, *255*
Metacarpal/hamate, fifth, fracture dislocation of,
    193
Metacarpophalangeal joints, finger, soft tissue
      injuries to, 193–194
  human bite injury at, 254, *255*
  thumb, ligamentous injuries of, 193–194

Metaphysis(ses), and pediatric knee fractures, 101–104, *102*
  fibrous defects of, 278–279, *280*
  of long bones, infection of, 47
Metastatic carcinoma, *286,* 286–287, *287*
Metatarsal(s), transverse proximal diaphyseal fracture of, 134–136, *135*
Metatarsal(s), 128
  fifth, fractures of, 133–134, 136
    stress fracture of, 238, *238*
  fracture(s) of, 133–136, *135, 136*
    internal fixation for, 134–135
    stress, 136, *137*
  fracture-dislocations of, 133, *134*
Metatarsal tuberosity, avulsion fracture of, *vs.* Jones' fracture, 135–136, *136*
Metatarsalgia, 299–300
Metatarsophalangeal joints, dislocations of, 138, *139*
  injuries to, 137–139, *139*
  palpation of, 28
  range of motion of, 30
Metatarsus adductus, 289, *291, 292,* 322
Methylprednisolone, in spinal cord injury, 207
Meyer and McKeever classification, of tibial eminence fracture, *104,* 105
MFH (malignant fibrous histiocytoma), *267,* 271, *273,* 283–284
Midfoot, anatomy of, 128
Midtarsal fracture subluxations, 132–133
Midtarsal fractures, 132–133
Milwaukee brace, *298*
Mitchell's causalgia, 261
Molding abnormalities, 305
Monteggia's fracture, 165, *166*
Monteggia's fracture-dislocations, 163, *164*
Mortality, and pelvic fracture, 38, 63
"Mortise view" of ankle, 124, *124*
Morton's neuroma, 219–220
Motor function, grading of, 51–52
Motor strength, grading of, 4
Motorcycle accidents, and pelvic fracture, 65
"Movie theater" sign, 99
MPFL (medial patellofemoral ligament), 89–90
MPML (medial patellomeniscal ligament), 89, 90
MPTL (medial patellotibial ligament), 89, 90
Multiple injuries, and spinal cord injury, 43
  with tibial fracture, 113
Muscle(s), deep wounds of, gas gangrene and, 43
  fatigue failure of, 237
  gastrocnemius, rupture of, *vs.* plantaris tendon rupture, 229
  injuries to, 227–235. See also specific injury or muscle.
  ruptures of, 227–228
  strains of, 227–228
  tumors of, 264t
Musculocutaneous nerves, 208, *209*
Musculoskeletal system, physical evaluation of, 4–6
  tumors of, 263–287, 264t
Mycobacterial infections, 254–255
  of hand, 250
Myelin, 199, *200*
Myeloma, 285–286
Myelomeningocele, 306–309, *309*
Myonecrosis, clostridial, clinical features of, 44
Myositis ossificans, 227
  vs. periosteal osteosarcoma, 282

Nail bed, 197, *197*
  in orthopaedic evaluation, 17
  infection of, *252,* 252–253
  injury to, 187–188, *188*
Nail fold, 197, *197*
  infected, *252,* 253
Nail matrix, of toe, 139
Navicular bone, dislocation of, in subtalar dislocations, 132
Neck, physical examination of, in spinal injury, 51
  rotational deformity of, *305,* 305–306
Neck pain, in spinal column injuries, 59–60
  with radicular pain, 60–61
Neonates. See under *Newborn.*
Neoplasms. See *Tumor(s).*
Nerve compression syndromes, 249
Nerve conduction studies (NCSs), 203
Nerve conduction (NC) velocity, 203
Nerve entrapment, 212–220. See also under specific nerve.
  causes of, 212
  differential diagnosis of, 213
  in lower extremity, 218–220
  in upper extremity, 214–218
  median, *214,* 214–215
  physical examination for, 212–213, *213*
  prevention of, 213–214
  symptoms of, 212
  treatment of, 214
Nerve function, tests for, 203, *204,* 262
Nerve injury, and causalgia, 261
  by blunt trauma, 205
  feigned, 261–262
  grading of, 199–201, *200*
  gunshot wounds as, 205
  mechanism of, 199
  pain from, 261
  traction, 203–204
  with tibial fracture, 114
Neural tissue, tumors of, 264t
Neural tube defects, 306
Neurilemmoma (Schwannoma), 269, *269*
Neurofibroma, 269–270
Neurofibromatosis, 325
Neurofibrosarcoma (malignant Schwannoma), 273
Neurologic examination, in spinal cord injury, 42–43
Neurologic level, defined, 207
Neuropraxia (grade I injury), 199, *201*
Neurotmesis (grade III injury), 199, *201*
Neurotrophic ulcers, in ankle injury, 124
Neurovascular examination, in femoral shaft fracture, 81
Newborn, birth (obstetric) palsies of, 210
  clavicle fracture of, 145
  developmental dislocation of hip in, 314
  glenohumeral joint dislocation in, 152
  humeral shaft fracture in, 157
  proximal humerus of, fractures of, 150
  ^{99m}Tc bone scintigraphy, in reflex sympathetic dystrophy, 259, *259*
  in tumor staging, 265
  of metatarsal stress fracture, 136, *137*
Nonossifying fibroma (fibrous cortical defect), 278–279, *280*
Nonpenetrating injuries, vascular trauma from, 45
Nonsteroidal anti-inflammatory drugs (NSAIDs), in arthritis, 332–333
Nonunion, in femoral neck fracture, 75
Nursemaid's elbow, 163

Obstetric (birth) palsies, 210
Occipital-C1 dislocation, 54
OI (Osteogenesis imperfecta), 325–326, *326*
Olecranon, medial, posterior, impingement of, 245
  palpation of, 15
Onychocryptosis (ingrown toe nails), 301, *301*
Open fracture(s). See *Fracture(s), open.*
Open reduction and internal fixation, for ischial avulsion, 243
  of ankle fractures, in children, 127
  of fractures about elbow, 162
  of tibial fracture, 114, *115*
Orthopaedic evaluation, 1–34
  history-taking in, 1–2
  neurologic examination in, 4
  of ankle, 27–31
  of arm, 15–17
  of cervical spine, 6–7
  of clavicular region, 11–14
  of elbow, 15–17
  of foot, 27–31
  of forearm, 15–17
  of hand, 17–20
  of hip, 20–24
  of knee, 24–27
  of leg, 24–27
  of pelvis, 20–24
  of shoulder, 11–14
  of thoracolumbosacral spine, 7–11
  of wrist, 17–20
  physical examination in, 4–6
  symptoms in, 2–3
Orthosis(ses), in spinal column injury, 50
  reciprocating gait, 309
  thoracolumbosacral, *297,* 298
Ortolani's test, 314, *315*
Os peroneum, 229
Osgood-Schlatter disease, 241
Osseous prominences, and flexor tendons of hands, 232
Osseous tissue, tumors of, 264t
Ossification, of clavicle, 145
  of humeral shaft, 156
  of proximal humerus, 149
  of scapula, 143
Ossification centers, of distal humerus, 158–159, *159*
  of radius and ulna, 165
  secondary, and pediatric knee fractures, 101–104, *102*
Osteitis, stress fractures of, 242
Osteoarthritis, 329–330, 330t, 332
Osteochondral fractures, acute, 91
Osteochondritis dissecans, 91–92, *92*
  of knee, 294–295, *296*
Osteochondromas, 275–277
Osteochondrosis(es), 292–297
  of capitellum of distal humerus, 296
  of head of second metatarsal, 295–296, *296*
  van Neck's, 296–297, *297*
Osteogenesis imperfecta (OI), 325–326, *326*
Osteoid osteoma, 275, *276*
Osteoma, osteoid, 275, *276*
Osteomyelitis, hematogenous, acute, 47–48
  radiographic studies in, 47
  subacute/chronic, 48, *48*
Osteonecrosis, in femoral neck fracture, 75
  of femoral head, in hip dislocation, 75
Osteoporosis, *302,* 302–303

Osteosarcoma, 279–280, *281*
  juxtacortical, 280–282, *282*
  secondary, 280
Osteotomies, 333
Overgrowth syndromes, *324,* 324–325
Overhead activities, impingement syndrome and, 243–244
Overhead lifting, and rotator cuff tendinitis, 231
Overuse syndromes, 236–257
  mechanism of failure of, 237
  of elbow, 244–245
  of foot, 237–240, *238, 240*
  of hand and wrist, 246–249, *247, 248*
  of hip, 242
  of knee, 241–242
  of leg, 240–241
  of pelvis, 242–243
  of shoulder (Little League shoulder), 243–244
  of upper extremity, 243
  of wrist and hand, 246–249, *247, 248*

Padding, in cast construction, 341, *341*
Pain, chronic, 258–260
  factitious, 261–262
  in spinal injury, 42, 51
  of compartment syndrome, 39
  of nerve origin, 261
Paint, and high-pressure injection injuries, 35, *36*
Palm, abscess of, 253
  acute suppurative tenosynovitis of, 253
Palmar arch, superficial, anatomy of, 223, *224*
Palmar slope, of distal radius, 169–170
Palpation, in orthopaedic evaluation, 4
Panclavicular dislocations, 148–149
Panner's disease, 296
Paralysis, evaluation of, 3
Paraplegia, defined, 206–207
Paraspinal muscles, and neck pain, 59–60
Paronychia, *252,* 252–253
Past medical history, 3
Pasteurella multocida, and hand infection, 250, 254
Patella, and jumper's knee syndrome, 241
  fractures of, *103,* 104, 108
    and rupture of knee extensors, 230
    in children, *103,* 104
    radiographic evaluation of, 107, *108*
  palpation of, 25
  subluxation of, 99
Patella alta, 98
Patellar ligament, avulsion of, *103,* 104
Patellar retinaculum, lateral, 90
  medial, 89–90
    tearing of, 98
Patellar tendon, and quadriceps tendon, 230
  reflex of, 27
  rupture of, 230
Patellofemoral joint, 88, 89, *89*
  dislocation of, 98–99
  injuries to, *98,* 98–100
Patellofemoral ligaments, 89–90
Patellomeniscal ligament, 89, 90
Patellotibial ligament, 89, 90
Pedestrians, and pelvic fracture, 63
Pelvic ring, 64, *64*

Pelvis, anatomy of, 63–64, *64*
fractures of, 38, *40,* 63–68
angiographic embolization of, 38
classification of, 65, *66*
evaluation and emergency management of, 65–68, *67–68*
force pattern(s) of, 64–65, *65–66*
radiographic evaluation of, 66, *68*
stabilization of, 66–68, *67–68*
unstable, 66, *68*
obliquity of, 7–8, 20
orthopaedic evaluation of, 20–24
overuse syndromes of, 242–243
palpation of, 20–21
Penetrating injury(ies), history and physical examination of, 250–251
of muscles and tendons, 228
vascular trauma from, 45
Percussion sign (Tinel's sign), 213, *213*
Perilunate dislocation, 174, *176*
dorsal, 178, *181*
Periosteal muscle, and shin splints, 240
Periosteum, juxtacortical osteosarcoma of, 280, 282
Peripheral nerve(s), anatomy of, 199, *200*
and scapula, 143
entrapment of, 212
in shoulder injury, 143
injuries to, 199–205, *200–204*
neurilemmoma in, 269, *269*
neurofibrosarcoma in, 273
pathway of, 199, *200*
Perkin's lines, 316, *317*
Peroneal nerve, entrapment of, *218,* 218–219
in fibular tunnel syndrome, *218,* 218–219
Peroneal spastic flatfoot (tarsal coalition), 291–292, *294, 295*
Peroneal tendinitis, 239
Peroneal tendon, 229–230
Peroneus brevis tendon, in metatarsal tuberosity fracture, 136
Perthes disease, 293–294, *295*
Pes cavus, 27, *28*
Pes planus (flatfoot), 27, *28*
posterior tibial tendinitis in, 240
Pes valgus, convex, congenital, 323, *323*
Peyronie's disease, 301
PFFD (Proximal femoral focal deficiency), 310–311, *311*
Phalanx (phalanges), distal, fractures of, 187–188, *188*
complications of, 189
reduction of, 189–190
fractures of, 187
middle, fractures of, 188–190, *189*
displacement of, 188, *189*
dorsal base avulsion, 195, *195*
palpation of, 18
proximal, fractures of, 188–190, *189*
Phalen's sign, for nerve entrapment, 213, *213*
reverse, for nerve entrapment, 213, *213*
Phalen's test, in carpal tunnel syndrome, 215
Philadelphia collar, in spinal column injury, 50
Physaliferous cell, 285
Physical therapy. See also *Rehabilitation.*
for chronic neck or back pain, 60
for injured knee, 90
for posterior cruciate ligament injuries, 98
for reflex sympathetic dystrophy, 260

Physis, and pediatric knee fractures, 101–104, *102*
fracture of, growth disturbances from, 104
of elbow, 160
of radius, 174
Pigmented villonodular synovitis, 271, *272*
Pilon fractures, 125, *127*
PIN. See *Interosseous nerve, posterior.*
PIP joints. See *Interphalangeal joint(s), proximal.*
Pisiform, fractures of, 183–184
Pivot shift test, for anterior cruciate ligament injury, 95, *96*
Pivot shifts, in sports injuries, 97
Plantar fasciitis, 239
Plantar fibromatosis, 301, *302*
Plantar flexion, 30, *30*
Plantaris tendon, 228–229
Plasma cystoma, 285–286
Plaster roll, in cast construction, 341–342, *342*
Plaster splints, construction of, 337–338, *338*
Polydactyly, of hand, 312–313
of foot, 323–324
Polymethylmethacrylate (PMMA), 286
Polytrauma, with pediatric femoral shaft fracture, 86
Popliteal artery, impingement of, in fracture of femur, *45*
in dislocation of knee, 45–46
injury to, 221
Popliteal region, palpation of, 25
Popliteus tendon, 89, 230–231
Posterior elbow long arm splint, 162, *162,* 163, 164
Posterior sag sign of Godfrey, 97, *97*
Post-traumatic arthritis, and distal radius fracture, 174
Posture, in orthopaedic evaluation, 4, *6*
Power tools, and ulnar artery thrombosis, 224
Preadolescent, osteochondritis dissecans in, 91–92, *92*
Pressure points, in casts, 345
Profunda brachii artery, and humeral shaft, 156
Pronation, defined, 1
of foot, 123, 239
of forearm, 16
Pronator syndrome, *214,* 214–215
Prone, defined, 1
Provocative maneuvers, in cubital tunnel syndrome, 216
in diagnosis of nerve entrapment, 212–213, *213*
in pronator syndrome, 215
in thoracic outlet syndrome, 225
Proximal femoral focal deficiency (PFFD), 310–311, *311*
Pseudoaneurysm, 222, *223*
Pseudoarthrosis, congenital, of clavicle, 311
of tibia (anterolateral bow), 318–319, *319, 320*
Pseudoepiphyses, of metacarpals, 185, *186*
Pseudomonas aeruginosa, and puncture wounds of foot, 256
Psoriatic arthritis, joints involved in, 330t
Pterygia, 324
Pubic ramus, fracture of, *66*
stress fractures of, 242
Pubis, 64, *64*
Pulled elbow, 163
Pulmonary embolism, 37–38, *39*
pulmonary angiography in, 38, *39*
Pulp abscess (felon), 251, *252*
"Pump bump," 240
Puncture wounds, to foot, 256
Pupil, constricted, in brachial plexus injury, 209, *210*
Pyogenic arthritis, 253–254

Quadriceps angle (Q angle), in patellofemoral joint injury, 98, *98*
Quadriceps femoris, 90, *90*
  in patellofemoral joint rehabilitation, 99
  spasm of, in femoral shaft fracture, 81
Quadriceps tendinitis, and jumper's knee syndrome, 241
Quadriceps tendon, rupture of, 230
Quadriplegia, *vs.* tetraplegia, 206

Racquet sports, and hamate fracture, 183
  and tendinitis, 248
Radial, defined, 1
Radial artery, anatomy of, 223, *224*
Radial head dislocations, reduction of, 164
Radial longitudinal deficiency (radial clubhand), 309–310
Radial neck fracture, 159, *161*
Radial nerve, 20, *21,* 208, *209*
  and elbow, 159, 160–161
  and humeral shaft, 156, 157
  entrapment of, *217,* 217–218
    vs. DeQuervain's tenosynovitis, 247
  function of, assessment of, 160–161
Radial nerve supply, 201, *202, 203*
Radial pulse, obliteration of, 225, *225*
Radial styloid process, fracture of, 172, *174*
Radial tunnel syndrome, *217,* 217–218
Radial wrist extensor tendons, and intersection syndrome, 248
  tendinitis of, 247–248
Radiation injury, to brachial plexus, 211
Radiation therapy, for soft tissue sarcoma, 274–275
Radicular pain, in spinal column injuries, 60–61
Radiocapitellar joint, palpation of, 15–16
Radiographic evaluation, 31–33
  in orthopaedic evaluation, 31–33
Radioisotope scanning, in tumor staging, 265
Radioulnar joint, distal, 159, 170
  dislocations of, 177–178, *180*
  fractures of, 177
Radioulnar synostosis, congenital, 312
Radius, dislocation of, 163
  distal, inclination of, 169
    length of, 169
  fracture of, distal, 169–174, *170–174*
    and extensor tendons of hands, 233
    and flexor tendons of hands, 232
    classification of, 169
    complications of, 169–174, *170–174,* 173–174
    imaging of, 169–170
    in children, 174
    measurement of, 169–170, *170*
  distal third, 165, *166*
Range of motion, active, defined, 4
  in orthopaedic evaluation, 4
  of cervical spine, 7, *9*
  of thoracolumbosacral spine, 10–11, *12,* 12–14, *13–14*
  passive, defined, 4
Raynaud's disease (primary Raynaud's phenomenon), 225–226
Raynaud's phenomenon, unilateral, in ulnar artery thrombosis, 224
Raynaud's syndrome (secondary Raynaud's phenomenon), 226

Reconstructive surgery, and pulmonary embolism, 37
  of knee, 92
Rectus femoris, 90, *90*
Reduction, closed, of ankle fracture, 126
    of calcaneus fracture, complications of, 130
    of elbow dislocation, 163–164
  open, and internal fixation. See *Open reduction and internal fixation.*
Reflex sympathetic dystrophy (RSD), 258–261, *259, 260*
  diagnostic tests for, 259
  edema of, 258, *259*
  in ankle sprains, 121
  multidisciplinary approach to, 260
  treatment of, 260
Reflexes, in spinal column injury, 52
  of ankle, 30–31
  of arm, 16–17
  of foot, 30–31
  of knee, 27
Rehabilitation. See also *Physical therapy.*
  for ankle sprain, of athlete, 118–119
  for lateral patellofemoral compression syndrome, 99–100
  functional, for ankle sprain, 118
  in patellofemoral joint dislocation, 99
  of anterior cruciate ligament injury, 96–97
  of collateral ligament injury, 94, *94*
  of glenohumeral joint dislocation, 154
  of knee, 90
  of meniscus injury, 93
Reiter's syndrome, joints involved in, 330t
Repetitive manual labor, and carpal tunnel syndrome, 249
Replantation, 198
  of fingertip, 198
  of traumatic amputations, 44, *44*
Respiratory system, in pelvic fracture, 65
Reticuloendothelial tissue, tumors of, 264t
Retrocalcaneal bursitis, 239–240
Reverse Bennett's fracture, 193
Reverse Phalen's sign, for nerve entrapment, 213, *213*
Rhabdomyosarcoma, 268
Rheumatoid arthritis, 330t, 330–331, *331*
  joints involved in, 330, 330t
Rocker-bottom foot, 323, *323*
Rolando's fracture, 191–193, *192*
Roos' sign, in thoracic outlet syndrome, 214
Rotation, external, of foot, 123
  of shoulder, 13, *14*
  spinal, evaluation of, 11, *12*
    quantification of, 10–11, *12*
Rotator cuff tendinitis, 231
RSD. See *Reflex sympathetic dystrophy (RSD).*
Runners, iliotibial band syndrome in, 241–242
  leg length and, 242
  Morton's neuroma in, 219–220
  sesamoiditis of, 137
Running, and foot malalignment, 239
  effect of, on foot, 237

SACH (soft ankle cushioned heel), 335
Sacral fracture, transforaminal, *66*
  transverse, *66*
Sacral wing fracture, *66*
Sacroiliac joint, diastasis of, *66, 67*
Sacroiliac ligaments, 64, *64*
Sacrospinous ligaments, 64, *64*

Sacrotuberous ligament, 64, *64*
Sacrum, 64, *64*
Sag sign of Godfrey, 97, *97*
Sagittal, defined, 1
Salter-Harris classification, of fractures, *32*, 34
    of distal radius, 174
    of pediatric knee, 101–103, *102*
Sarcoma(s), adjuvant systemic chemotherapy for, 275
    brachytherapy for, 275
    epithelioid, 272–273
    Ewing's, *284*, 284–285
    radiation therapy for, 274–275
    soft tissue, 268
        malignant, 271–273
    synovial, 272
"Saturday night" palsy, 205, 218
Scaphoid, fractures of, 179–180, *182*
    and distal radius fracture, 173–174, *175*
Scaphoid wrist fractures, with capitate fractures, 182–183
Scapholunate advanced collapse (SLAC) wrist, 176, *179*
Scapholunate angle, normal, 175, *179*
Scapholunate ligament tears, 175, 176, *177*
    and distal radius fracture, 173–174
Scapula, congenital elevation of, 311–312
    dislocations of, 143–145, *144, 145*
    fractures of, 143–145, *144, 145*
        classification of, 143
        injuries associated with, 144–145
            vascular, 145
        radiographic evaluation of, 144, *144*
        treatment of, 145, *145*
    in brachial plexus injury, 209–210
    winging of, 14, *14*
Scapular nerve, dorsal, 143
Scapulothoracic dissociation, 143
Scheuermann's kyphosis, *298*, 298–299
Schwann cells, 199, 269
Schwannoma, malignant (neurofibrosarcoma), 273
Schwannoma (neurilemmoma), 269, *269*
Sciatic nerve, 203, *204*
    in acetabular fracture, 68
    in posterior hip dislocation, 68
Scintigraphy, skeletal, in tumor staging, 265
Sclerae, blue, 325
Scoliosis, adolescent, idiopathic, *297*, 297–298
    congenital, 306, *307, 308*
    spinal examination for, 7–8, *10, 11*
Segmental innervation, of muscle groups, 51–52, 52t
    sensory distribution of, 52, *53*
Segond's fracture, 95, *97*
Sensation, evaluation of, 4, *5*
Septic arthritis, 46–47
    joints involved in, 330t
Sesamoiditis, treatment of, 137
Sesamoids, and great toe, dislocations of, 138
    bipartite, 137, 239
    bone scan of, 137, *139*
    fracture of, 136–137, *138, 139*
        stress, 238–239
Sever's disease, 239, 295
Sharp-dull discrimination, 201, *201*
Shenton's lines, 316–317, *317*
Shin splints, 240
Shock, hypovolemic, in pelvic fracture, 65–66
Shoe, wear pattern of, 27
Short arm cast, 343, *343*
Short leg cast, *343*, 343–344

Shoulder, abduction of, 12, *13*
    arthritis of, surgery and, 333–334, *334*
    dislocations of, 151–154, *152, 153, 154*
    extension of, 12, *13*
    flexion of, 12, *13*
    fractures and dislocations of, 142–154. See also
        under *Clavicle; Glenohumeral joint; Scapula.*
        active range of motion in, 142–143
        history of, 142
        inspection of, 142–143
        neurovascular examination of, 143
    immobilization of, 145, *145*, 151, *153*, 153–154
    orthopaedic evaluation of, 11–14
    osteoarthritis of, 333–334, *334*
    overuse syndromes of (Little League shoulder), 243–244
    range of motion of, 12–14, *13–14*
    rotation of, 13, *14*
    rotator cuff tendinitis of, 231
Shoulder/hand syndrome, 258–261, *259, 260*
"Silver fork" deformity, 171
Sindig-Larsen-Johannsen disease, 241
Single gene mutations, 304
Skeletal scintigraphy, in reflex sympathetic
        dystrophy, 259, *259*
    in tumor staging, 265
    of metatarsal stress fracture, 136, *137*
    three-phase, in acute hematogenous
        osteomyelitis, 47
Skiing, and ulnar collateral ligament injuries, 194
Skin, and casting, 345
    and congenital scoliosis, 306
    in reflex sympathetic dystrophy, 258
    necrosis of, in metatarsal fractures, 133
Slab splint, *340*
SLAC (scapholunate advanced collapse) wrist, 176, *179*
Slipped capital femoral epiphysis, 290–291, *294*
Smith's fracture, 171–172, *172*
Social history, 3
Soft ankle cushioned heel (SACH), 335
Soft tissue(s), in human bite injury, 254, *255*
    in metatarsal fractures, 133
    in spinal injury, 52–53
    of hand, injuries to, 185–198. See also under
            specific injury or part of hand.
        evaluation of, 186
        management of, 186–187, *187, 188*
    of wrist, palpation of, 18
    sarcoma of, 268
    tumor-like lesions of, 268–273
    tumors of, 264t, 267–268
        benign, 269–270
        biopsy of, 266–267
        malignant (sarcomatous), 271–273
            radiation therapy for, 274–275
        vs. tumor-like lesions, 268–273
Spastic flatfoot, peroneal (tarsal coalition), 291–292, *294, 295*
Spinal column. See also *Spinal cord injuries; Spine.*
    injuries to, 50–62
        history of, 50–51
        low back pain in, 59–60
        motor examination of, 51–52, 52t
        neck pain in, 59–60
        neurologic examination of, 51
        of lower cervical spine, *57*, 57–59, *58*
        of lumbar spine, 59, *59, 60*
        of thoracic spine, 59
        of upper cervical spine, 54–57, *54–57*

Spinal column *(Continued)*
    physical examination of, 51–52, 52t, 54t
    radicular pain in, 60–61
    roentgenographic evaluation of, 52–54, *54–55*
    sensory examination of, 52, *53*
    spondylolysis and spondylolisthesis in, 61–62
Spinal cord injuries, 41–43, 206–207. See also *Spinal column; Spine.*
    clinical syndromes of, 207
    diagnosis of, 42
    grading of, 206
Spinal deformities, in myelomeningocele, 308
Spinal flexion, quantification of, 11, *12*
Spinal rotation, evaluation of, 11, *12*
Spine. See also *Spinal column; Spinal cord injuries.*
    arthritis of, surgery and, 335–336
    cervical. See *Cervical spine.*
    congenital deformities of, 304–309. See also specific deformity, e.g., *Klippel-Feil syndrome.*
    curvature of. See *Kyphosis; Scoliosis.*
    flexion of, quantification of, 10, 11, *12*
    lumbar. See *Lumbar spine.*
    osteoarthritis of, 335–336
    postural alignment of, 4, *6, 7*
Spin-echo imaging, 265
Spinous process fracture, 58
Splinting, of tibial fracture, 111–112
    of tibial plateau fracture, 107, *108*
    vs. casting, 338
Splinting techniques, 337–340, *338–340,* 346
Splints, digit, 339, *340*
    three-sided, 340, *340*
    types of, 337
Spondylolisthesis, degenerative, 61–62
    in spinal column injuries, 61–62
    isthmic, 61
    traumatic, 57, *57*
Spondylolysis, in spinal column injuries, 61–62
Sprain(s), of finger carpometacarpal joints, 193
    of metatarsophalangeal joints, 137–139, *139*
Sprengel's deformity, 311–312
Stab wounds, and brachial plexus injury, 210, 211
    vascular trauma from, 45
Staging, radiographic, of tumors, 265–266
Stance phase, of gait, 5, *8*
Staphylococcus aureus, and felon, 250
    and hand infection, 250
    and paronychia, 252
    in osteomyelitis, 47
    infection of diabetic foot, 256
Sternoclavicular (SC) joint, in clavicle dislocation, 147, 148, 149
Sternoclavicular ligaments, in clavicle fracture, 145
Sternocleidomastoid muscle, contracture of, *305,* 305–306
    palpation of, 7, *9*
Steroid injections, intra-articular, in arthritis, 333
Stinson's reduction maneuver, 74
Stockinette, of cast, 340–341, *341*
Street fighter's fracture, 190, *190*
Streeter's dysplasia, 324
Strength, motor, grading of, 4
Streptococcal infection, anaerobic, 43
Stress fracture, 237
    Jones' fracture as, 135, *135*
    metatarsal, 136, *137*
    of sesamoids, 137

Stress injury, musculoskeletal, anatomic malalignments and, 236–237
    mechanism of failure in, 237
    nonoperative treatment for, 237
    training errors and, 236
Stubbed toe, 139
Stump, care of, 44
Subluxation(s), 34
    cervical, 54
    defined, 34
    of knee, congenital, 318
    of peroneal tendons, 229
Subperiosteal aspiration, 47
Substance abuse, and thrombosis of ulnar artery, 223
Subtalar dislocation, 131–132
    complications of, 132
Subtrochanteric fractures, 78–79
    radiographic evaluation of, 79
Sudeck's atrophy, 259
Sugartong splint, 167, *167,* 338, *339*
    for Colles' fracture, 170
"Suitcase" injury, 205
Supination, of foot, 123
Supine, defined, 1
Supracondylar fracture, of distal humerus, *159*
    injuries associated with, 160–161, 162
Supracondylar process, fracture of, 159
Suprascapular nerve, 143
Surgery, and arthritis, 333–336
    for ankle fracture, 126, *127*
    for anterior cruciate ligament injury, 96
    for dislocated elbow, 164
    for elbow fracture, 162
    for gas gangrene, 44
    for glenohumeral joint dislocation, 154
    for hand fractures, 187, *188*
    for humeral fracture, 157
    for osteochondral lesions of talus, 121
    for posterior cruciate ligament injuries, 98
    for tibial plateau fracture, 107, *108*
    limb-sparing, 273–274, *274*
        for sarcoma, 273–274, *274*
Swan neck deformity, 195, 196, *196,* 234, *234*
Swelling, and splints, 345
Swimming motions, and rotator cuff tendinitis, 231
Swing phase, of gait, 5, *8*
Sympathectomy, in reflex sympathetic dystrophy, 260
Sympathetic nervous system, and reflex sympathetic dystrophy, 258
Symphysis, diastasis of, *66*
Symphysis pubis, 64, *64*
    fracture at, 38, *39*
Syndactyly, 312
    of foot, 323, *323*
Syndesmotic ligaments, in Maisonneuve's fracture, 123, 125
    injury to, 123, 125
Synostosis, radioulnar, congenital, 312
Synovectomy, 331
Synovial fluid, in arthritis, 332
Synovial tissue, tumors of, 264t
Synovitis, acute, 47
    villonodular, pigmented, 271, *272*

Talar neck fractures, 130, *131*
    and avascular necrosis, 131
    treatment of, 131
Talar tilt test, 117, 119, *121*

Talipes equinovarus (clubfoot), 320–322, *321, 322*
Talocalcaneal angle, in clubfoot, 321, *322*
Talofibular ligament, 117
    anterior, in ankle sprains, 118, *118*
Talonavicular joint, in subtalar dislocations, 131–132
    injury to, 132–133
Talus, fractures of, 130–131, *131, 132*
    osteochondral lesions of, 120, *121*
        radiographic evaluation of, 120, *121*
Tapezium, fractures of, 181–182
Tarsal coalition (peroneal spastic flatfoot), 291–292, *294, 295*
Tarsal tunnel syndrome, 219, *219*
Tarsals, stress fracture of, 238
Tarsometatarsal fracture-dislocations, 133, *134*
"Teardrop" fracture, *vs.* teardrop fracture-dislocation, 57–58
Tendinitis, DeQuervain's, 246–247, *247, 248*
    diagnosis of, 246
    extensor carpi ulnaris, 248
    extensor pollicis longus, 248
    flexor carpi ulnaris, 248
    intersection syndrome, 247–248
    of foot and ankle, 239
    of hand and wrist, 246–249
    peroneal, 229
    rotator cuff, 231
Tendon(s), fatigue failure of, 237
    injuries to, 227–235. See also specific tendon, e.g., *Plantaris tendon.*
    ruptures of, 227–228
Tendon sheath, giant cell tumor of, 270–271
Tennis, and gastrocnemius muscle rupture, 229
Tennis elbow, 245
Tenosynovectomy, 331
Tenosynovitis, DeQuervain's, 246–247, *247, 248*
    peroneal, 229
    suppurative, acute, 253
TENS (transcutaneous electrical nerve stimulator), 205
Teratogens, 304
Tetanus, 114, 255, 256
Tetraplegia, *vs.* quadriplegia, 206
TFCC (triangular fibrocartilage complex), 177, *178*
Thermal injuries, in casting and splinting, 337–338, 340, 345
Thermography, in reflex sympathetic dystrophy, 259, *259*
Thigh, upper, physical examination of, in femoral shaft fracture, 81
Thomas test, for hip flexion contracture, 21, *22*
Thompson's test, 228, *228*
    for Achilles tendon continuity, 31
Thoracic injuries, associated with clavicle fracture, 146
Thoracic kyphosis, 4, *6*
    increased, 7, *10*
Thoracic outlet syndrome (TOS), 214, 225, *225, 226*
Thoracic spine, injuries to, 59
Thoracolumbosacral spine, neurologic examination of, 11, 14, *14*
    orthopaedic evaluation of, 7–11
    palpation of, 10
    range of motion of, 10–11, *12,* 12–14, *13–14*
Three-phase bone scan, in diagnosis of osteomyelitis, 47
Thromboembolism, 37–38, *39*
Thrombosis, arterial, in upper extremity, 223–226
    of vascular trauma, 45
Thumb. See also under *Finger(s).*
    felon of, 251, *252*

Thumb *(Continued)*
    flexion of, 19–20, *20*
    palmar abduction/adduction of, 19–20, *20*
    range of motion of, 19–20, *20*
Thumb interphalangeal joints, dislocations of, 196
Thumb metacarpal joint, fractures of, 191–193, *192*
Thumb metacarpophalangeal joint, dorsal dislocation of, 194
Thumb spica cast, 342–343, *343*
"Thurston-Holland" fragment, 103
Tibia, anterior unicortical stress fractures of, 240
    displacement of, in cruciate ligament injuries, 95, *95, 96*
    fractures of, 110–115. See also *Tibial plateau, fractures of.*
        causes of, 111
        closed, 111–112
        consequences of, 114
        eminence of, in children, *104,* 105
        in children, 114–115
            radiographic evaluation of, 115
        location of, 11, *113*
        open, *112,* 112–114, *113, 115*
            compartment syndrome in, 114
            early care of, 113–114
            infection in, 113, 114
            nerve injury in, 114
            physical examination of, 114
            radiographic evaluation of, 114
        patterns of, 111, *111*
        proximal, in children, *103,* 104–105
            metaphyseal, 115
        splints for, 339–340, *340–341*
        tuberosity of, in children, *105,* 106
    in knee dislocation, 45, *46*
    metaphyseal, proximal, 115
    palpation of, 25
    posteromedial bowing of, congenital, 319, *321*
    proximal, epiphysis of, displacement of, *103,* 104–105
        fractures of, 108
    pseudoarthrosis of, congenital, 318–319, *319, 320*
Tibial artery, anterior, injury to, 221
Tibial muscle, anterior, strength of, 6
    posterior, and shin splints, 240
Tibial nerve, in ankle injury, 124
    posterior, in tarsal tunnel syndrome, 219, *219*
Tibial plateau, fractures of, 107–108, *108,* 109
    lateral, avulsion of anterior cruciate ligament from, 95, *97*
Tibial stress syndrome, medial, 240
Tibial tendinitis, posterior, 239, 240
Tibial tendon, posterior, 230, *230*
Tibial torsion, internal, with femoral anteversion, 290, *292, 293*
Tibiofemoral joint, 88, *89*
    injuries to, 90–92
Tibiofibular joint, 88, *89*
Tibiofibular ligament, anterior, *118*
    anteroinferior, in inversion ankle sprain, 121
Tibiotalar subluxation, anterior, 119, *120*
Tinel's sign, 203, *204,* 213, *213*
    in carpal tunnel syndrome, 215
    in thoracic outlet syndrome, 214
Tinel's test, 18
Tobacco use, 223
Toddler(s), developmental dislocation of hip in, 317–318
    femoral fracture in, 86
    knock-knees in, 289, *290*

Toddler(s) *(Continued)*
  tibial fractures in, 115
  toeing in/out in, 290, *292, 293*
Toe(s). See also *Great toe; Lesser toes.*
  fracture of, 139–140, *140*
  great, neurologic examination of, 25, 26
    sesamoids of, fracture of, 136–137, *138, 139*
  lesser, deformities of, 300–301, *301*
    neurologic examination of, 26
  polydactyly of, 323–324
  syndactyly of, 323, *323*
  tendons of, extensor and flexor, rupture of, 235
Toe flexor tendinitis, 239
Toe nails, ingrown, 301, *301*
Toeing in/out, 290, *292–293*
Tomography, computed, in tumor staging, 265
"Too many toes" sign, 230, *230*
Torsion, of blood vessels, by fracture fragments, 45
Torticollis, muscular, congenital, *305,* 305–306
TOS (thoracic outlet syndrome), 214, 225, *225, 226*
Total hip arthroplasty, and fat embolism, 37
  and femoral neck fracture, 75, *78*
Total knee replacement, 92
Traction apophysitis, of calcaneus, 239
  of iliac crest, 242–243
  of tibial tubercle, 241
Traffic accidents, and pelvic fracture, 63
Transcutaneous electrical nerve stimulator (TENS),
    205
Transfer lesion, of metatarsal fracture, 133, *135*
Translation, of fracture, *32, 34*
Transverse, defined, 1
Trapeziometacarpal joint, of thumb, osteoarthritis of,
    333
Trapezium, fractures of, 181–182
Trapezius muscle, and neck pain, 59–60
Trapezoid, fractures of, 182
Trauma, evaluation of, 2
  high-energy, and acetabular fractures, 68
    and open tibial fracture, 113
    and shoulder injury, 143–144
    and subtrochanteric fractures, 78
    in spinal column injury, 50–51
    open fracture from, 41
    pelvic fracture from, 38, *40, 63*
    tarsometatarsal fracture-dislocations from, 133,
      134
  multiple, with pediatric femoral shaft fracture, 86
Trauma management. See also *Emergency care.*
  of amputations, 44, *44*
Traumatic arthritis, joints involved in, 330t
Trendelenburg lurch, 6, *9*
Trendelenburg test, 23, *24*
Triangular fibrocartilage complex (TFCC), 177, *178*
Triceps, 159
  reflex of, 17
Triggering, 232
Trimalleolar fractures, 125, *126*
Triquetrolunate dissociation, 177, *178*
Triquetrum, fractures of, 181, *184*
Triradiate cartilage, 64, *64*
Trochanters, in hip fracture, 75–78, *79*
Trunk shift, in Trendelenburg lurch, 6, *9*
Tumor(s), 263–287, 264t
  biopsy of, 266–267
  bone, 263–267, 264t, 275–287. See also specific
    tumor.
    benign, 275–279
    biopsy of, 266–267

Tumor(s) *(Continued)*
    history and physical examination of, 263–267
    malignant, 279–287
  giant cell, 278, *279*
    of tendon sheath, 270–271
  history and physical examination of, 263–267
  magnetic resonance imaging of, 265–266, *267*
  malignant, treatment of, 273–275
  radioisotope scanning of, 265
  soft tissue, 264t, 267–268
    benign, 269–270
    biopsy of, 266–267
    malignant (sarcomatous), 271–273
      chemotherapy for, systemic, 275
      radiation therapy for, 274–275
    vs. tumor-like lesions, 268–273
  staging techniques for, 265–266, *266*
Turf toe, 137
Two-point discrimination, 186, 201, *201*

Ulna, 165
  dislocation of, 163
Ulnar, defined, 1
Ulnar artery, anatomy of, 223, *224*
  thrombosis of, 224–225
Ulnar gutter splint, 338, *338*
Ulnar negative wrist, 180–181
Ulnar nerve, 20, *21,* 208, *209*
  and carpometacarpal joint injuries, 193
  and elbow, 159
  and hamate fracture, 183
  function of, assessment of, 161
  in cubital tunnel syndrome, *216,* 216–217
  in Guyon's syndrome, 217
Ulnar nerve supply, 201, *202*
Ulnar shaft, proximal, fracture of, and proximal
    radial head dislocations, 163, *164*
Ulnar styloid, fractures of, 170, 177
Unicameral bone cyst, 277
Upper cervical spine, 54–57, *54–57*
Upper extremity(ies), casts for, 342–343, *343*
  motor innervation of, 201, *202, 203*
  overuse syndromes of, 243–249. See also specific
    part; specific site, e.g., *Shoulder.*
  splints for, 338–339, *339–340*
Urethra, in pelvic fracture, 38
Urologic injury, in pelvic fracture, 38
U-shaped plaster splints, 157, *157*

Valgus, 34. See also *Genu valgum.*
  defined, 1
Valgus stress test, in collateral ligament injury,
    94, *94*
van Neck's osteochondrosis, 296–297, *297*
Varus, 34. See also *Genu varum.*
  defined, 1
Varus stress test, in collateral ligament injury, 94, *94*
Vascular damage, from frostbite, 226
  in dislocation of knee, 46
  management of, 44
Vascular examination, in orthopaedic evaluation, 4
Vascular injuries, 221–226
  associated with fractures and dislocations,
    44–45, *45*
Vascular tissue, tumors of, 264t
Vasospastic conditions, primary, 225–226

Vastus intermedius, 90, *90*
Vastus lateralis, 90, *90*
Vastus medialis, 90, *90*
Vastus medialis obliquus, in patellofemoral joint
    rehabilitation, 99
  of quadriceps, 90
Velpeau shoulder immobilizer, for clavicle injury, 147,
    148
Vertebra, in congenital scoliosis, 306, *307*
Vertebral body, compression fractures of, calcaneus
    fractures and, 128
  fractures of, 57, *57*
Vesicles, of herpes simplex, 250, 253, *253*
Vibrating tools, and carpal tunnel syndrome, 249
  and thrombosis of ulnar artery, 223
  and ulnar artery thrombosis, 224
Volar fracture, and avulsion of profundus tendon, 196
Volar intercalary segment instability, *178*
Volar plate injury, in dorsal dislocation of
    metacarpophalangeal joint, 193–194
Volar tilt, *170*
Volleyball, and jumper's knee syndrome, 241
von Recklinghausen's disease, 269, 273
von Volkmann, Richard, 38

W position, 290, *293*
Water temperature, for plaster splints and casts,
    337–338, 340, 345

Watson-Jones classification, of tibial eminence
    fracture, *105,* 106
Web space abscess, 253
Wedge fracture, *66*
Wedge vertebrae, 307
Weight-bearing, after metatarsal fractures, 133, *135*
  foot and, 128
  in arthritis, 333
  in sesamoiditis, 137
Weight-lifters, osteolysis of distal clavicle in, 243
Whiplash, 59–60
Wrist, anatomy of, 174, *176*
  and hand, overuse syndromes of, 246–249, *247, 248*
    tendinitis of, 246–249
  arthritis of, 176
  extension of, 16, 19–20, *20*
  flexion of, 16, 19–20, *20*
  fractures of, 169–184
  ligamentous injuries of, 169–184
  orthopaedic evaluation of, 17–20
  palpation of, 17–18
  radiographic evaluation of, *170–173,* 174–175,
    175–184
  range of motion of, 19–20, *20*
  tendinitis of, 247–248
Wrist ligaments, injuries to, stages of, 174

Xanthoma, synovial, 271, *272*

ISBN 0-7216-5436-3

90038